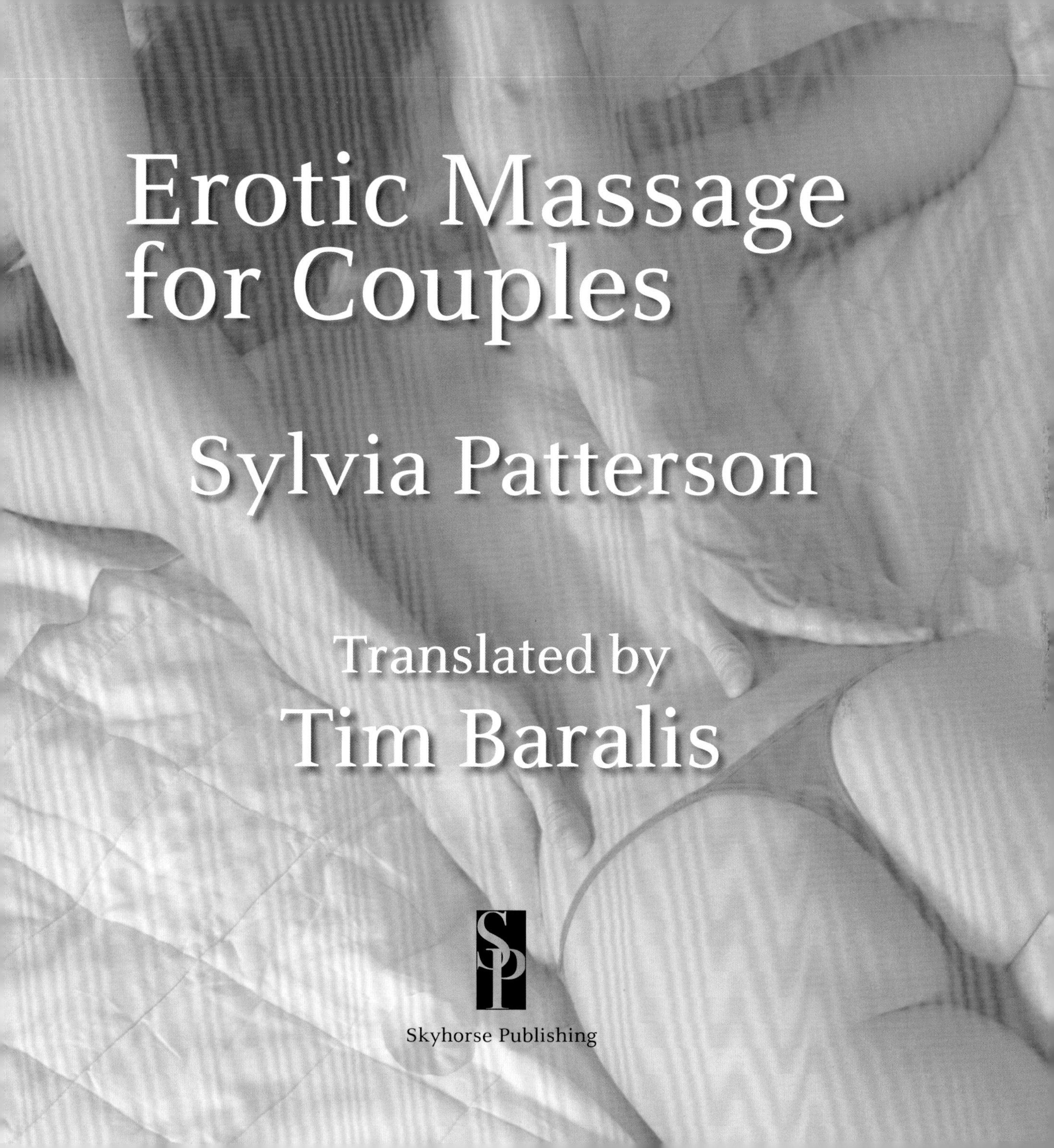

Erotic Massage for Couples

Sylvia Patterson

Translated by

Tim Baralis

Skyhorse Publishing

Original title: MASAJE ERÓTICO PARA PAREJAS

Photographs: Johann Wolf, Becky Lawton, Archivo Océano
Models: Alfonso Marín, Ivona Laluhova

10 9 8 7 6 5 4 3 2

Library of Congress Cataloging-in-Publication Data is available on file.

Cover design by Qualcom Design
Cover photo credit Thinkstock

ISBN: 978-1-62914-469-6

Printed in China

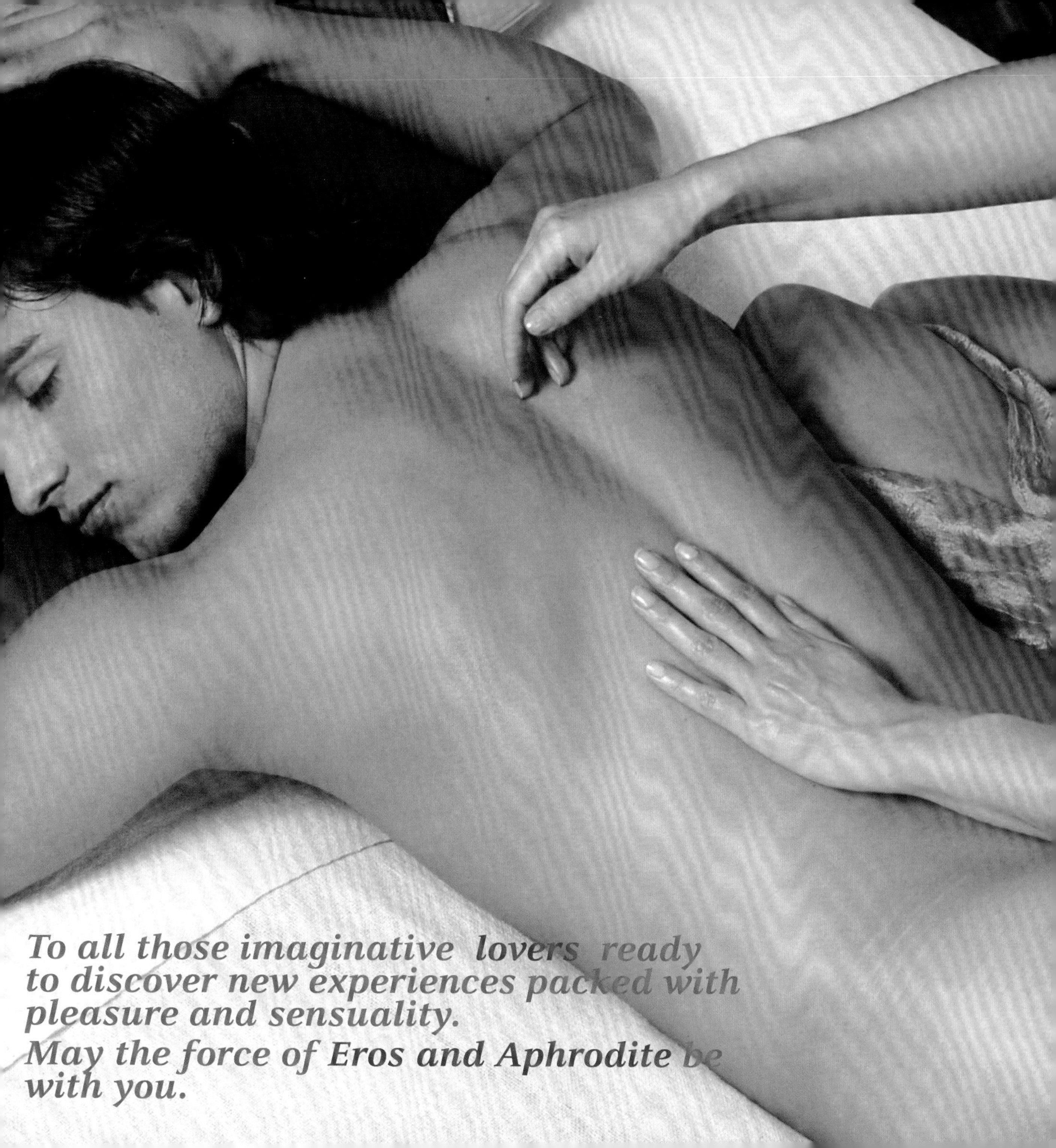

To all those imaginative lovers ready to discover new experiences packed with pleasure and sensuality.
May the force of Eros and Aphrodite be with you.

Contents

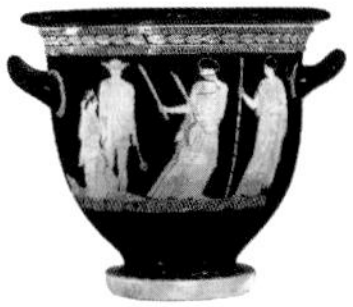

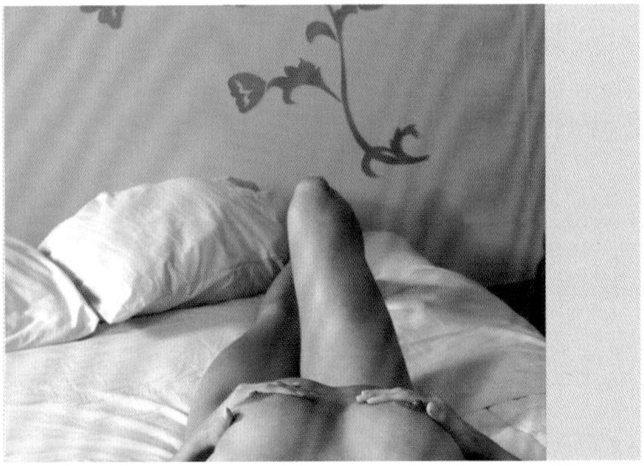

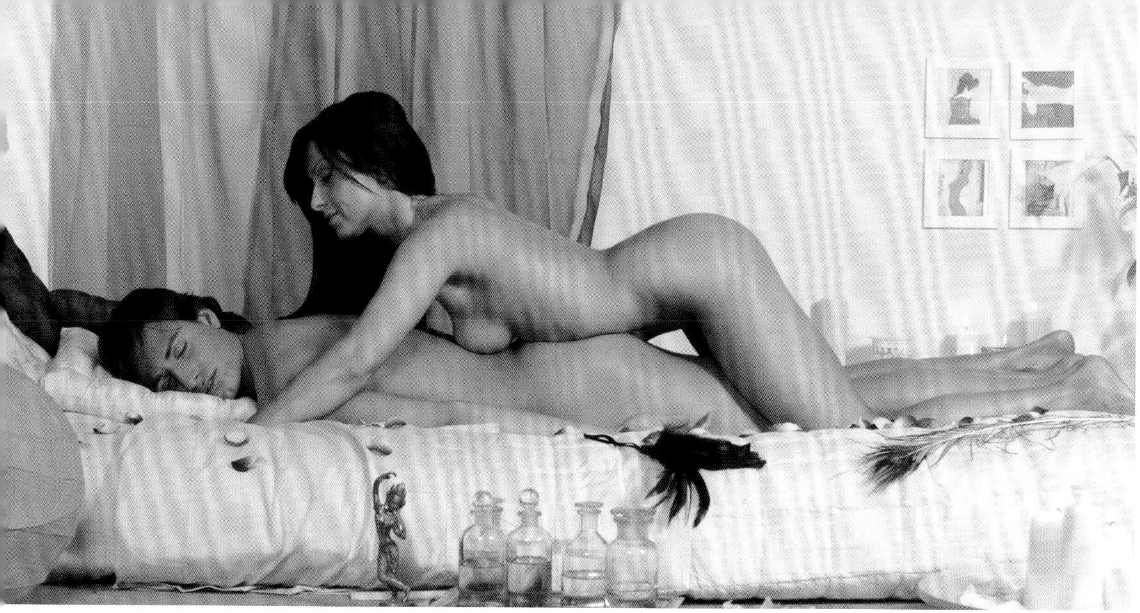

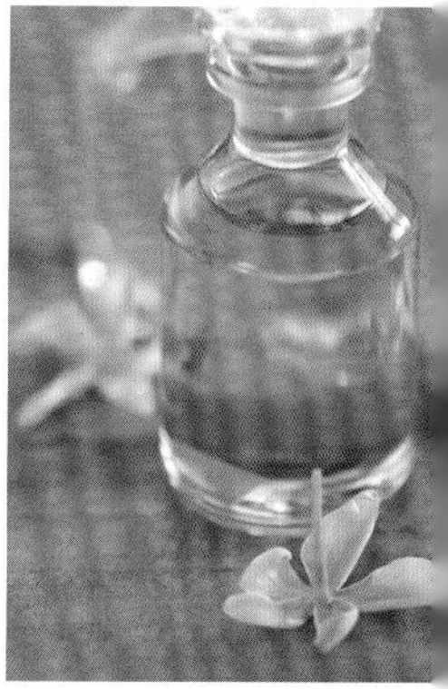

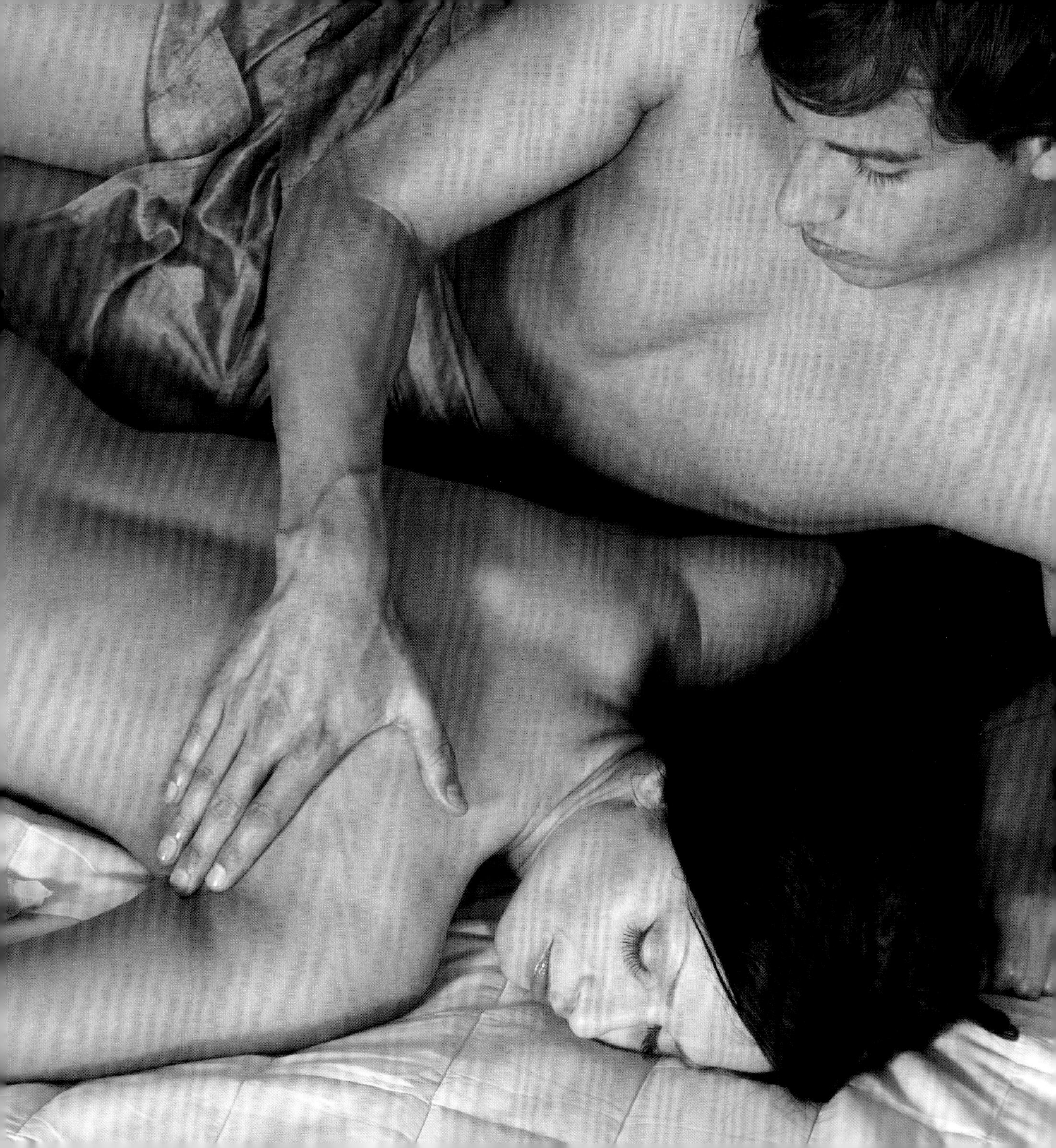

A Refined Touch

To caress is the most simple and natural way to show affection using touch. Each caress is a message of love and erotic massage is nothing less than the most seductive and refined way of showing this love. In this book we invite you to undertake a wonderful journey of exploration across your lover's skin. It is a journey that will take you to the center of their soul.

The skin protects us from the outer world and also puts us in contact with it. It is our biggest and most important sexual organ. It is a gateway to sensuality and deep emotion.

Dare to awaken your body, and that of your partner, to new experiences of sensual love and pleasure. Have fun experimenting with the abundant know-how offered in this book: seductive aids, aromatic oils, tempting aphrodisiac drinks, and, above all, a good massage. Such a combination will prove irresistible to your partner.

The type of massage you will learn here offers more intimate, profound, and mindful contact than that proffered by mere sex. And, of course, it provides much more pleasure.

It is a marvelous, unforgettable experience to realize what effect the slightest touch of our hands can have on our partner, and how it is possible to share the excitement and pleasure they are capable of giving. It is equally wonderful to let ourselves go by putting ourselves in our lover's hands, so they may awaken our body to the endless possibilities of unexpected, extraordinary feelings and sensations.

Discover, here, a new way of getting in touch with your body, a new way of erotic encounter with your beloved, a path full of sensuality, pleasure, and partnership.

SYLVIA PATTERSON

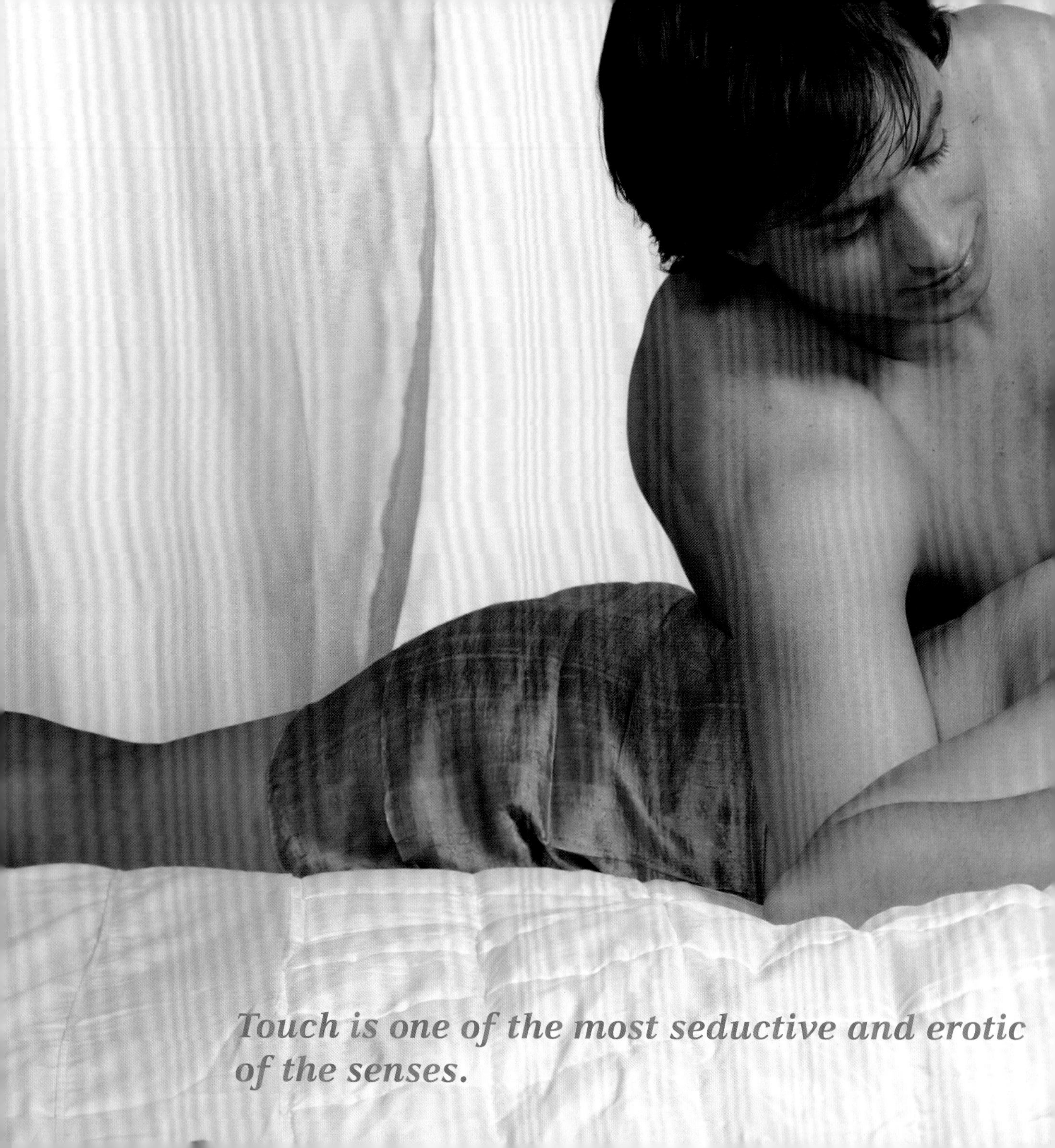

Touch is one of the most seductive and erotic of the senses.

Physical Contact

THAT WONDERFUL NEED

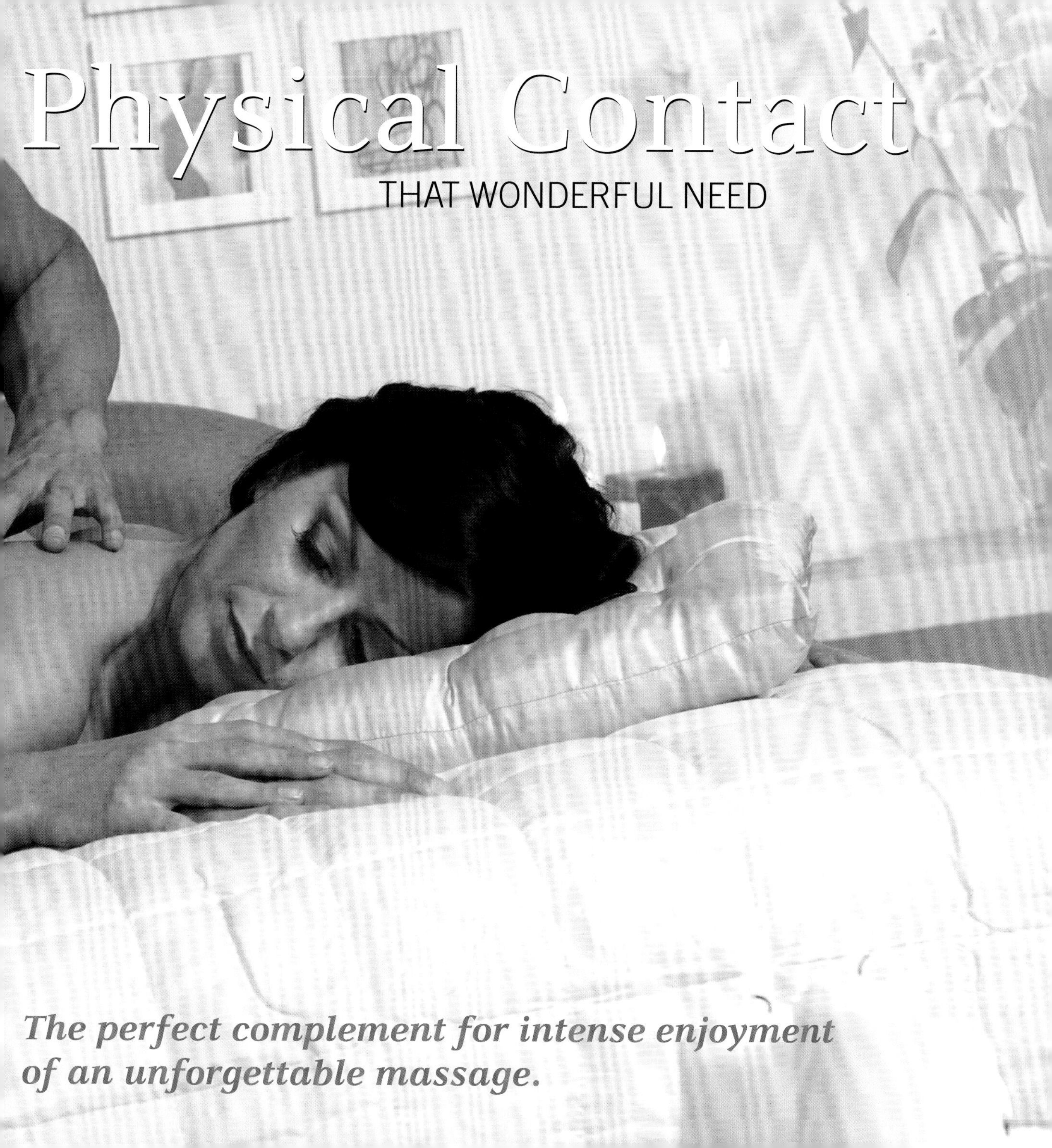

The perfect complement for intense enjoyment of an unforgettable massage.

Touch: Our Greatest Consolation

The greatest consolation and most beautiful way we tell each other "I love you" every day comes from learning the language of touching, that language lovers use to send subtle, passionate messages.

We use the word "touch" not only to refer to caresses. We also use it when talking about something that has moved, inspired, or made a deep impression on us. We say "we are touched," and in this way our language reflects to what extent this contact is essential to us.

Physical contact is also our greatest comfort, the best way to undo a hurt, to soothe a wound, to **revive love.** In this sense, couple's massage, that wonderful way of giving and receiving, is our best means of caring for a relationship, to enrich it and strengthen its weak points, to make it more profound and more substantial each time.

When we are gently touched, **our self-esteem is strengthened** and we feel, as a result, happier and more valued as persons. When our partner bestows their gentle touch on us, they give us all kinds of pleasant sensations, and we feel reborn in our love for them and immediately experience the desire to return the same delight to them.

Couple's massage can **revive** a stuck relationship and it can bring two people who are drifting apart to feel **renewed love.** It can bring back **passion** to a loving relationship that has become routine. This can happen for any couple, whatever their age, for there are no limits to the power of touch.

Stress: Our Greatest Threat

Why do so many people, with the passing of time, lose interest in touching and being touched? Why do they seem too tired for love?

Today, the majority of us are subjected to stress and we should be aware this is the principal enemy of sensuality and erotic love. Stress causes us to be permanently stuck in our problems, it

A simple touch of the skin can cause us to quiver with pure delight.

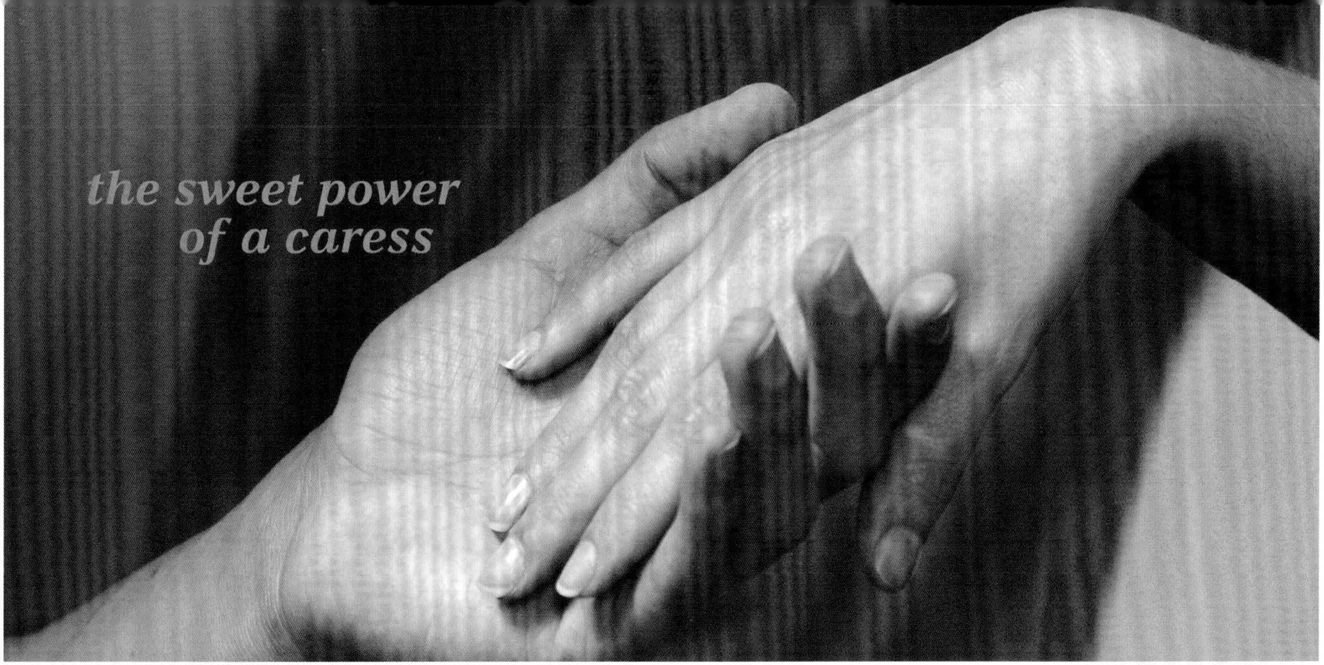

makes us feel mentally strung out and causes enormous muscular tensions in our bodies. It makes sense that insofar as we are its victims, we will have little desire for fulfilling our love fantasies, nor will we have any energy for love play. Nevertheless, a good sensual massage is our **best weapon** to fight against stress and its terrible effects, since it will bring about the relaxation we need to ready our body and mind for sensual love and sex.

The next time your partner comes home tired or preoccupied after an exhausting day at work, you don't have to do anything more than put the **sure-fire benefits of touching** to the test. Greet him/her affectionately, have them sit a while on the sofa. **Take their hand, gently,** and begin stroking their arm. Invite him/her to lie back and relax while you give them a soft, loving foot massage. You can also gently stroke and caress his/her face. Whatever you do, the most important thing is to fully enjoy the sense of intimacy that you feel growing between the two of you. It is quite possible this affectionate attention will arouse your mutual **sensual desire.** Plan on including these little "love getaways" in your daily round and you will see, before long, how your sexual relations will greatly improve.

With touch we communicate love, desire, and friendship. . . . Say it with your hands.

The Power of Touch

It might seem like an exaggeration, but it isn't; if we were willing to give our partners just ten minutes a day of affectionate caressing, a minimum of three times a week, it would save thousands of marriages. It would also save millions of dollars in visits to doctors and therapists, so great is the potential of gentle touch and so little does it demand of us.

Insurance companies have proved that the risk of getting into a traffic accident on the way to work is dramatically reduced by a morning "goodbye" kiss. It would seem **a kiss is a type of anti-stress vaccine** that protects us, calms us, and affords us the wonderful experience of being loved and valued by someone. It has been shown that men and women who receive daily hugs and kisses live an average of five years longer than those who receive them only on occasion. **Touch** is, therefore, seen to be a fundamental factor when it comes time to rate the quality of our life. We are speaking here of touch in the wider sense, including those small shows of affection exchanged at any time, so simple and much to be encouraged, as well as a good massage, a massage given just to help our partner relax, or a sensual massage which may or may not turn into a pleasurable sexual encounter. The important thing to understand is **all affectionate touching is powerful and essential.**

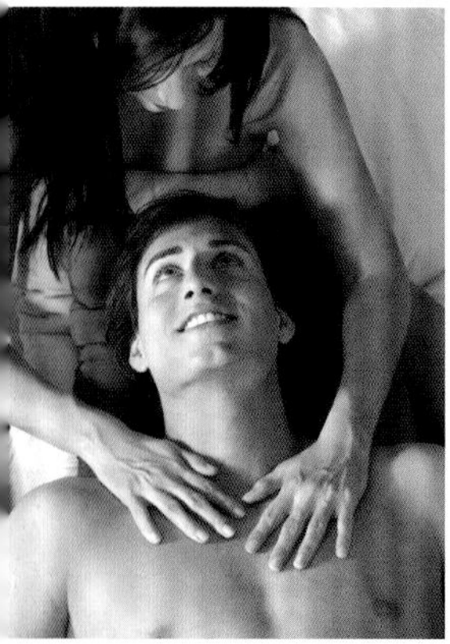

A Blurred Line Between Relaxation and Pleasure

When we talk about couple's massage, it is actually quite difficult and unnecessary to establish a clear boundary between a massage given simply for comfort and one that awakens that excitement that turns into a potent erotic impulse. The couple will draw that line. It is easy to convert a comforting massage into an erotic event by just changing the intensity of the hand pressure.

Tactile sensations capture all of our attention and allow us

For example, we can go from applying intense pressure that loosens the muscles to the most gentle stroking that allows us to be sensitive to the feeling of our partner's skin and the contours of their body. The most important thing is for the massage to unfold spontaneously and not according to some plan, or be overly controlled.

Skin Deep

Our dominant senses are sight and hearing. For massage, however, **touch** is the most involved sense. During couple's massage, tactile sensations will draw our total attention and allow us to discover new ways of experiencing and knowing our bodies. It is an experience where intimacy, pairing, and sensuality take on the major role.

Were you aware that fingertips and lips contain almost countless nerve endings directly connected to our brain? For this reason, an erotic massage is a **pleasure involving all five senses** and no part of the body should be excluded. Caressing can do it all. Just as with the sexual act, massage involves the entire skin.

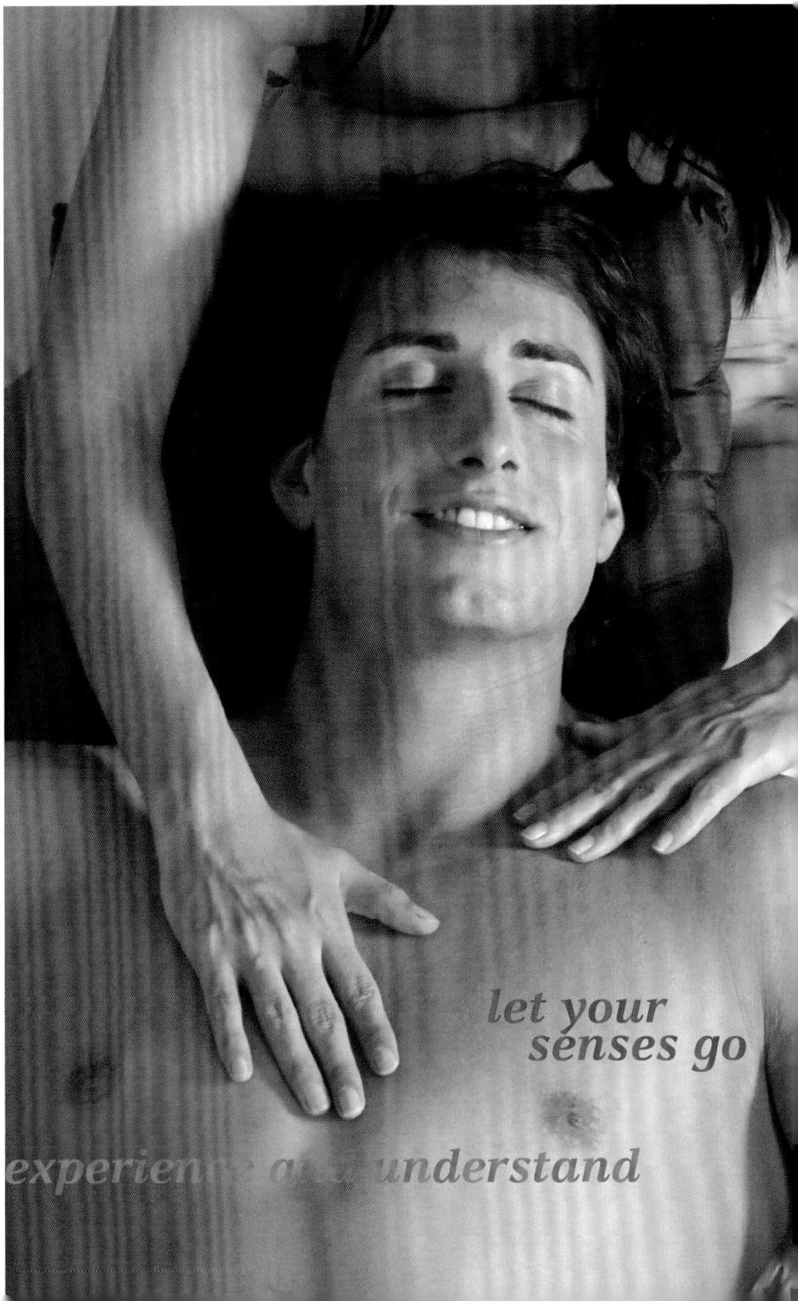

to discover new ways to experience and understand our bodies . . .

The Importance of Smell

It might sound strange, but **when it comes time to choose a mate, the sense of smell rules.** Whether we are aware of it or not, we are always sensing the odor of others and when we are "skin to skin" the body of the other person gives off scents, which act directly on our unconscious mind. Whether we know it or not, smell helps us choose our mate.

Both erotic massage and massage for relaxation share the objective of becoming more attuned to olfactory experience. In line with this, we can choose a special blend of aromatic oils before we begin. These oils will increase our pleasure and help us reach a greater degree of intimacy with our partner.

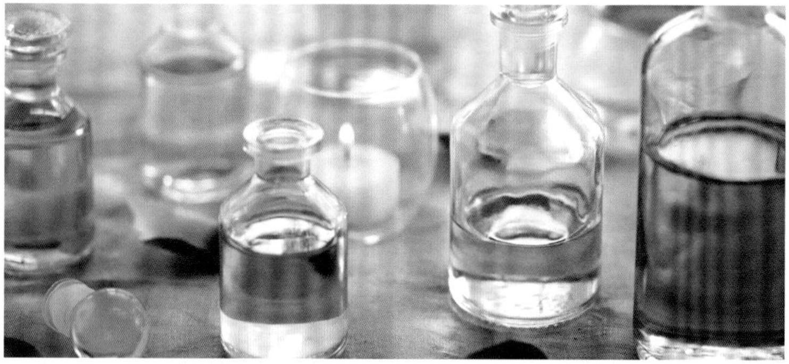

Marvelous Aromas

Even the faintest exposure to a pleasant fragrance can raise our spirits. **Aromas awaken memories and feelings** and can greatly stimulate creativity, focus, and sense of well-being. For this reason, the secret of aromas and their wonderful effects has captivated humanity for generations.

Today almost all of us know there are scents that can greatly help us to relax. It's been proven for quite some time that beta brain waves, which indicate the presence of stress, can be changed to beneficial alpha waves by means of meditation and relaxation exercises. The same effect can be realized using pleasant aromas.

Making a blend of scents that pleases both partners can foster **deep relaxation,** equivalent to that experienced during sleep. These aromas can also help us when it's time to elicit and wake up **sexual desire.**

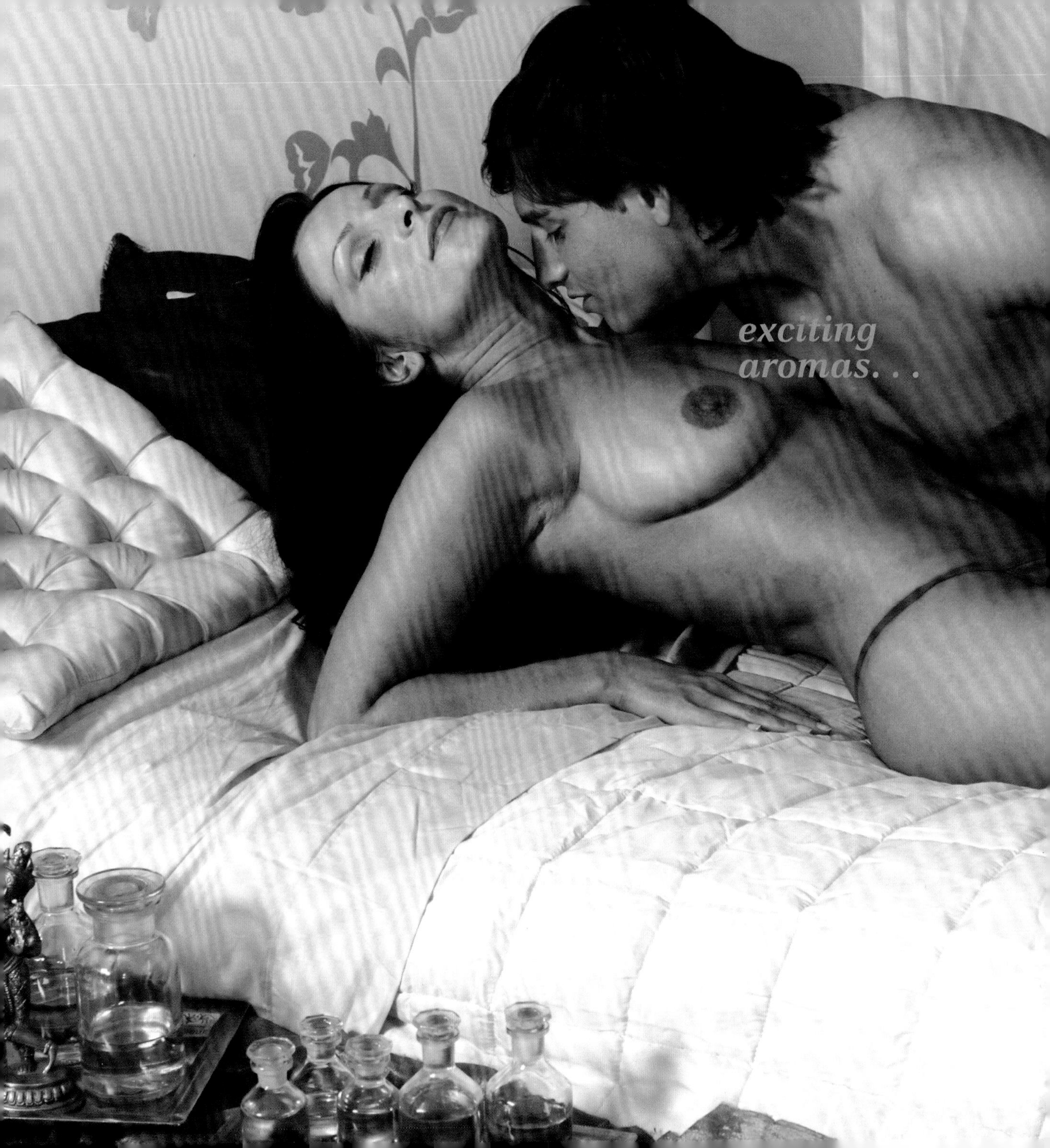
exciting
aromas. . .

A Brief History of Massage

Aroma and Seduction

Different cultures of antiquity knew very well to what extent taste and smell can be stimulated by massage. Immersing themselves in a world of sensual eroticism, they made use of aromatic baths, oils, and ointments. In Greece and Rome, love, eroticism, and sensuality were represented mainly by female gods. Aphrodite is the Greek goddess of love and Venus is her Roman equivalent. Aphrodite was highly venerated in ancient Greece with festivals dedicated to her, particularly in Athens and Corinth. Her name derives from the Greek word "aphros," which means foam.

In India, on the other hand, the masculine principle was strongly associated with sensuality and eroticism. In any event, all of these ancient cultures were closely linked by their common interest in sensual aromas, symbolized by images of plants. We are fortunate that their knowledge has been fully preserved up to the present day.

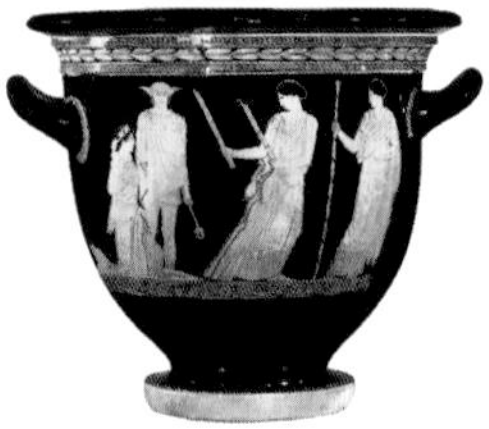

Greek vase with images of the goddess Demeter.

The Greek Gods

The first Greek philosophers represented the feminine archetype with six goddesses:

Demeter is the goddess of sustenance, **Hera** is the one who seeks power, **Athena** represents a shrewd and prudent woman, **Artemis** is lover of nature and freedom, **Persephone** represents intuition, spirituality, and emotional intelligence and, of course, **Aphrodite** is the goddess of love and represents supremacy of sensuality and beauty.

Aphrodite is the one who interests us the most when it comes to erotic couple's massage. She is sovereign over scents, sensuality, massage, caressing, love play, cosmetics, beauty, and everything concerning aesthetics and pleasure. The Greek god Apollo, who symbolizes life, immortality, harmony, beauty, and good would be Aphrodite's masculine equivalent.

The history of all the Mediterranean peoples is closely related to the goddess Aphrodite, who is the great representation of love, beauty, sexuality, and passion. She is the goddess of all lovers and represents the power of the feminine role in art and sex. According to legend, Aphrodite was born in the foam of the waves and when she became aware of her nakedness she covered herself with a branch of flowers of the **myrtle bush.** It is for this reason the leaves of the myrtle are compared to the form of the vagina, whose outer lips resemble the myrtle's leaves and whose inner lips resemble the fruit of the myrtle. Aphrodite rules sensuality and is the divinity with total knowledge of the stimulating effects of aromatic plants. The adjective "aphrodisiac" is derived from her name and refers to everything that excites and prepares us for love and sensual pleasure.

Similarly, Eros, the name of that other god, refers to eroticism and love's dalliance. According to Greek mythology, the art of perfuming was introduced by the nymph Oenone, an attendant of Aphrodite and lover of Paris.

Rome and Venus

The art of perfuming, invented by the Greeks, arrived in Rome when the Greeks colonized Italy and men and women began to bathe themselves several times a day using scented bath water.

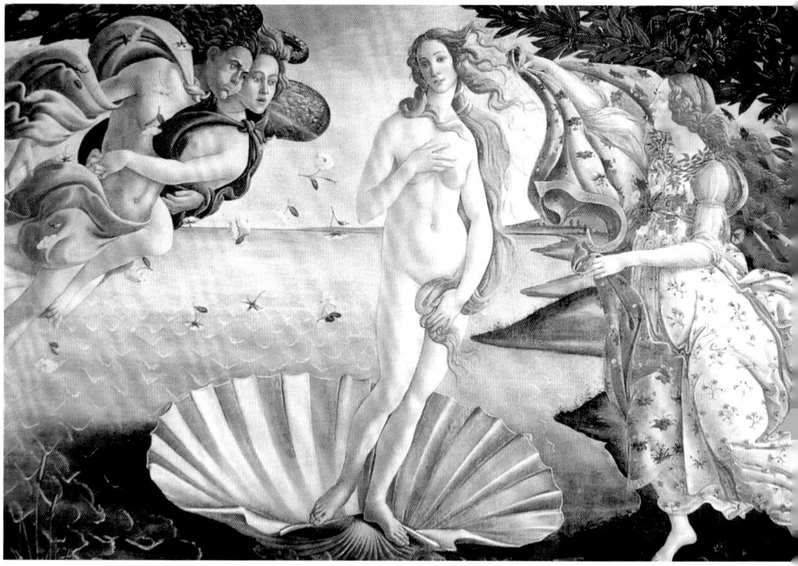

Birth of Venus (1485), by *Alessandro Botticelli.*

The Roman goddess of love and sensuality was named **Venus.** She, also, is described as having arisen from the foam of the waves and also covered her nudity with myrtle leaves. **The Three Graces**, who served her and her son **Cupid,** equivalent to the Greek's **Eros**, are often shown wearing garlands of myrtle. Roman temples were always adorned with roses, the essence of which was considered to be the "blood of Venus." As for the "Mount of Venus," this is another name for a woman's *mons pubis*, the pubic mound. And certainly, the name of Venus is carried on in the legendary name of the city of Venice that is known, even today, as the "city of lovers."

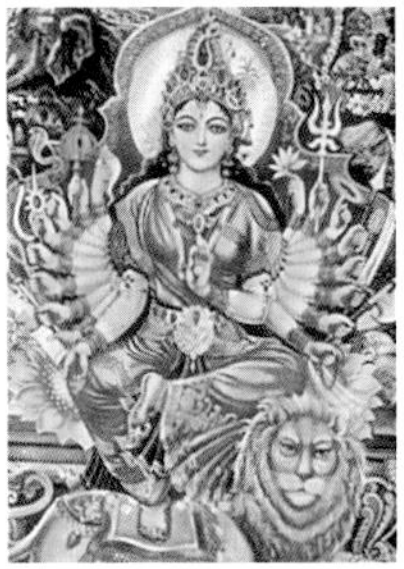

Shakti symbolizes the creative power of nature. She is feminine, active, and changeable.

The Romans were very aware that sensual aromas possessed medicinal properties. The most popular recipes were chiseled on marble plaques and displayed in the temple of Venus. Following the example of the Egyptians, the Romans instituted public baths of water perfumed with fine, aromatic additives. Romans would go to the baths daily. During the reign of Nero, Rome had over a thousand public baths using aromatic waters. Nero's wife, Popea, bathed every day in donkey milk, a practice recommended by the erotic tradition of India.

The Tradition of India

The most famous book about sex in the world, the **Kama Sutra,** has come down to us from India. In this ancient text, aromas (especially sandalwood) permeate everywhere from temple to bedroom. The Kama Sutra contains precise instructions about aromatic substances and blends that form an essential component of sexual play.

In the Hindu tradition we see the god Indra always appearing with sandalwood paste anointed on his chest.

Another important Hindu god is Kama, who is equal to the Roman god Cupid. He always appears armed with a bow made of sugar cane and arrows tipped with jasmine, known for its aphrodisiac qualities.

Kama's arrows are intended to reach the "victim's" heart through one of the five senses.

The Ritual of the Five Essences

Shakti is the Hindu deity who represents the creative force. In tantric practice, the woman is venerated before coitus as the personification of this force/deity. According to the ritual, the woman's body is anointed and massaged with different aromatic essences to honor her role as creator and to raise her spirit so as to manifest her divine nature. In the "ritual of the five essences" that is used to stimulate the five senses, jasmine oil is spread over her hands, patchouli oil over her face and neck, amber perfume or musk on her breasts, oil of ox musk on her genitals, sandalwood oil on her thighs, and saffron oil on the soles of her feet. For his part, the man is anointed only with oil or paste of sandalwood on his forehead, neck, chest, navel, genitals, arms, thighs, hands, and feet.

It's only natural that the aforementioned treatises that talk of how to prepare the

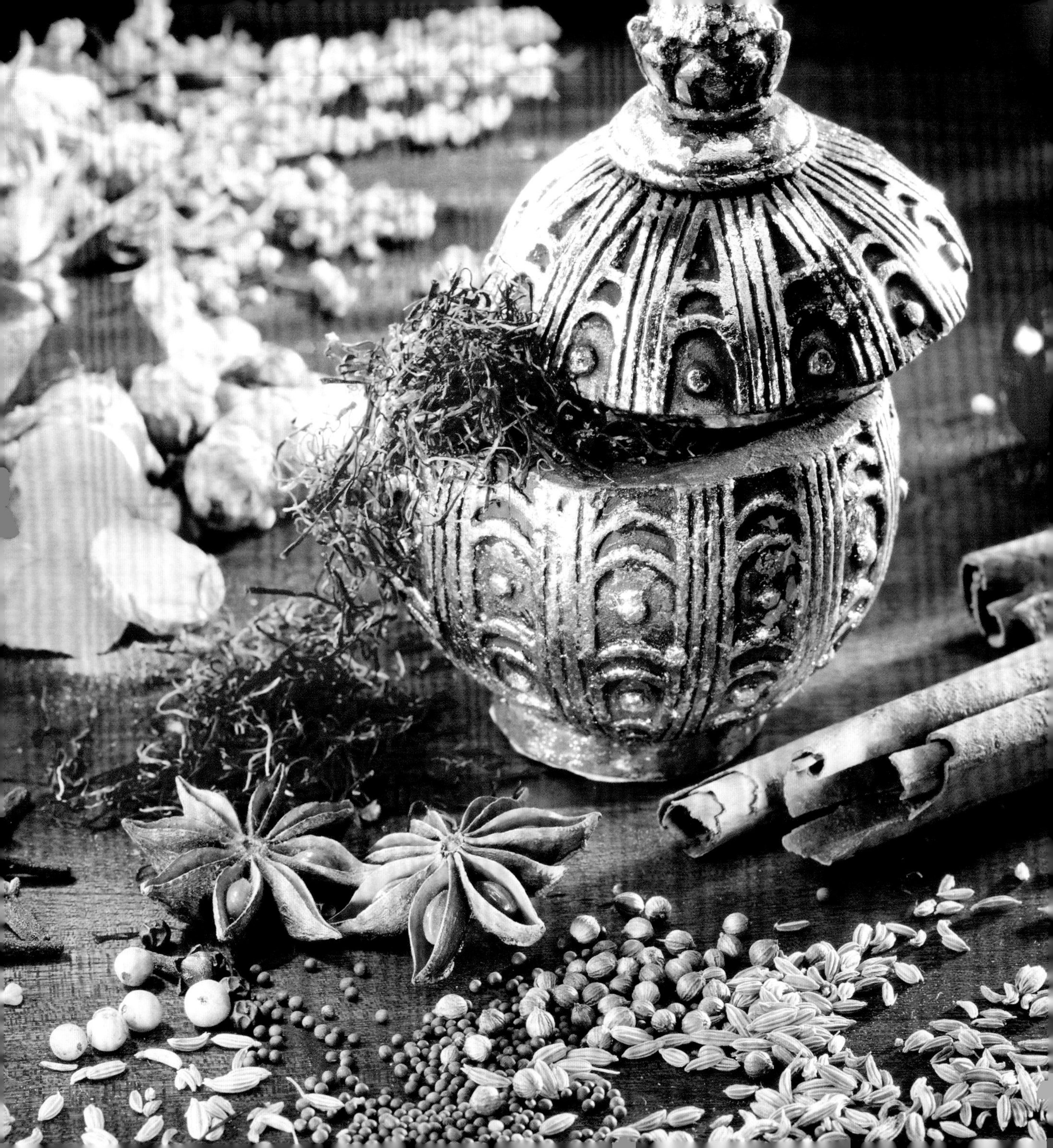

body for love making were written in a part of the world where there are daily celebrations dedicated to the sun as a symbol of life and sexuality, where rose water is produced in abundance, where sandalwood trees abound, and where hundreds of aromatic plants grow and flowers and herbs are part of the rituals and daily life of the people.

The Egyptian Tradition

One of the most long-lived love stories still with us today has come down from Egypt. It deals with the passionate, intense, and ultimately tragic love between **Marc Antony** and **Cleopatra.** Tradition tells how their meeting took place on the banks of the Tiber and that the beautiful queen captivated Marc Antony by soaking the sails of her barque in jasmine oil and other substances loaded with sensual aromas and powerful aphrodisiacs. **Shakespeare,** in his tragedy *Anthony and Cleopatra* writes "the winds were lovesick with them," referring to the aroma of Cleopatra's perfumed sails.

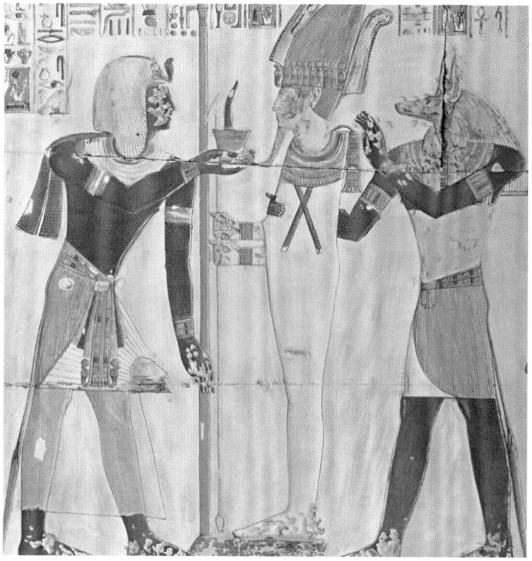

Incense ceremony represented on a fresco found in the tomb of Sethi I.

From the Renaissance to Today

For a period of time the Christian tradition, with its rejection of sensuality and bodily pleasure, put an end to the cultivation of the senses developed by the Greeks and Romans and the use of aromatics and aphrodisiacs in daily life.

It wasn't until the Middle Ages, with the Crusades, that aromatic substances were rediscovered along with their power of sensuality. Thanks to the discovery of new, exotic perfumes,

Egyptian men and women would use fine oils and perfume

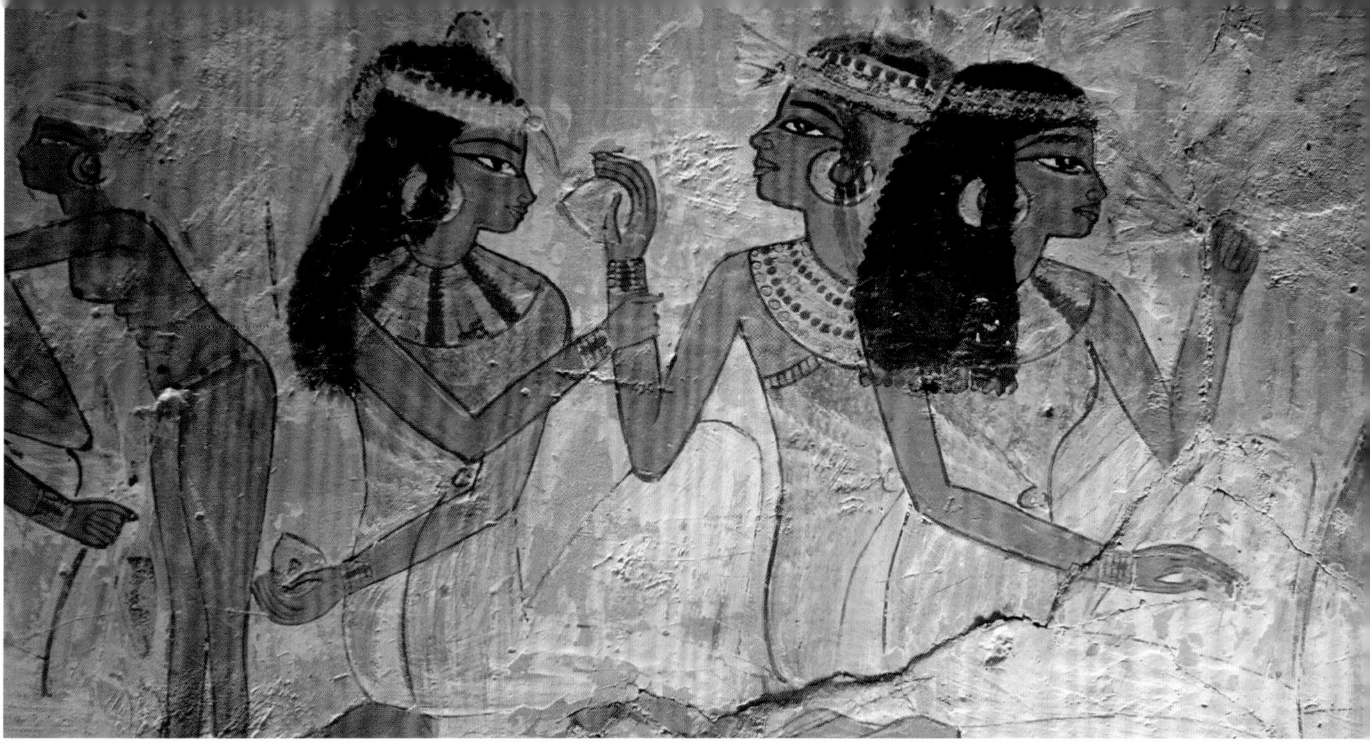

the body again began to be valued and attended to and cared for as it deserved. A primary aid in this was rose oil, mixed with camellia seed, that tasted and smelled divinely and was used to moisten the lips. Different parts of the body came to be perfumed and anointed with aromatic oils, each with its particular virtue, and so the first massage rituals made their appearance in our culture.

Many of the practices coming down from ancient cultures are still completely valid and easy to follow today. We can fill the bathtub with salts and take a romantic candlelight bath, or anoint our bodies with aromatic oils and essences and adorn our bedroom with seductive accessories. All of this will help to bring partners closer together and encourage their tenderness and communication. If we are not used to these simple practices, then one member of the couple will have to take the first step. Usually, it will be the woman who dares to do it. Apparently, a woman's capacity to take the initiative is as old as the techniques of massage itself.

In ancient Egypt using unguents and oils was a common practice.

for both personal care and sacred rituals.

The Pleasure of Touching and Being Touched

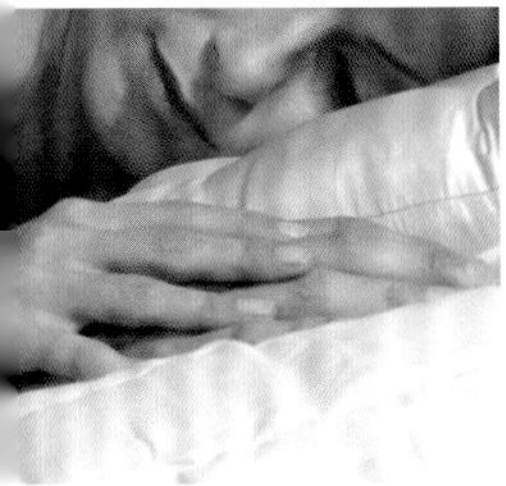

Perfect Reciprocity

When we speak of erotic massage being a technique used to obtain intense pleasure for all our senses and even capable of serving as a viable alternative to orgasm, it is evident we have the idea of reciprocity in our minds. Couple's massage should always be characterized by a **perfect balance of giving and receiving.** It is probable that if one always gives without receiving in kind, that person will lose interest.

We are not suggesting that it is necessary to get a massage immediately after having given one, though giving and getting in the same session can be extremely pleasant. It's likely that during a session of sensual massage harmonious giving and receiving will flow naturally, but it is also possible and equally recommended to change roles on different days and sessions. The important thing is that both partners have the opportunity to enjoy the experience of both giving and receiving a massage.

It is also important to understand that when one gives one is also receiving, since giving a caress is not just giving pleasure but also receiving it *through the giving.*

But what about when your companion seems reluctant to participate, or if they snicker at all the oils, perfumes, and erotic paraphernalia? Maybe they find the feathers and silk handkerchiefs you want to experiment with a bit weird. This often happens with "accessories." It also happens quite often that a man will be pleased to get a massage, but afterwards is not inclined to give one due to its relaxing effect. If this has happened to you, be patient. Don't get upset, **keep indulging him, from time to time, with sensual massages**, and don't set aside the "accoutrements." Let your imagination fly. Don't give up and you will see very soon that **your partner will realize how much those items enrich your sex life.** With your persistence, affection, and a bit of time, you will get him to change his old patterns and habits.

The delicate touch of your partner's fingers, their naked skin upon your back . . .

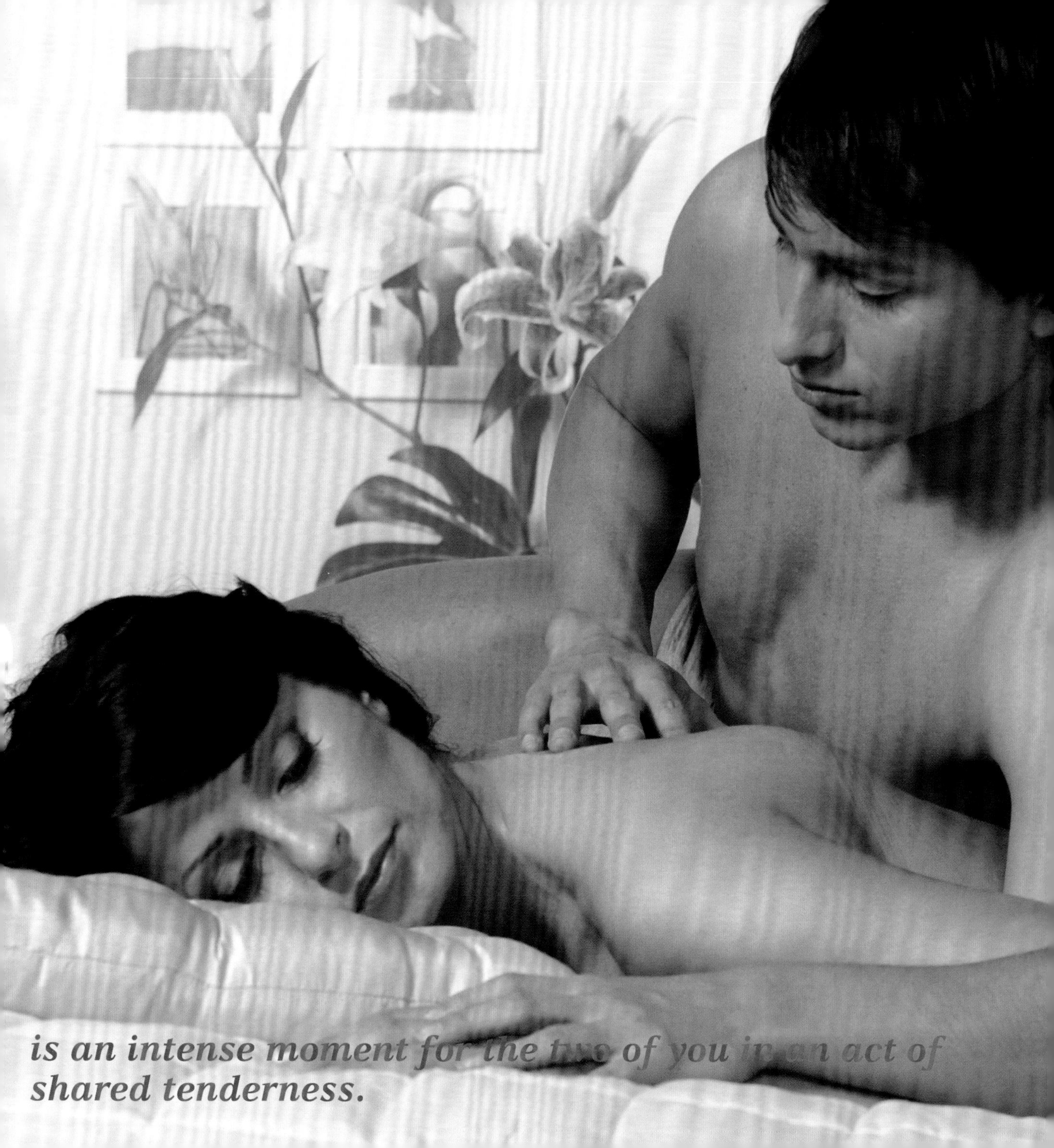

is an intense moment for the two of you in an act of shared tenderness.

Taking the Initiative

Over the centuries in the West, women have been considered as beings devoted to nature. It has always been their responsibility to take care of the family and today it continues to be the norm that the woman bears most of the couple's burden; she must be patient, affectionate, she must take care of him . . .

Nevertheless, women often complain that their partners do not caress them tenderly, unless they want sex, and that the man's affectionate touching always carries this end in sight. For their part, it is the men who usually take the initiative and assume the active role regarding sex. Men often complain about this and say they would like their companion to seduce them and show their desire in a more direct way.

A couple's massage can become the perfect remedy to address this desire for mutuality expressed by both sexes. For the men, massages provide a way to learn to be sensitive to and pamper their partner, as well as surrender to her and receive from her. For women, when they give the massage, they can take advantage of assuming the active role that is usually deferred to the men. In this way, both learn to strengthen their respective masculine and feminine aspects.

man and woman: two energies opposed yet complementary

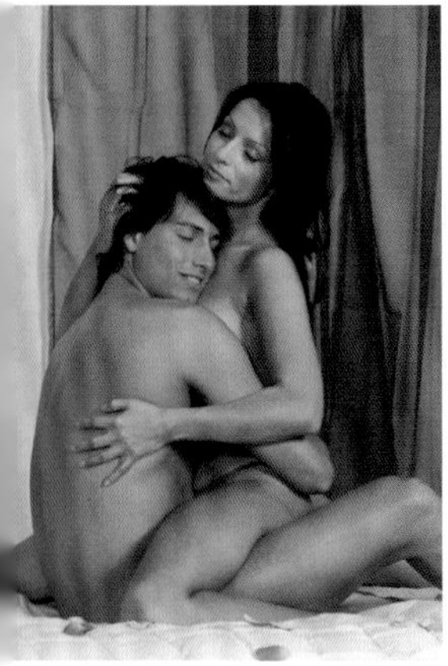

Yin and Yangs

In this book, when we speak of "male" or "female," we are referring to the archetype of the two forces, the energies the Chinese Taoists knew as "Yin" and "Yang." **Yin would come to be known as the receptive, feminine force, and Yang the active, energetic masculine.** The Yin/Yang symbol embodies the unity of both forces and the fact that one doesn't exist without the other. Both are part of constant change and alternation such as day and night that, though mutually exclusive, also give rise to each another.

Men and women throughout the ages have always embodied this constant contest between the two forces. Man searches for woman and woman searches for man. Like the androgynous beings Plato described that were part man and part woman joined back-to-back, and later condemned to be apart, we constantly search for the other, who is our own missing half.

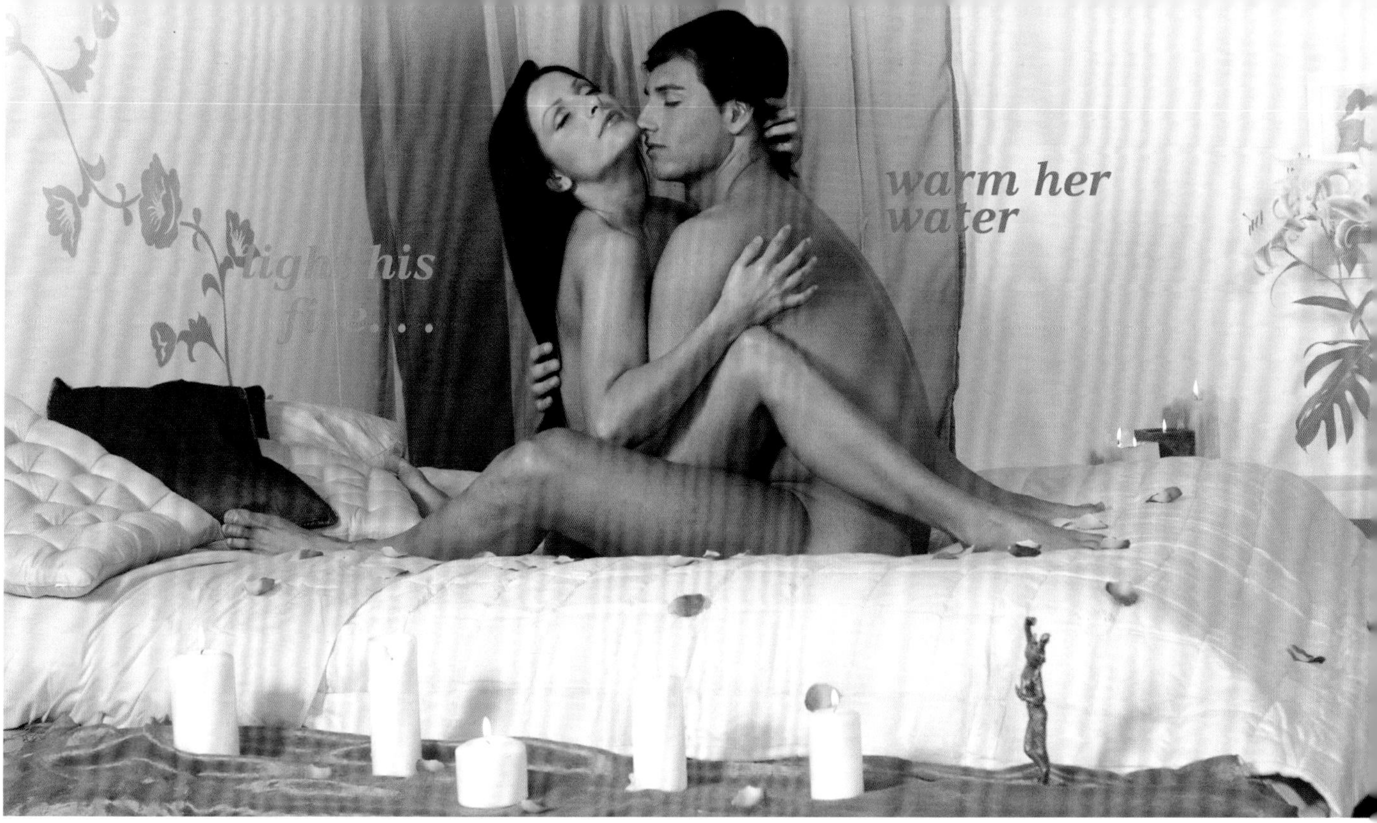

Union

In sexual union, man and woman realize the perfect blending of Yin and Yang, those two vital energies that are opposed and antagonistic and simultaneously complementary.

To better satisfy his woman, Chinese tradition advises the man to practice the "Tao of Love" that will excite her and make her reach orgasm more slowly, but with greater intensity. The Tao of Love teaches that **woman is like water and man is like fire. Fire burns quickly and extinguishes quickly, while water heats up slowly and once hot, takes a long time to cool down.** Man, therefore, is the fire that ignites instantly and goes out quickly, and the woman is the water that gets hot and takes a while to cool off. Fire is put out by water, and water is heated by fire.

Chinese culture, as well as other Eastern cultures, teaches that a man has a feminine aspect and a woman a masculine aspect. These cultures have made massage and erotic sport keys to attaining a fulfilled and happy love life.

The chapters that follow are filled with suggestions designed to achieve this end. Letting yourself be inspired by them and using your five senses, practice everything from the gentlest touching and stimulation to full-blown, exciting sensual massage.

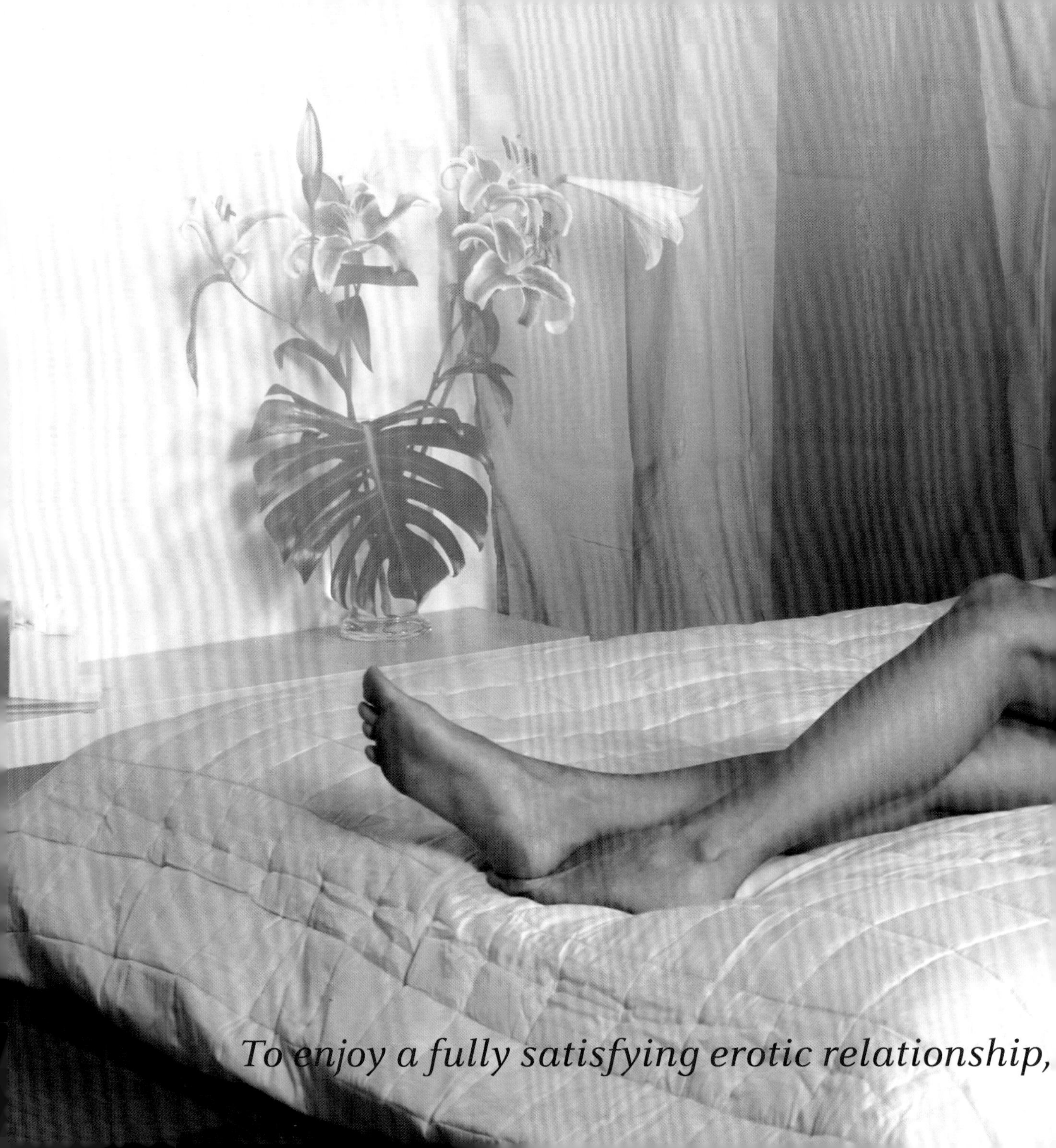

To enjoy a fully satisfying erotic relationship,

Knowing and Loving Yourself

THE SECRET TO PLEASURE

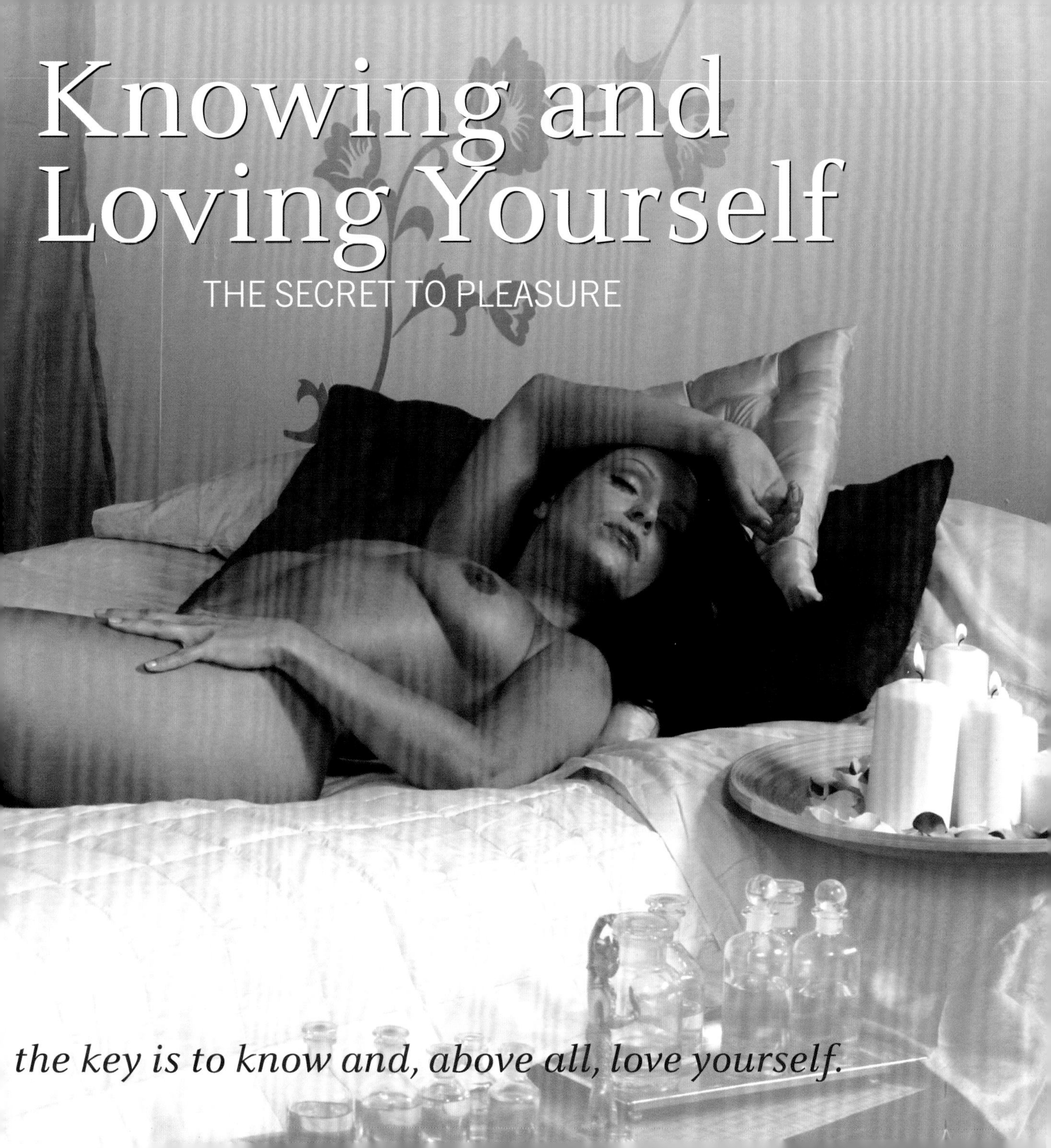

the key is to know and, above all, love yourself.

The Enemies of Sensual Love

The desire to totally attend to your partner's body, to lavish him or her with caresses, cuddles, and care is often lost due to routine and exhaustion. That pleasant thrill of love's enchantment extinguishes and gives way to an apathy and weariness, which cause love making with our partner to become more sporadic and less intense.

In the first chapter we saw how stress can be the chief enemy of sensual love. Routine is another unwelcome guest. It is that weariness that entices us to sit comfortably in front of the TV instead of preparing a nice bath with our partner and enjoying a full massage. Sure, sitting in front of the tube can be more comfortable, but remember that this excess of "comfort" can end up impoverishing our sex life and having very negative effects on the relationship with our partner.

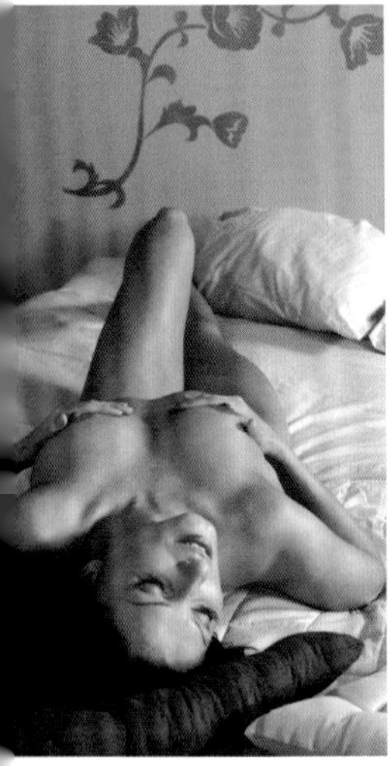

Sometimes our own inhibitions hold us back from touching our partner freely or giving ourselves to their caresses without reservation. It is usually women who have more hang-ups about their bodies and feel dissatisfied with them. The urge to be as "perfect" as the models in ads prevents them from totally enjoying physical relations.

Self-Acceptance

The first, irrevocable requirement for being able to enjoy sex fully and richly is to lay aside all hang-ups and accept yourself just as you are. Just as to love and be loved by others requires us to love ourselves first and consider ourselves worthy of love, so does sensual pleasure with our partner proceed from liking our own body and being able to relax and feel sexy.

Women often have problems along these lines. Excessive publicity, movie stars, super-models, etc. all set an impossibly high standard of beauty that weakens and quashes their self-esteem.

To enjoy pleasuring yourself is the key to learning to

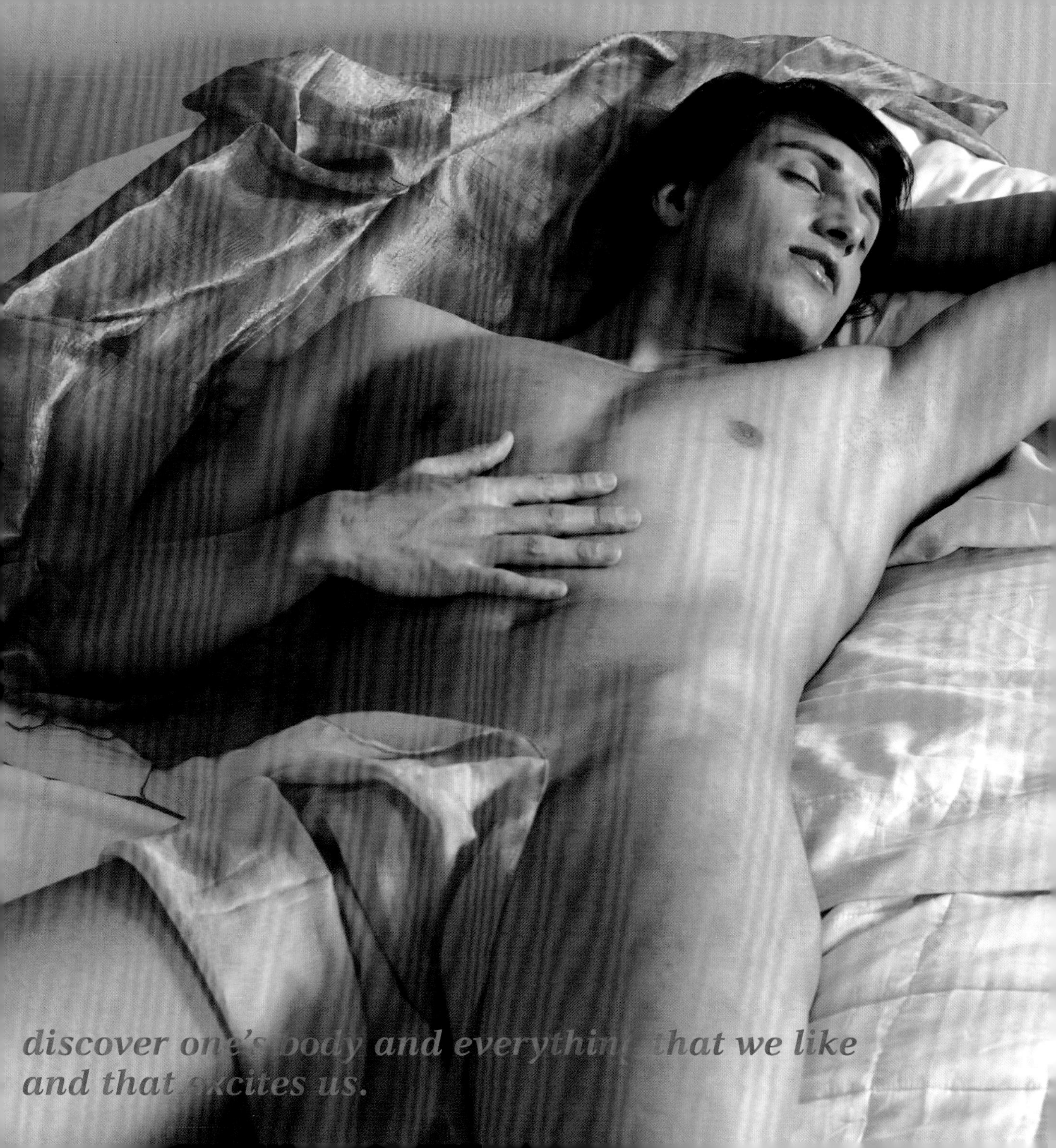

discover one's body and everything that we like and that excites us.

It is likely that their breasts will seem to be too big or too small, or their thighs too chubby, or their hips excessively wide. They become obsessed by an ideal that, in the majority of cases, has absolutely nothing to do with their actual physical makeup and so they forget their own unique, individual beauty. They ignore the most important and most effective secret of seduction: that when we feel satisfied with our own body we become more sensual in the eyes of others.

Among the different cultural traditions there are various rituals and useful exercises to help us better know our bodies. In the famous Hindu tradition of Tantra that profusely and precisely describes all types of sexual techniques and practices, first place is given to completely knowing your own body and how it functions. All those cultures that have concerned themselves with the body and eroticism have taken the view that first and foremost it is necessary to know and accept yourself just as you are.

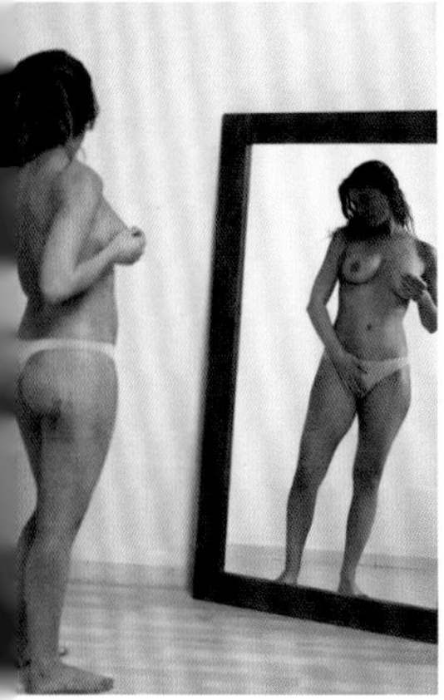

To Be Able to Love, Love Yourself

Our long Christian tradition has given us the wise and significant words of Jesus: "Love your neighbor as yourself."

Simply analyzing the structure of this sentence makes it evident that to love oneself is an indispensable condition for loving others. What sense would the word "as" have if I don't love myself? How am I going to know how I should love?

Psychologists do not tire of repeating that those who don't love or accept themselves are incapable of loving and accepting others. For this reason, one of our first and prime tasks must be to examine ourselves and our own capacity for self-love. Only if we become aware of our own complexity and individuality will we be able to understand, forgive, and correct ourselves. And only then will we be able to understand and love others and accept them as they are with all their faults and virtues, just the same way we accept ourselves.

Erich Fromm, in his fascinating work *The Art of Loving,* dedicates a whole section to the importance of self-esteem and self-love, showing to what extent both are indispensable to learning to love.

How do we take the first step in loving and knowing ourselves? Beginning with the body would be the best way. It might sound strange, but pleasuring ourselves is a great way to learn how to give pleasure to others.

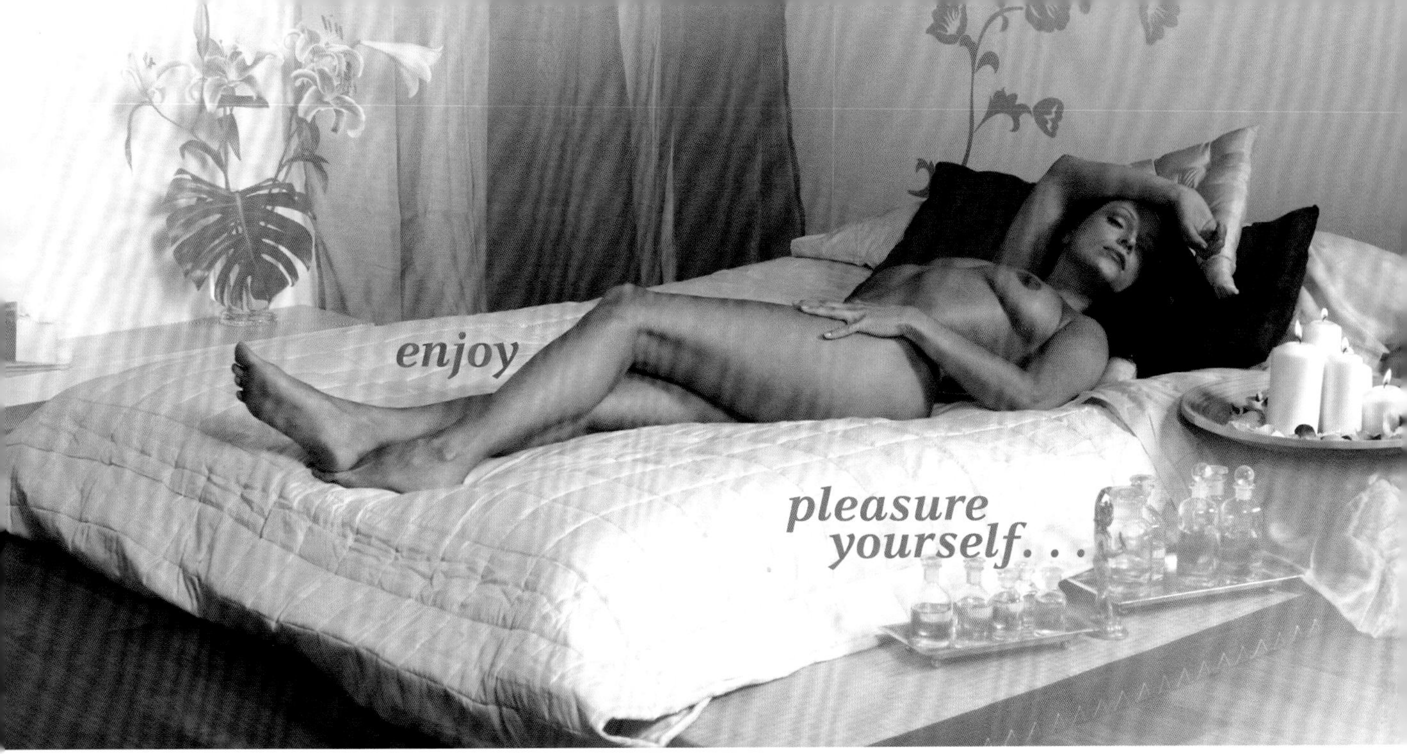

Exploring Our Own Body

What is the secret? How can we arrive at feeling at ease in our own skin? How can we get rid of our hang-ups and give ourselves totally to pleasure? The first thing is to consider the whole body, and not just certain parts of it, as one enormous erogenous zone which can be stimulated thousands of different ways using our imagination. Put your hands to the task and don't skimp when it comes time to choosing and using those items that seem "naughty" to you (feathers, scarves, brushes, etc.) and begin by massaging yourself; it is the best way to come to know your own body and its needs.

We are going to provide you with instructions on how to caress your body in three sessions. We suggest you choose three successive days around evening time and after a light supper. Find an intimate space where no one will bother you and begin by making it pleasant and exciting to be in. The bedroom or bath is the usual choice, just make sure it's warm enough and illuminate the space with candles. Put on your favorite music and prepare a blend of aromatic oils that you find most seductive (later on you will find a text box with three suggestions). Keep a feather, scarf, or brush nearby.

First Session

Begin with a hot and relaxing aromatic bath. Toward the end of this book we will recommend a number of essences you can use.

Once you're in the bath, anoint your body with the oils, slowly and gently. While you are doing this, pay attention to those parts of your body you usually neglect, for example, the backside of your knees or between the toes of your feet.

Next, **dry yourself with a soft towel** (give yourself a treat and heat it on the radiator beforehand). But don't dry yourself thoroughly. Leave yourself a bit damp and go to the bedroom, where it should be pleasantly warm and decorated with nice things.

Choose an aromatic massage oil and apply it gently over your still-moist skin. Don't worry about using any special massage techniques, just **move your hands delicately and spontaneously,** improvising as you go and paying attention to the different areas and nuances of your entire skin, examining the muscles and shapes of your body.

You don't have to hurry; take your time, **enjoy the tactile sensations,** and rest easy. Pay attention to the areas you like the most and later give more time to those parts that are less attractive to you. Try to approach them with a good mindset and in a positive way. Don't get fixated on anything you consider to be a defect, rather concentrate on the more agreeable features. For example, instead of repeating to yourself that your belly is a little bit bigger than you would like, notice how smooth it is and how good it feels to touch it.

And one more important detail: on this first day, don't stimulate your genitals.

Second Session

In this second session you will proceed exactly as you did with the first, the difference being **this time you will include your genitals in the massage.**

Put massage oil on this area with the same gentleness you use for the rest of your body. Notice where it's most pleasant to touch. Trust your sensations and let your body tell you what it wants and give it what it is asking for.

Choose a quiet time, turn off your cell phone and TV.

Third Session

Begin as you did the previous two days, but focus specifically on your erogenous zones. Caress those parts of your body that stimulate you the most. Vary pressure and motion of the strokes. Experience how pleasurable this is to your genitals and go deeper in your exploration of this area. **Imagine how much pleasure you would give another person by caressing them this way.**

Do whatever suits your fancy to turn yourself on. Music and erotic texts can certainly help. *Delta of Venus,* by Anaïs Nin, is highly recommended.

"Palpable" Results

Repeat these pleasant sessions of self-massage as often as you can. If you allow your body to get used to pleasure, you will learn what you like and succeed in feeling more comfortable in your own skin. You will also get used to physical contact with others and get over your hang-ups. **You will realize the pleasure your body can provide and with this you will enrich all facets of your life.**

Blends of Essential Oils for Intimate Moments

Relaxation Blend
½ glass of almond oil
5 drops of lavender essence
5 drops of pink geranium essence (Pelargonium asperum)
3 drops of rosewood essence (Aniba roseadora) or
3 drops of petitgrain essence (Citrus amara).

Sensual Blend
5 tablespoons of almond oil
1 tablespoon of musk rose essence
3 drops of sandalwood oil
3 drops of Ylang Ylang

Invigorating Blend
½ glass of almond oil
3 drops of vanilla
3 drops of benzoin resin
1 drop of essence of Damask rose, either Turkish or Bulgarian
5 drops of orange essence

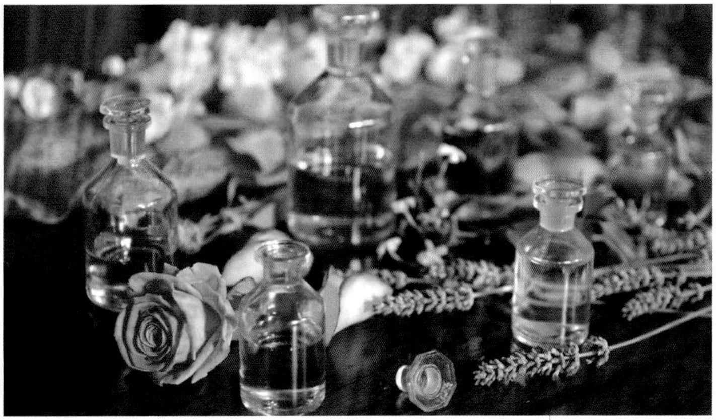

Make a nice, hot bath using aromatic oils and salts.

Massages for Two

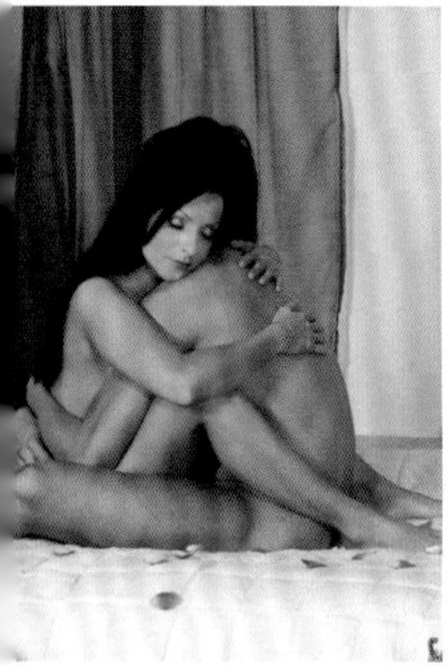

To be able to communicate our own desires to a partner and also commit ourselves to fulfilling theirs, it is necessary to have a good relationship with our own body. Only then will the couple be ready for mutual pleasuring.

Further on we will share a series of massages that don't require special techniques or specific manipulations. They will be presented in greater detail later; right now we would like you just to work on your harmony as a couple. One thing only is necessary: **great sensitivity and a delicate touch,** since the simple, affectionate movements of loving hands are guaranteed to bring about the best results. Approach your partner with **interest and curiosity** and join with him/her in a sensual journey of mutual exploration.

No Haste

No matter how busy your partner may be, he or she will not say "no" to a nice massage of the **head and nape,** neither will they deny you giving them an attentive **back rub**, or massaging their legs and butt, or **caressing** their breast and belly, or even their feet. At this first stage, the only thing you need to do is give each other more time. I know you're rushed for time, but it doesn't take a lot. And the little time you devote to this will pay off handsomely if you take advantage of exploring the possibilities of physical contact.

Preparing the Space

Begin by suitably arranging your environment.

- The first thing to keep in mind is to maintain a **pleasant temperature.** This is an essential condition for feeling comfortable during the massage. If the weather is unpleasant and it's a bit chilly, turn on the radiator or use a small heater, even if it's summertime. It is impossible to enjoy your body when you feel cold. Also, if it's too hot, turn on the air-conditioning.
- Don't forget to use essential oils whenever you can. You already know how these suggestive and captivating aromas can turn any massage into

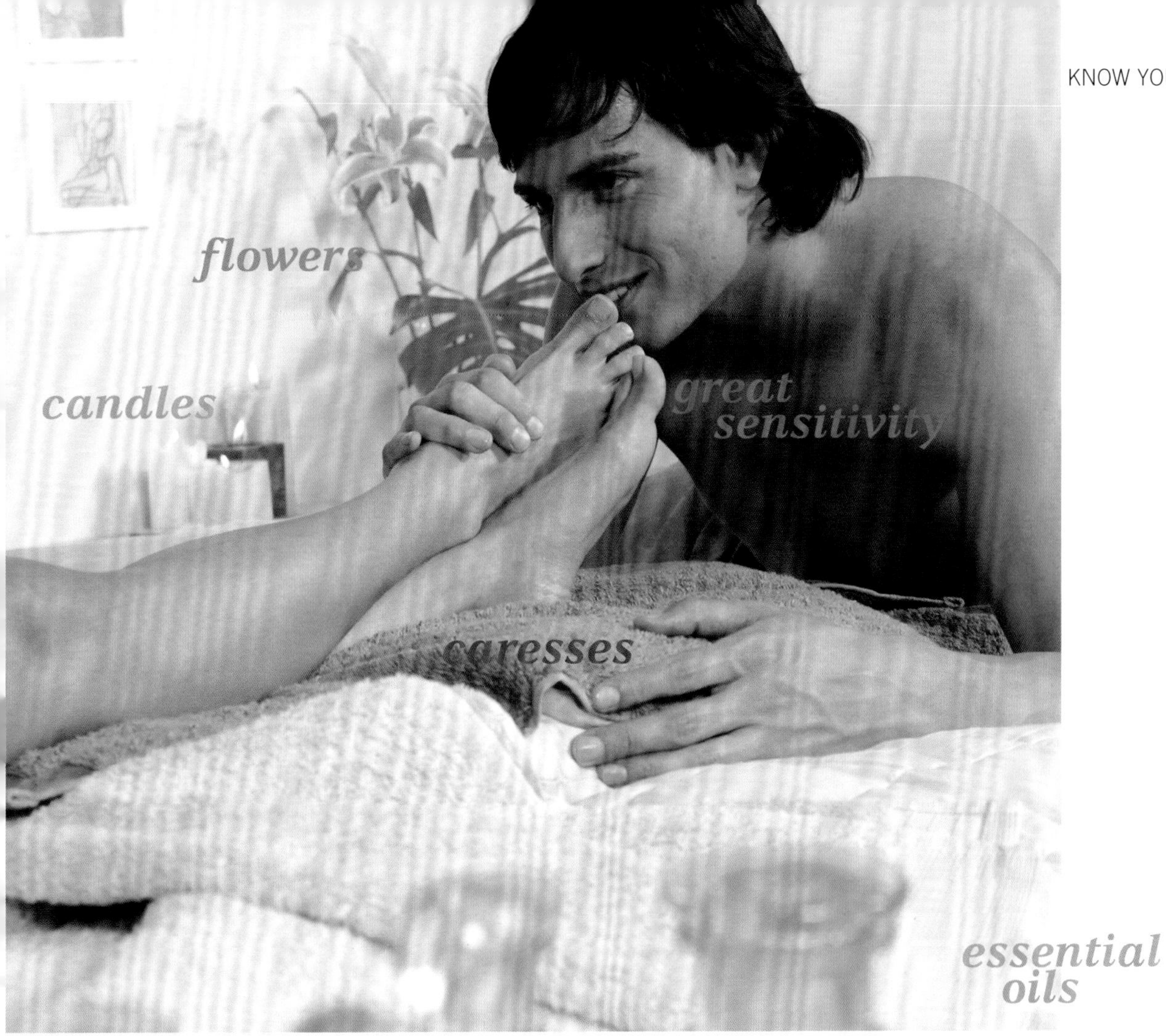

a voluptuous delight. Essential oils usually come in small, expensive bottles. Just keep in mind that you only need to add a couple of drops to your regular massage oil base to obtain spectacular results. You can also pour a few drops into an oil heater and enjoy the whole room permeated with the delightful and sensual fragrance.

- **Visual stimuli, such as flowers, beautiful paintings, colorful walls, candles, or plants** can help to create a seductive atmosphere. You only have to let your imagination go, take your time, and enjoy the ritual of preparation as you anticipate the pleasures to come.

Head Massage

There is no better way to begin your initiation into the art of massage than giving a head massage, ideal for helping your partner relax and overcoming his or her tensions.

It is not necessary to undress for this type of massage. But don't get the idea this has to be something simply chaste and innocent. If you do it, you will quickly discover that it is a very intimate form of contact and can quickly turn into something quite sensual.

The initial movements of the head massage are devoted to working the area between the forehead and the nose, the energetic center also known as the "third eye." Without realizing it in the slightest, we daily accumulate a lot of tension in this area. You should know that once we manage to alleviate this, a great sense of serenity and well-being will immediately overtake us. Just holding our partner's head can sometimes result in such a great release that time and space seem to disappear and all tensions along with them.

Step by Step

Have your partner lie comfortably on his/her back, either on the bed, a sofa, or even on the floor, using a yoga or exercise mat for cushioning.

Sit in a comfortable position (make sure your back is not bent) behind your partner. Have his/her head rest on your lap. Supporting it on a pillow is best.

1. Begin by placing both hands on the forehead, carefully, and massage the area running from the eyebrows to the edge of the scalp, alternating your hands rhythmically.
2. Repeat this motion at least 10 times. Change pressures and ask your partner which he/she prefers.
3. Next, place your hands on their forehead with palms resting on their temples. Your fingertips should lie right in the center of their forehead, on the area between the eyebrows, commonly known as the "third eye."
4. Keep your hands in this position for a couple of minutes and let your partner experience the energy that flows from them. He/she will feel completely relaxed and protected.

Use some massage oil with a smooth texture and captivating aroma.

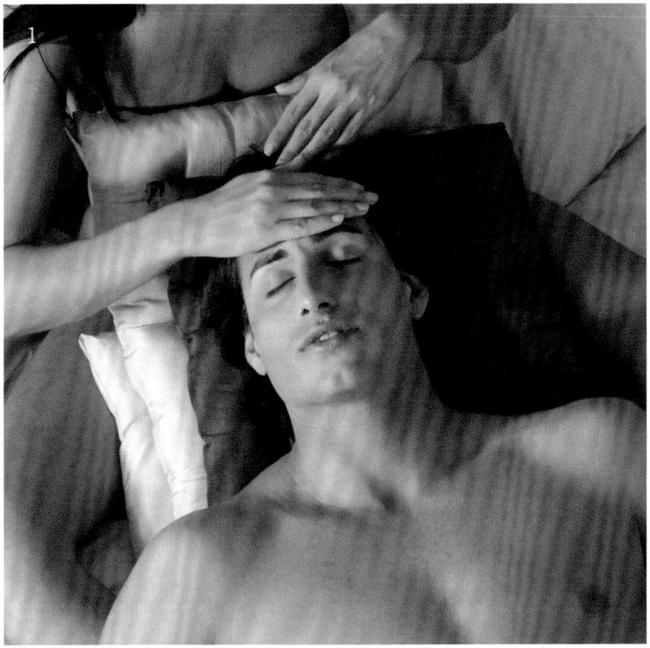
1

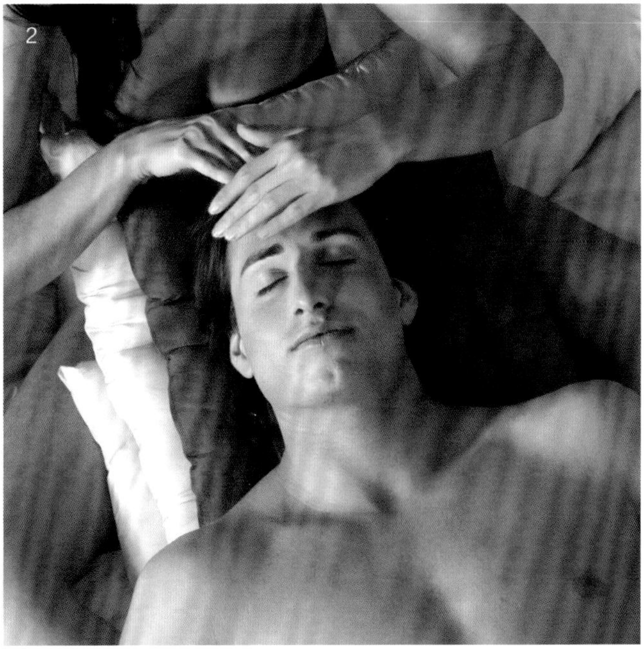
2

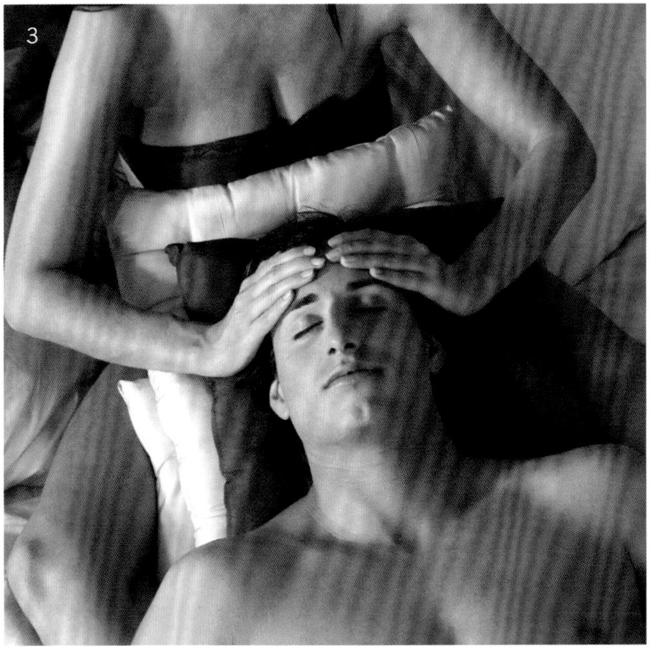
3

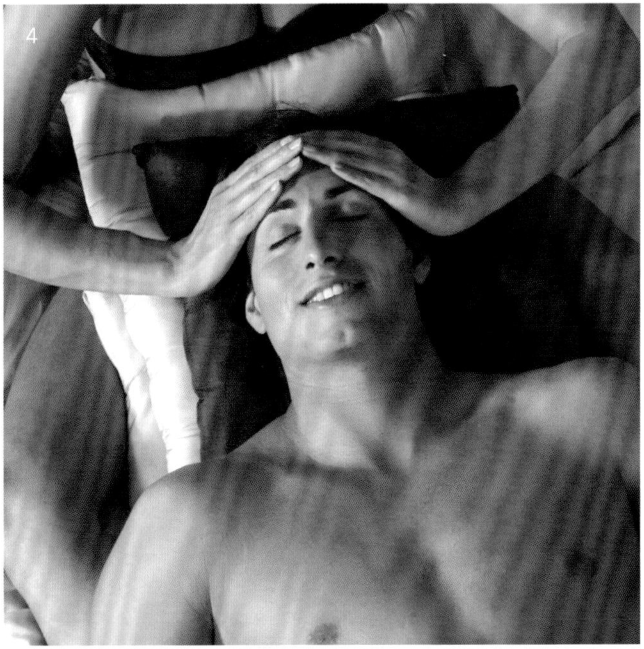
4

Scalp Massage

You are probably already aware that there are points of sexual stimulation located all over the body, but you might be surprised to hear that some of these are located on the head and, more specifically, on the scalp. When these sensitive areas are stimulated with rhythmical movements, the result is profoundly relaxing and, at the same time, somewhat surprising, since by using the tips of the fingers, or just the thumbs to make small circles on the scalp, we can bring our partner to sexual arousal in record time.

Step by Step

Let your partner remain comfortably on his/her back.

Remain seated or kneeling behind them and let their head rest in your lap on a cushion.

Begin by covering the contours of his/her head with little circles made with your fingertips, the palms of your hands, or your thumbs.

Ask your partner if he/she likes what you are doing and if the pressure and intensity are right.

1. Gently explore the contours of your partner's head.
2. Softly, use your fingertips to go over their forehead and temples.
3. Then slow down the circular movements and use just one hand. Gently support the back of your partner's neck with your other hand.
4. Now put the hand you were using to make the circles on the crown of their head and rotate their skin to the right in a circular motion. Note if their scalp moves easily or if it is tense. If it is tense that means your partner needs to relax a bit more. Go back to making the small circles on their forehead and ask him/her if they like it.
5. Finally, make little circles with your fingertips on your partner's scalp. While you are doing this, make sure not to tug on their hair.

A scalp massage is particularly exciting for men

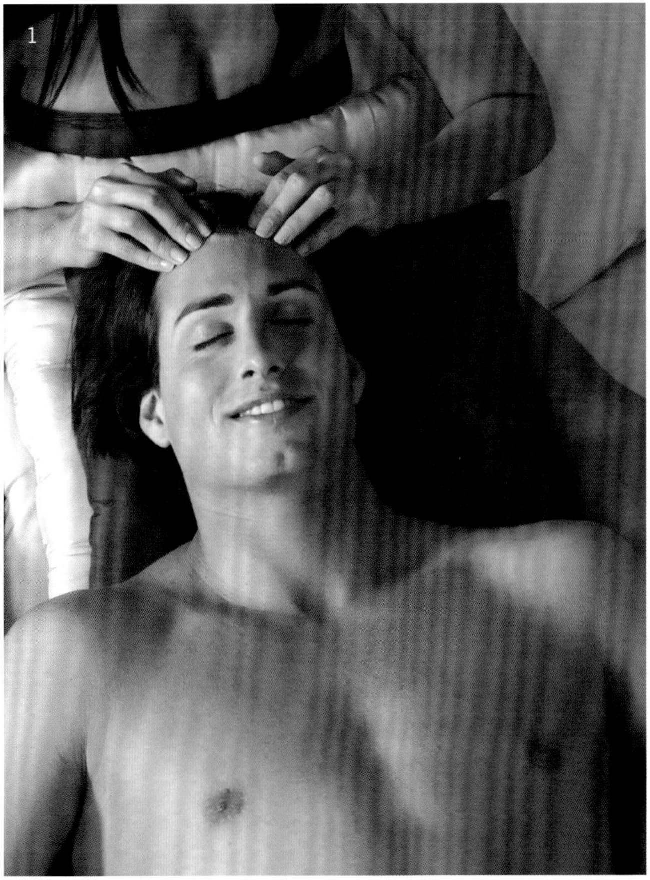
1
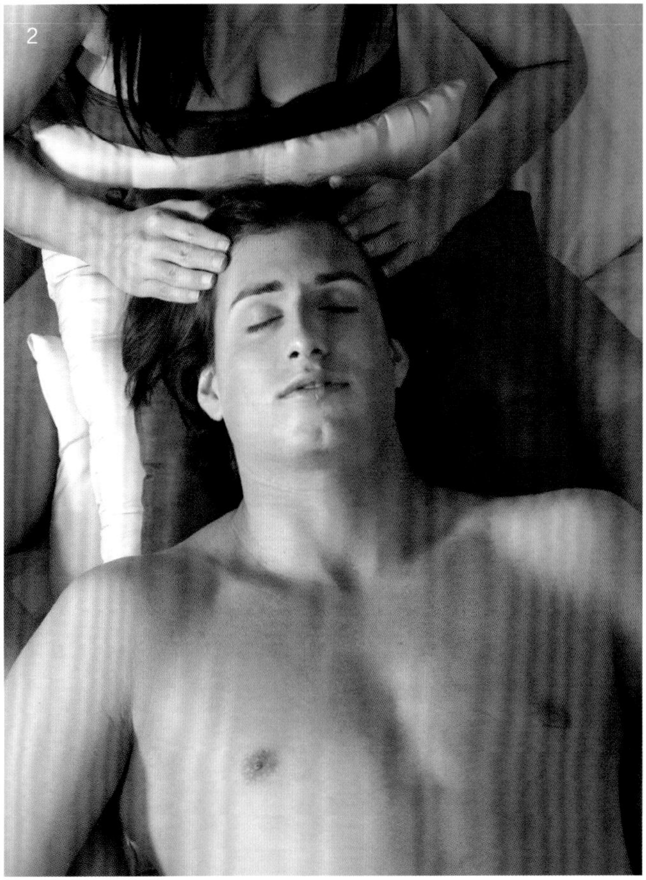
2
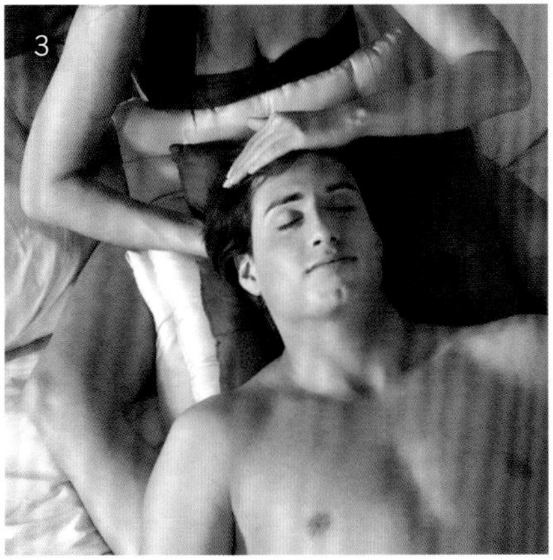
3
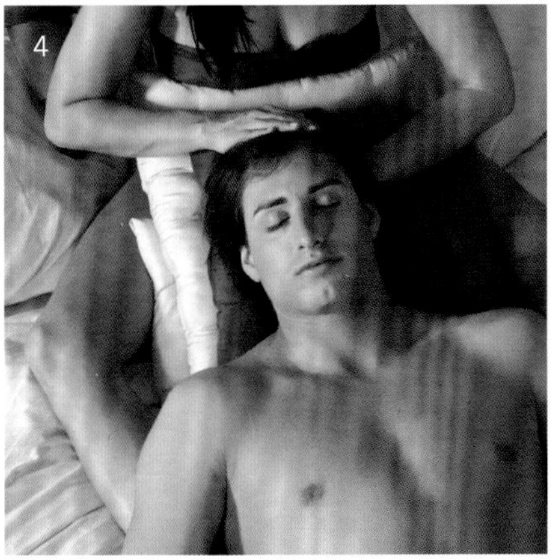
4
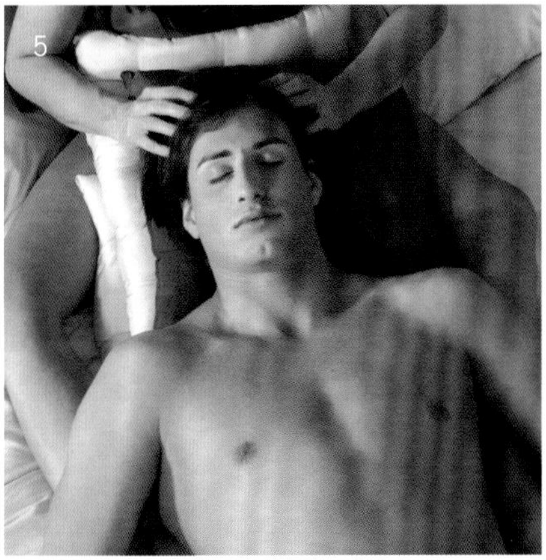
5

Massaging the Back of the Neck

The following massage of the back of the neck (nape) is an ideal way to end the gently stimulating head massage we just described.

Watching for Signals

You will have noticed that when we described how to perform these initial massages, we often stressed the importance of asking your partner if he/she likes what you are doing and what type of stimulation they prefer. Understand that massage is a special form of contact that possesses its own intimate, private language. That is to say, you must learn to interpret the expressions, sighs, and other bodily signals your partner gives which express what he/she likes and what they don't like. This is as true for a couple with easy communication as well as for a more reserved couple.

In any event, you must learn to communicate beyond just words. Constantly asking your partner if he/she likes what you are doing is liable to put a damper on creating a sensual atmosphere.

Step by Step

Have your partner lie comfortably on his/her back. As before, kneel behind him/her and have his/her head resting on your thighs, delicately.

1. Begin making small circles with your thumbs from the inside of the nape to the outside (use your fingertips if that is more comfortable for you).

2. Begin at the base of the skull and draw circles to the right and left of the spinal column. Then do the same with your fingertips. Start with 2 or 3 fingers, then finish using 4 at a time.

3. Continue downward with these motions, following the line of the spinal column until you reach the shoulders. Change the pressure and ask your partner what intensity he/she prefers. Repeat this movement at least five times and pay attention to and pace your partner's rate of breathing.

4. To finish, gently grasp a tuft of hair in each hand using the thumb and index finger and tug delicately. This will give your partner a subtle and erotic tingle.

Don't forget to ask from time to time if your partner likes the pressure you are exerting. Modify it to his/her preferences.

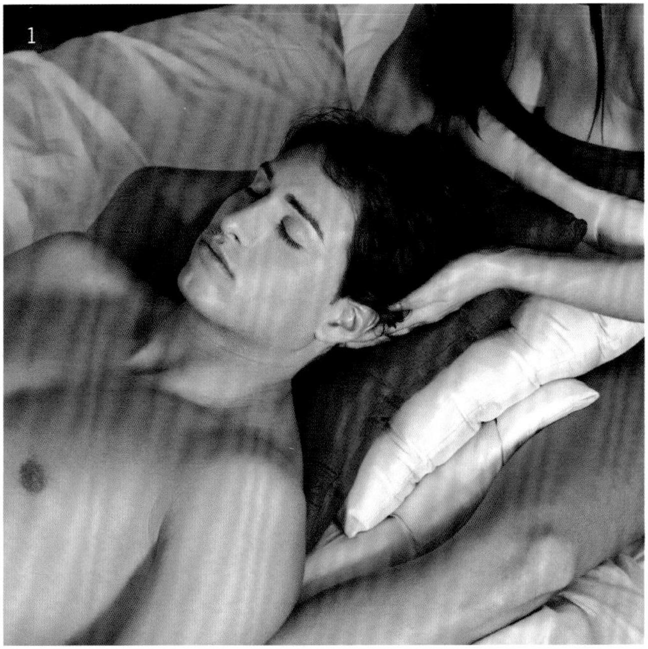
1
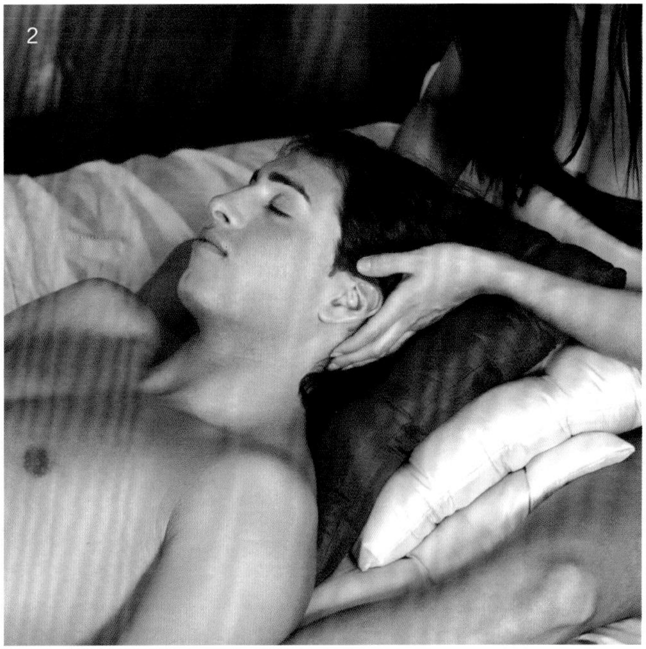
2
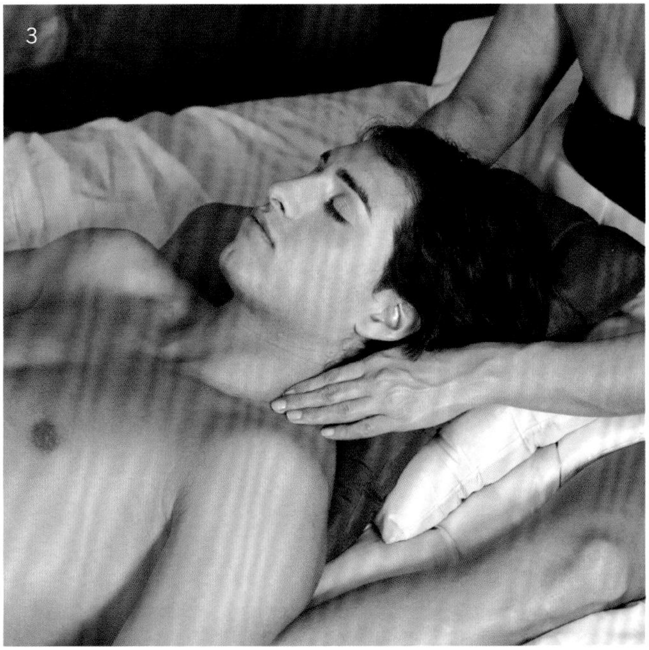
3
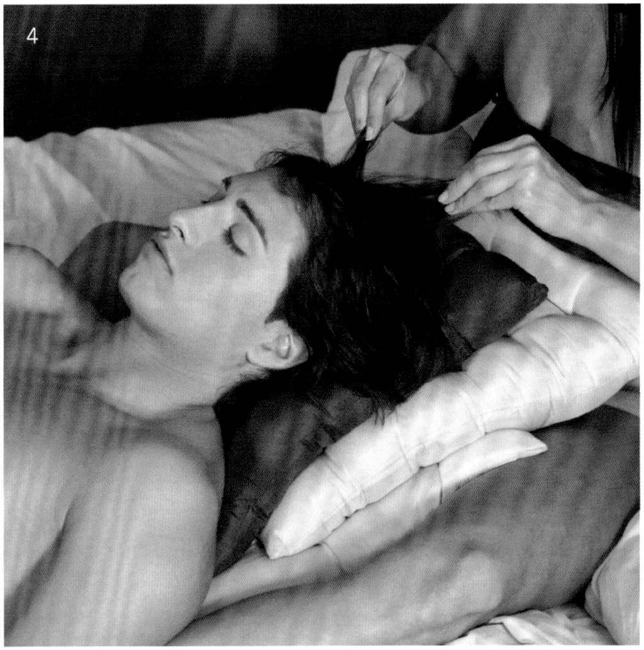
4

Facial Massage

According to recent studies, **men and women possess different sensory proclivities starting from infancy.** Women are more responsive to tactile stimuli, while men are more responsive to the visual. A good way to make both sexes happy is to employ both forms of stimulation in a facial massage, since this involves not only the softness of touching but also the facial expressions of the partner. The facial massage also provides a wonderful way of getting to know the loved one's face more intimately. As we all know, the face is the mirror of the soul.

Facial massage also induces extreme relaxation of the facial expression. In this regard, it is like a back massage, whose effects are evident throughout the whole body. So don't put it off any longer; choose a scent you both like and you will be ready to begin.

Step by Step

Sit with your legs apart and place a cushion between them so your partner can rest his/her head.

Put a bit of massage oil on your hands and rub them together to warm the oil.

Place a hand on each side of your partner's face and gently keep them there while you both breathe in sync a few times, relaxing. Focus on your partner's breathing and let yourself get totally into its rhythm.

1. Gently massage the area that runs from the chin to each side of the jaw. Repeat this stroke 10 to 15 times.

Ask your partner if the pressure and intensity of the stroke are OK for them.

2. Next, use your fingertips to caress the nose, cheeks, ears, and chin of your companion.

This time, don't count how many reps you are doing, just take your time and enjoy the sensation of rubbing his/her skin.

Make sure he/she likes it, but this time don't ask, simply pay attention to his/her expression, sighs, and any other sounds they make.

3. Put some more oil on you hands and go over their forehead again, a few more times.

The secret of this massage is to do it slowly,

Check to see if your partner relaxes with these delicate manipulations.

4. Next, continue by massaging the area around the mouth and use your fingertips to caress the area that runs from the tip of the nose to the upper lip. This part of the face is especially sensitive.

Don't forget to ask your partner what pressure they want applied to this most sensitive spot.

Finish by stroking the forehead, the cheeks, and the chin, and finally use both hands to cover the face for a few moments.

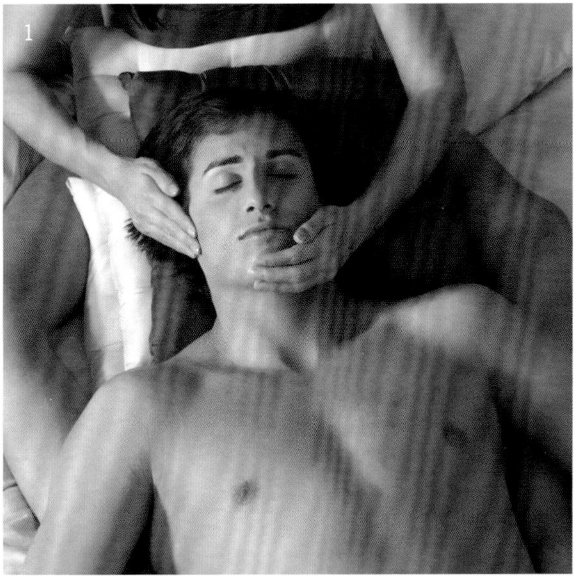

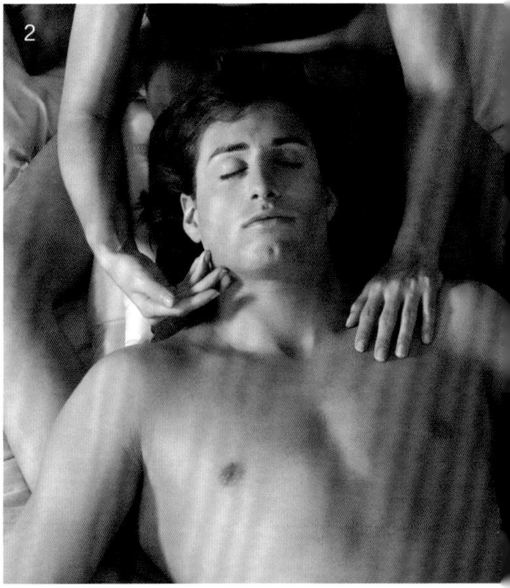

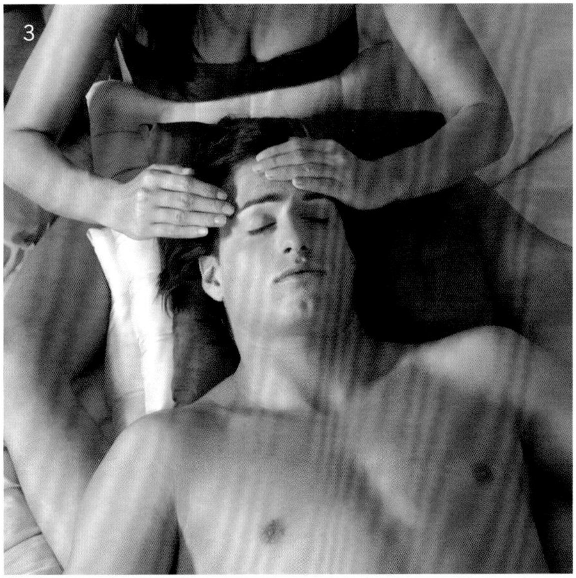

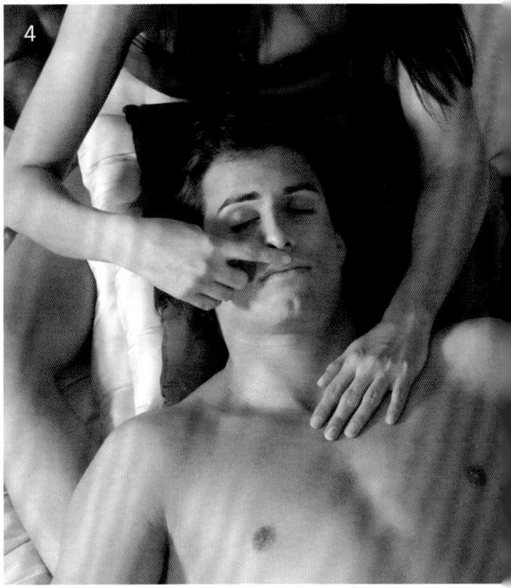

gently, and with utmost sensitivity.

Give Your Partner a Magical Ritual of Love

This delicate, sensitive massage can become its own little love ritual as a way of giving and receiving a special greeting that bit by bit wakes up your desire. You can do it either **dressed or undressed,** without making a big fuss, but making sure to do it with enthusiasm and sensuality.

The Practice of Self-Love

set the scene for a magical moment

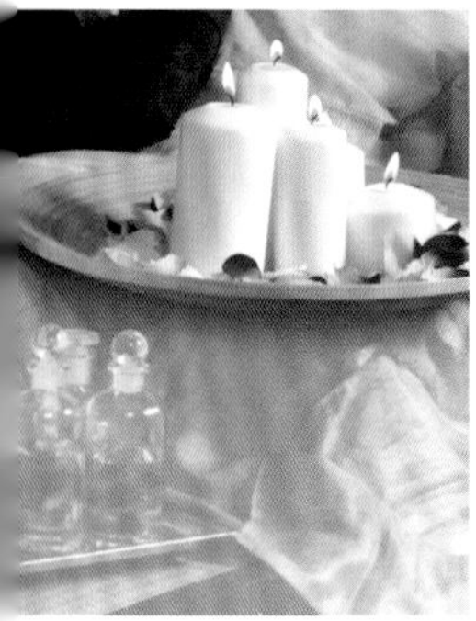

Below are some tips that can help make couple's massage a much more important part of our lives.

- It is important to turn the space where you do the massages into an intimate, warm, little **love nest.** It should be a special place where you are surrounded by **sensual and inviting** aromas, lighting, and music.
- Choose together and blend your own oils and fragrances. In nature, odors play an important role in seduction. If your couple's massage is identified with a particular scent you both like, this aroma will create a special bond between you that will serve to strengthen your relationship. You will unconsciously associate this specific smell with the desire you feel for your partner. In the future, just the smell of it will trigger that desire and bring back the memory of those pleasant experiences you shared.
- Take advantage of every session to **explore** a different part of your lover's body and enjoy how their skin is charged with erotic sensitivity, how their body hair stands up, how their sexual parts become aroused and a thrill runs through their entire body.
- Get used to **giving as well as receiving** massages and how nice it is to enjoy caressing and seeing to what extent our own caresses are exciting to the one who receives them.
- **Totally surrender** to the sensual encounter. Use your hands, your hair, the tips of your fingers, your forearm, feet, or even rub your whole body against your partner's.
- **Try new things**. For example, you can begin each erotic massage with a

The fine essential oils, the flowers, fabrics, candles, the soft light of the

A Nice Touch . . .

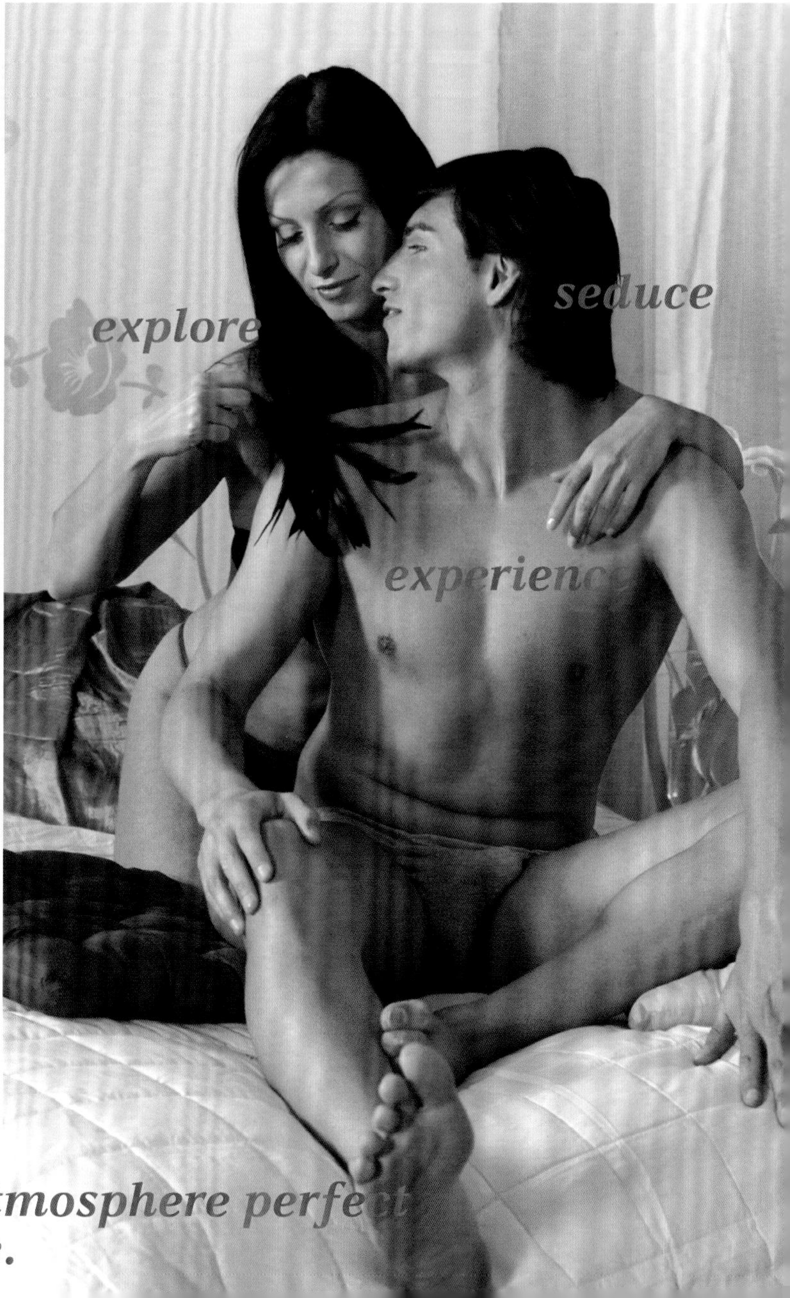

welcoming ritual which strengthens bonding and heightens anticipation.

- Make sure you **stay open to new experiences,** especially once you have gotten into a rhythm and gained a certain confidence. You can keep up the excitement by using unexpected surprises such as **silk scarves, feathers, brushes, gloves, masks,** and all those things which get your imagination going. In the "Magic Moments" chapter (p.109), you will find a number of suggestions if inspiration fails.
- Not everybody is psychic and so it is important for each partner to state his or her preferences. **Talk frankly** and openly about them with your partner or write him/her little notes if that makes you feel more comfortable. Never cease enriching your relationship.

all create a seductive atmosphere perfect for giving in to pleasure.

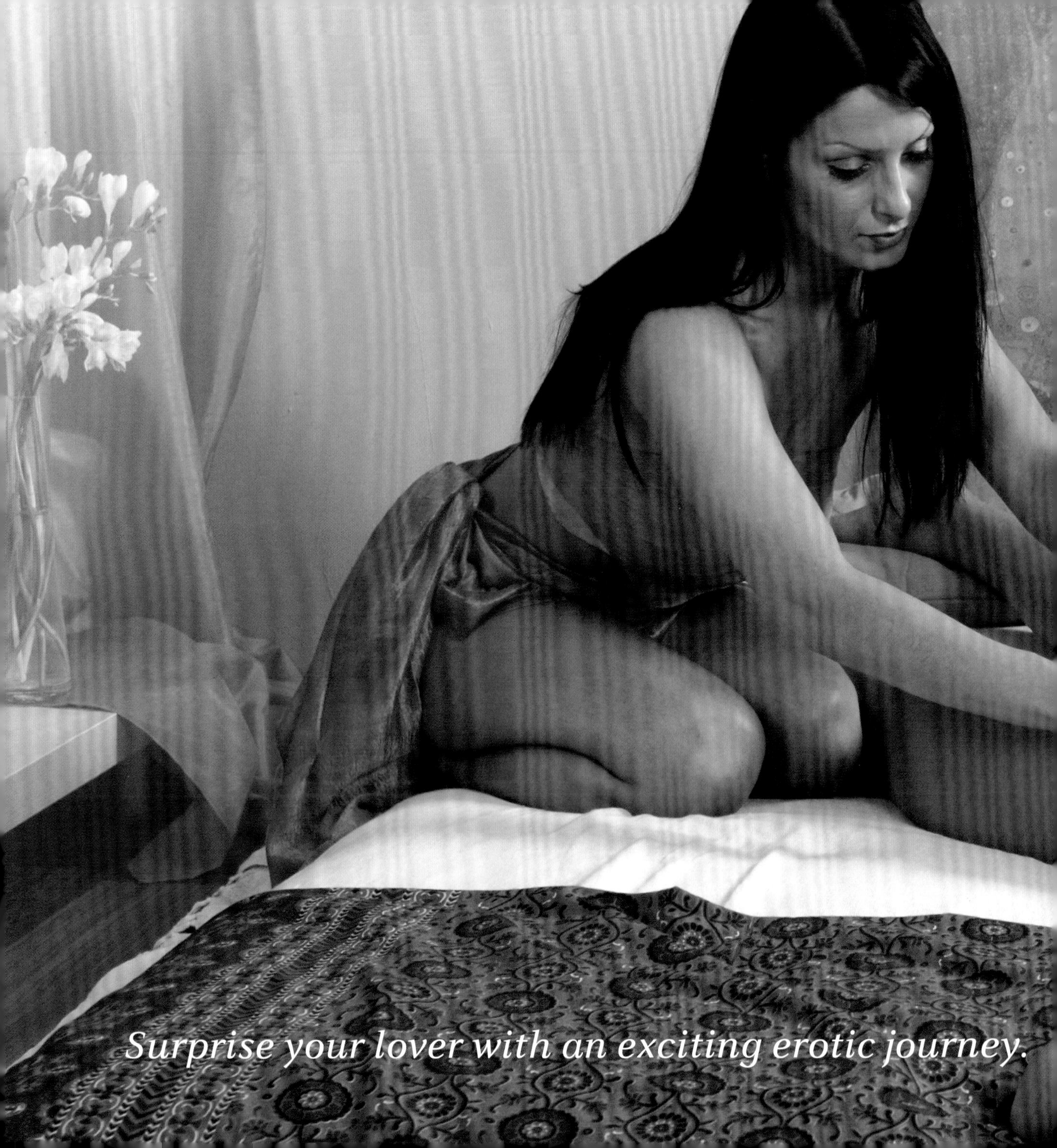
Surprise your lover with an exciting erotic journey.

With Great Pleasure

DISCOVERING YOUR PARTNER'S EROGENOUS ZONES

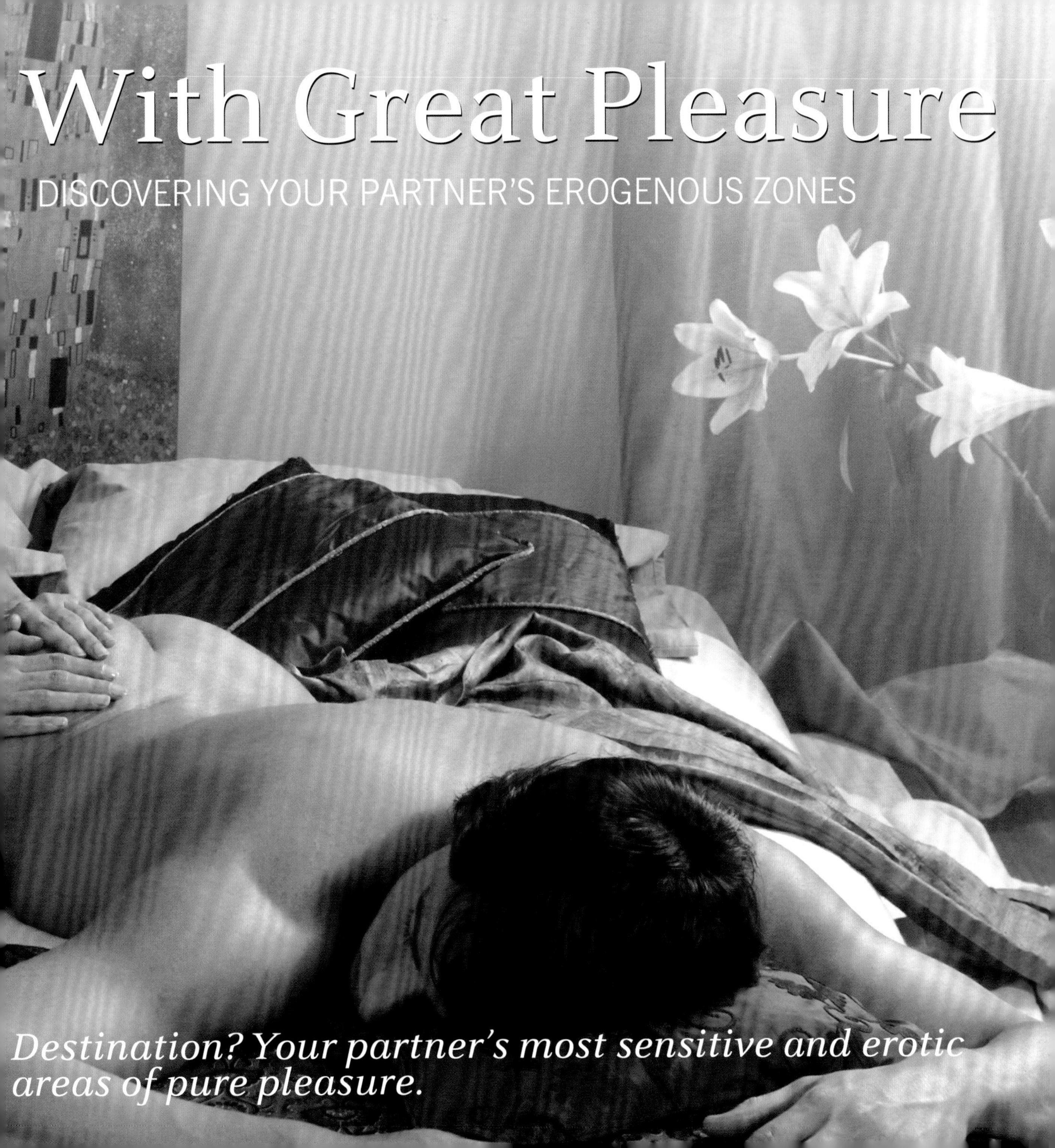

Destination? Your partner's most sensitive and erotic areas of pure pleasure.

The Erogenous Zones

If we were guided solely by the practices of our Western culture and kept in mind only conventional scientific criteria, the principal erogenous zones would be the clitoris and nipples for a woman and the penis for a man. The Oriental traditions, which increasingly assert their presence in our culture, offer us a much different and more open-minded perspective. Their valuable experience provides a permanent source of inspiration for us.

Energy and the Meridians

Oriental medicine describes a complex system of energy lines known as **meridians.** These are considered to be invisible "circuits" that are not identifiable with any specific anatomical features. **Qi (or Chi), the energetic force that maintains the harmony and equilibrium of our bodies,** flows along these meridians. If the flow of Chi is disrupted because of stress or any other cause, the body's energy flow will be impeded and the person will experience apathy or tiredness, even becoming ill as a result.

The image on the right shows various erogenous zones for a woman (lumbar points, points for buttocks and coccyx) according to Shiatsu massage.

Massage and stimulation of certain points along the meridians can help free up the energy flow.

According to traditional Chinese medicine, energy circulates down the posterior part of the body and ascends up the anterior part. Each meridian is assigned to a specific bodily organ or function. Along these energy lines that run from the top of the head to the tips of the feet, there are numerous points involving sexual stimulation. Stimulating these points with massage can affect the functioning of the sexual organs and endocrine glands, thus producing an increase in sexual vitality.

Acupuncture, Acupressure, and Shiatsu

The Taoist philosophy of China maintains the existence of a balanced relationship between the "Yin" and the "Yang," that is the feminine (Yin) and masculine (Yang) energies. This balance is the basis of health, well-being, and sexual desire. For approximately five-thousand years, humankind has been served by

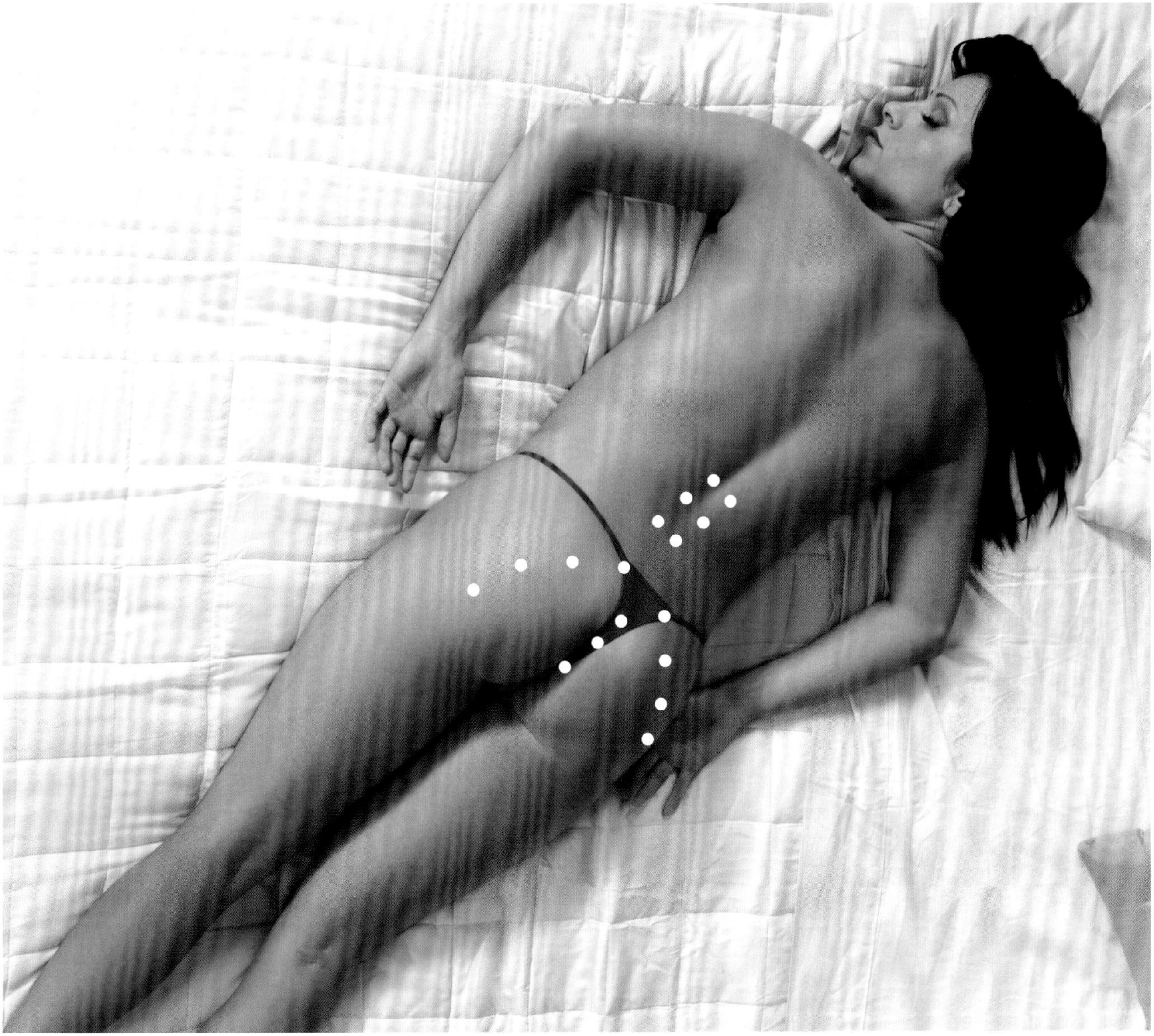

the ancient practices of acupuncture and acupressure to achieve perfect equilibrium of body, soul, and spirit.

Acupuncture involves stimulating certain energy points on the body's surface using needles. There are hundreds of these points which can be stimulated. To be able to do this requires exact knowledge of the energy points and special training. Using **acupressure,** in contrast, is much easier and involves thumb pressure on the energy points applied for seconds or even a few minutes.

When we're talking about couple's massage, the touch we use has much more in common with Shiatsu than acupressure, since we don't massage the points only, one by one, but also the entire area around them. The Japanese technique of Shiatsu helps to restore a balanced energy flow. To do it you don't just pressure the points separately, but you work along the energy meridians as well.

The Two Main Meridians

There are two principal meridians which encompass the body and are responsible for healthy sexual function. They are named the **"governing vessel" and the "conception vessel."** The governing vessel begins in the coccyx, goes up the spinal column over the cranial dome, and ends at a point in the middle of the upper lip of the mouth. The conception vessel begins in the perineum, the area between the anus and genitals. It passes through the sexual organs, the navel, and goes up the center of the chest, continuing upward by way of the neck until it reaches the center of the edge of the lower lip. There are a number of points along both meridians which positively influence the sexual organs when stimulated.

The skin's electrical conductivity is greater at the points along these meridians since these energy lines carry an especially energetic charge.

A Stimulating Trip

Below we offer a seductive itinerary of your partner's body. We will visit the erogenous points and parts of both the woman and the man. Though you can massage these points and the areas around them as much as you want, it is not necessary to concentrate exclusively on them. It is best to consider them "stops along the way" as you meander about your companion's body, lingering from time to time at those special locales.

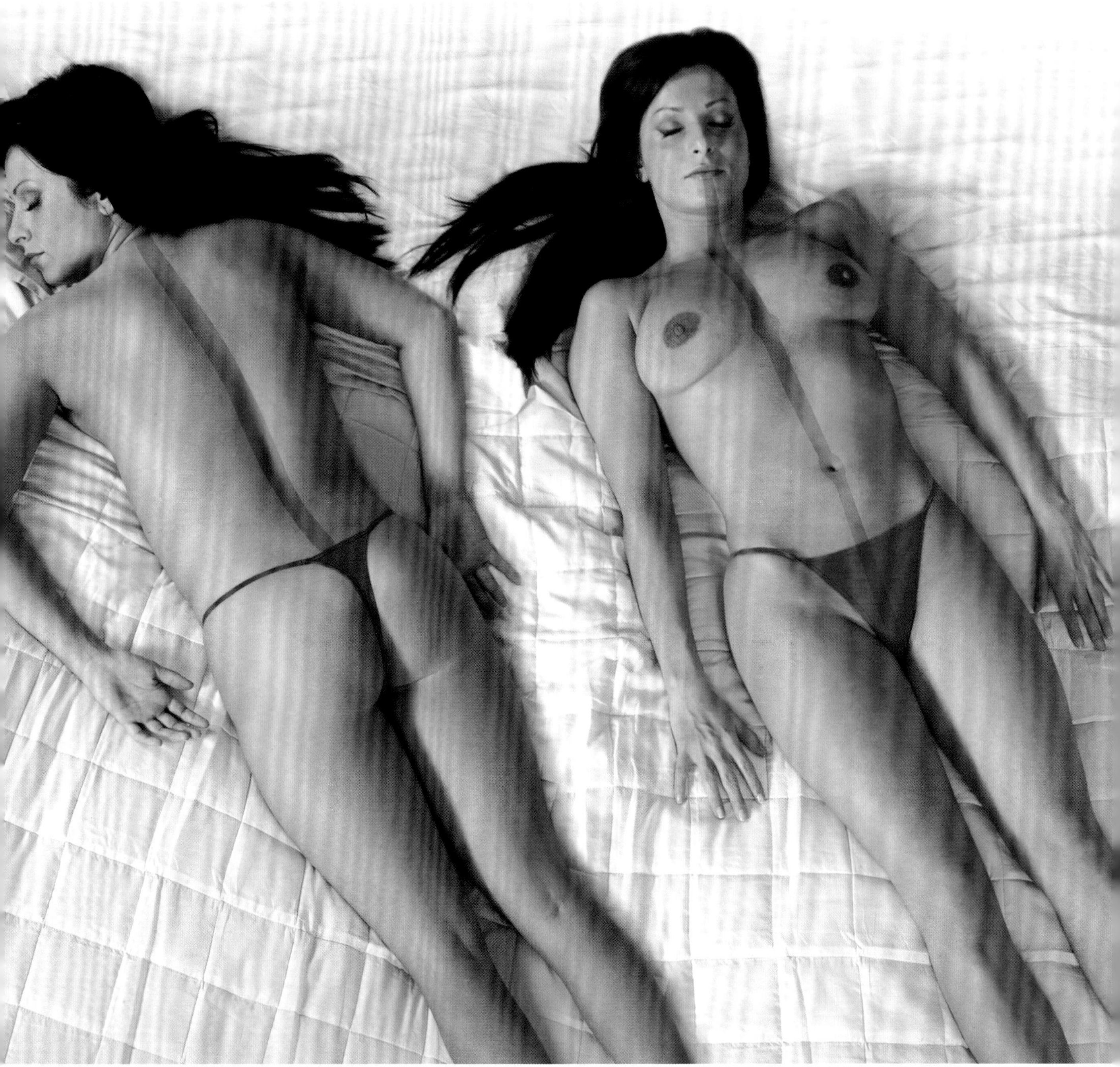

Erogenous Zones of the Man

In the area that runs from **the navel to the pelvis,** there is a great concentration of highly charged sexual energy. This region spans approximately 4 inches (10 cm), or four fingers in width, and includes a point which lies just below the navel, with another at the upper edge of the pubic bone and one that lies between them. All three points are to be considered as one unit when you massage there.

- There is also great sexual charge at the **lower edge of the pubic bone,** from both sides of the root of the penis to the hips.

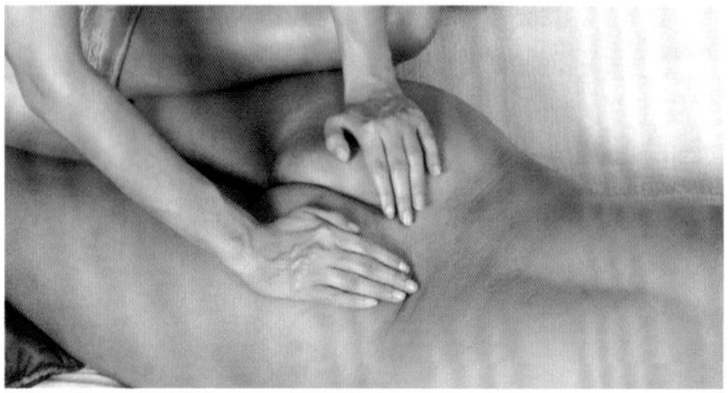

- Located on the man's back, approximately **2 inches (5 cm) above the coccyx** at both sides of the buttocks there are two points that, when massaged, stimulate the prostate and cause secretion of testosterone.
- There are two big lines in the **groin area.** These are very easy to stimulate.
- From where the **legs start to the tip of the kneecap,** along the inner part of the thighs, is a highly sensitive zone whose stimulation wakes up sexual desire.
- There are also points of sexual stimulation on the **head,** in the area of the **nape of the neck,** just in the center of the base of the skull, **right above the upper lip,** and at the center of the **edge of the lower lip.**

The area around the masculine genitals is very sensitive

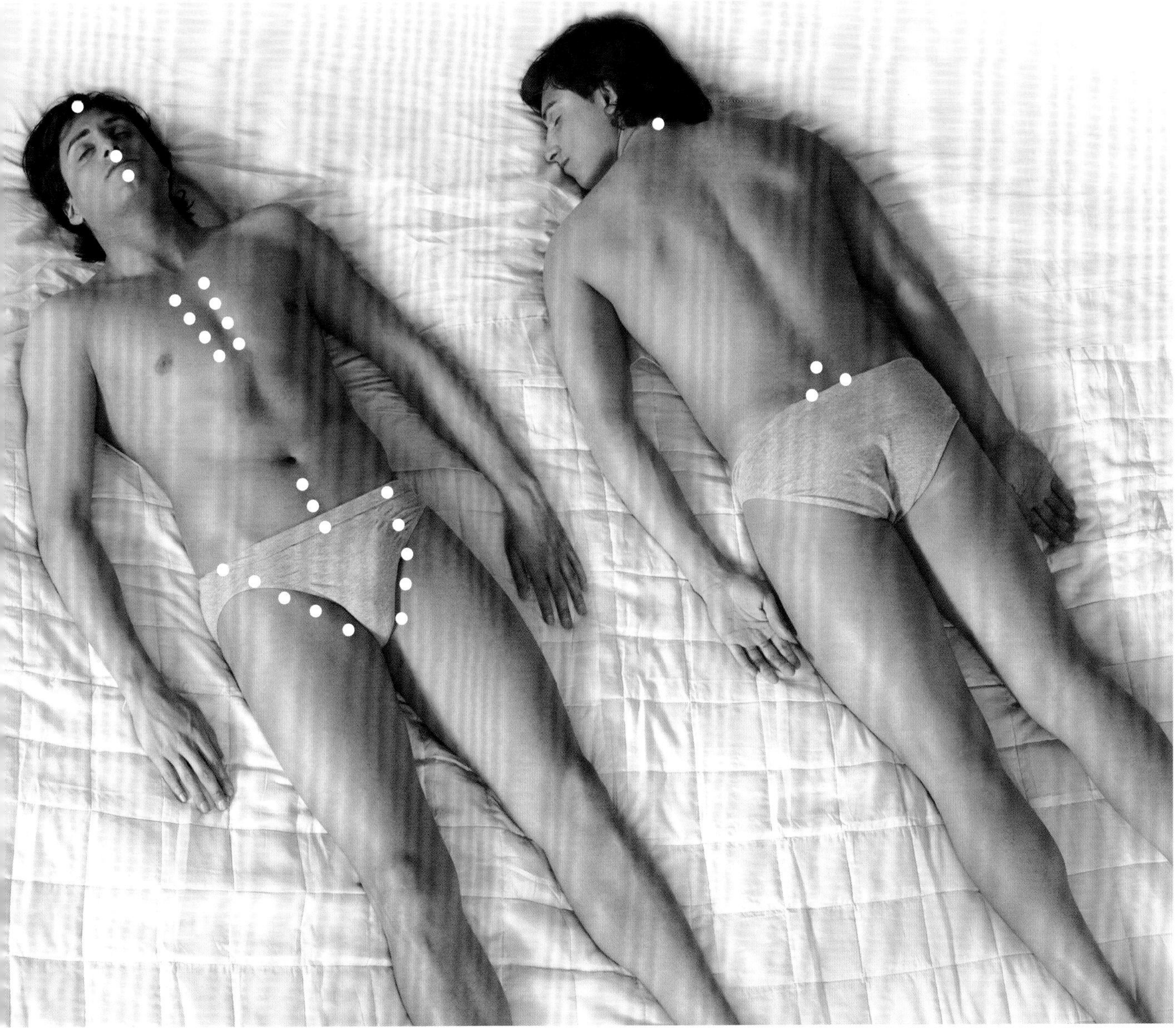

nd erogenous, especially between the navel and pelvis.

Erogenous Zones of the Woman

Here we will examine those points of sexual stimulation for a woman which differ from those for a man.

- Approximately 2 inches (5 cm) above the pubic bone there is a point which strongly activates the sexual energy and firms up the vagina.
- On the back, about 2 inches (5 cm) above the start of the coccyx is a point that, when stimulated, increases a woman's sexual desire.

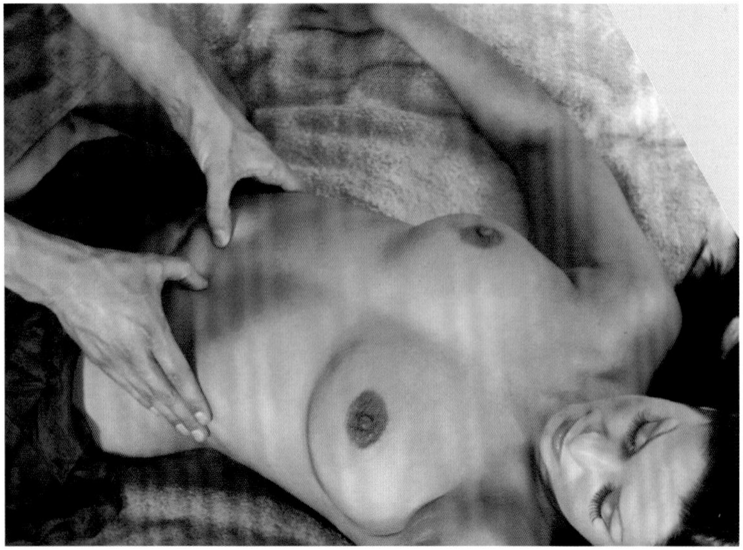

- On the abdomen, on the upper border of the pubic hair, there are several energy points that stimulate the ovaries and uterus.
- As with the man, the groin area harbors numerous points and areas of stimulation.
- From the pubic hair up to the sternum we can draw a line running through the center of the body. Stimulating the points that lie on this line produces intense sexual arousal.
- The nipples, and two parallel lines between the breasts and along the upper part of the sternum, are also susceptible to sexual arousal.
- We find another especially sensitive and erotic area on the back along the spinal column from the coccyx to the waist.
- As with the male body, the inner part of the thighs, the face, and head also contain important points of stimulation.

Women feel special pleasure when they are massaged along the abdomen.

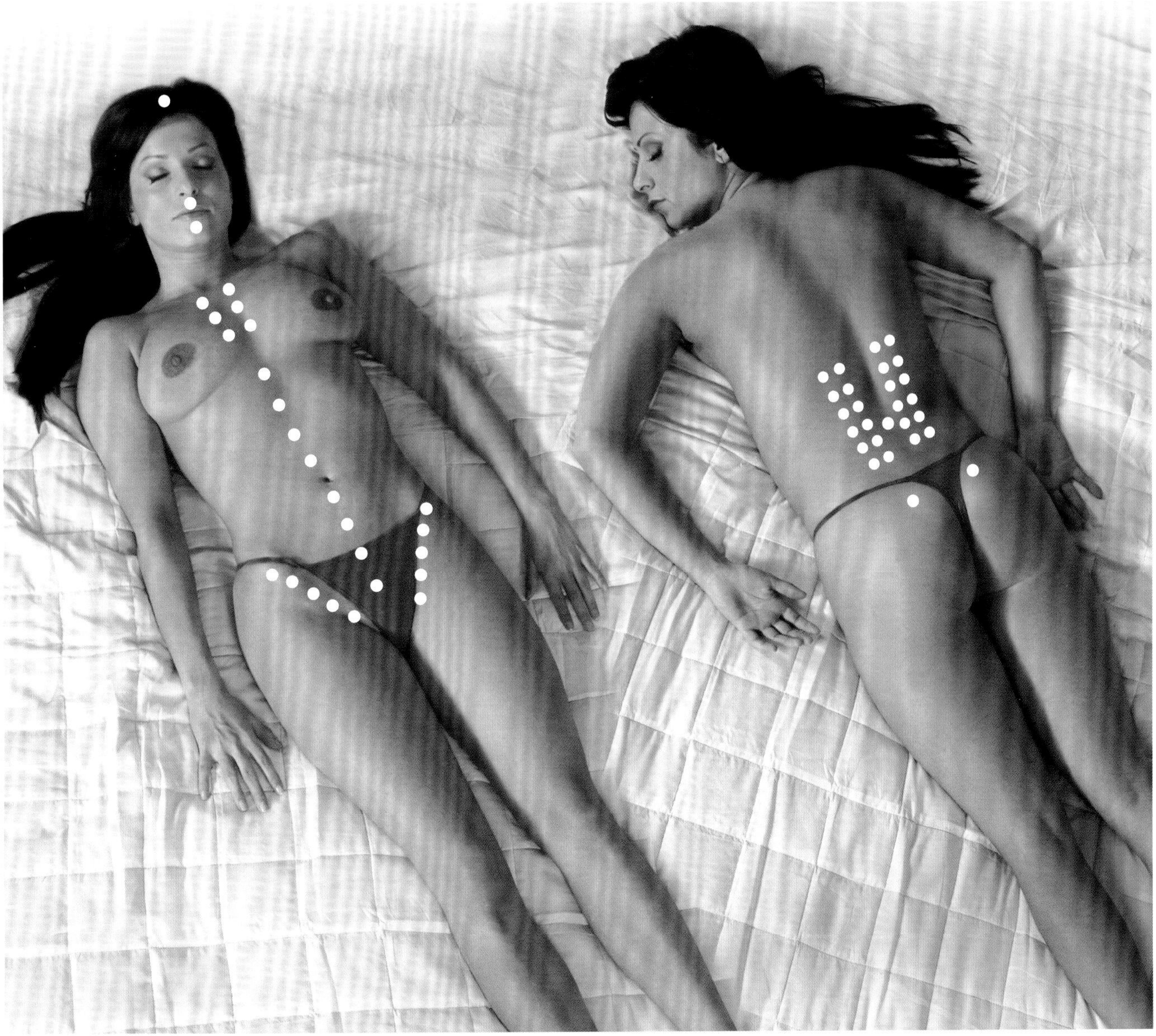

The loins and lower back are also important erogenous zones.

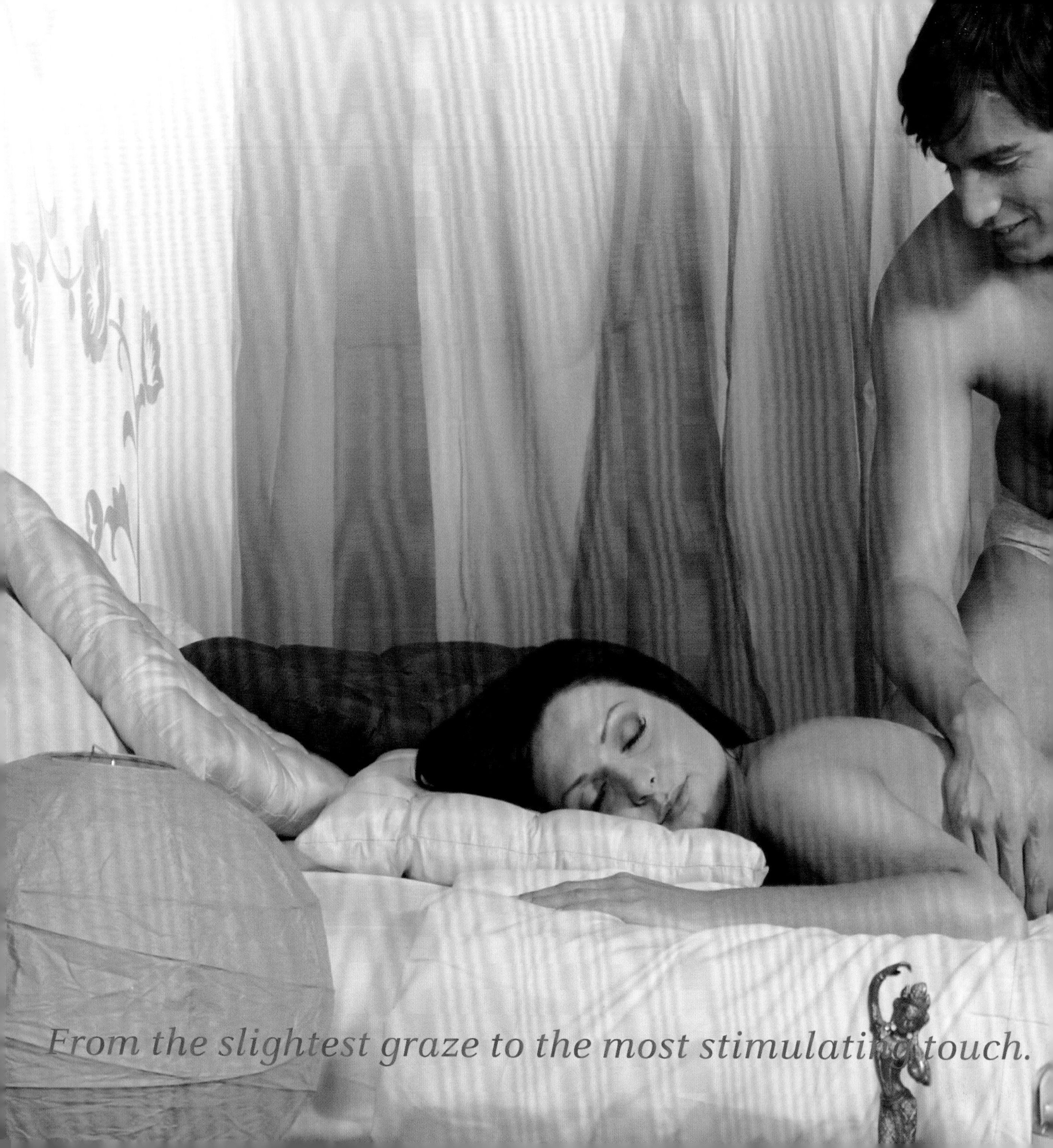
From the slightest graze to the most stimulating touch.

Basic Techniques

TO START OFF RIGHT

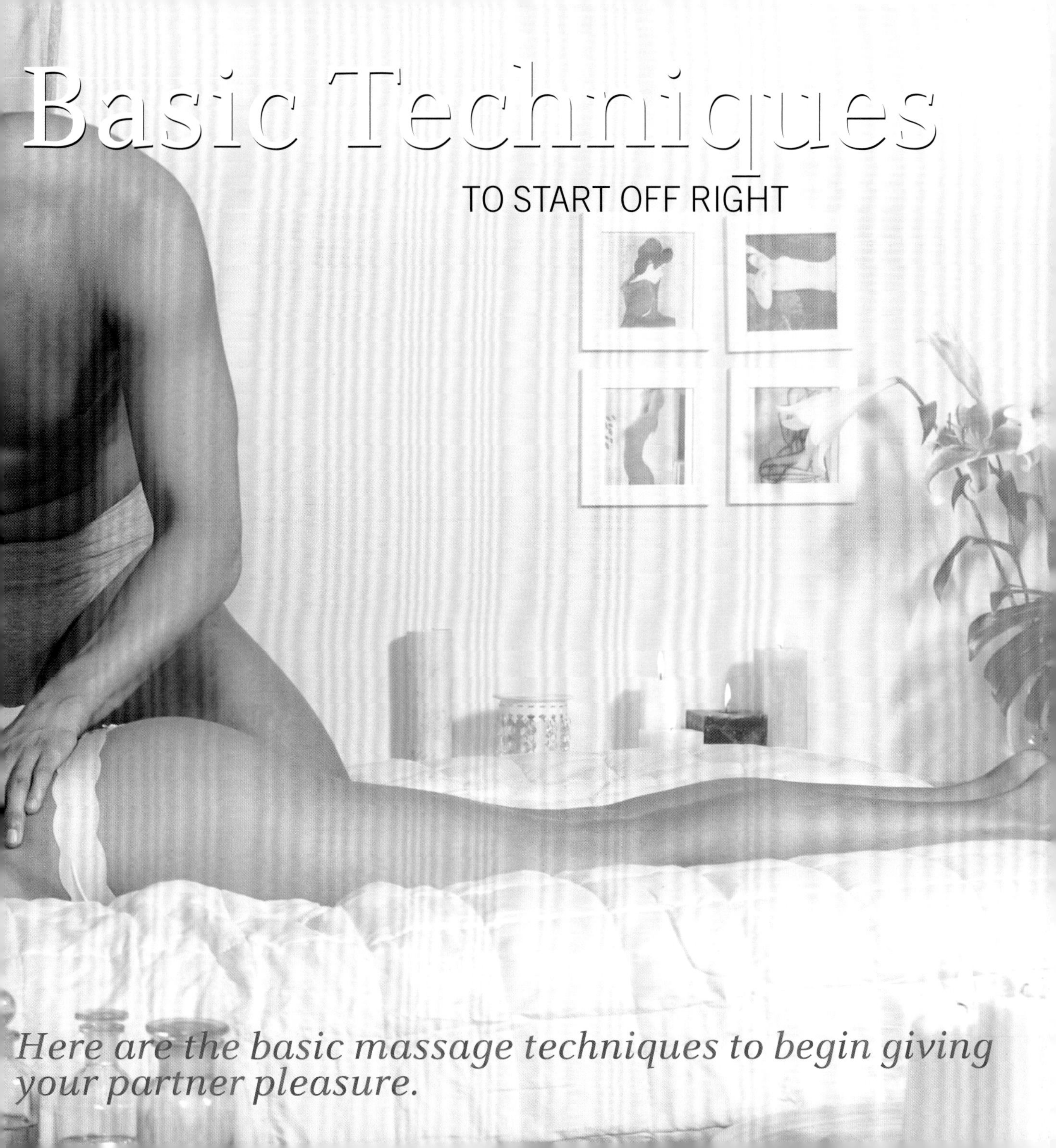

Here are the basic massage techniques to begin giving your partner pleasure.

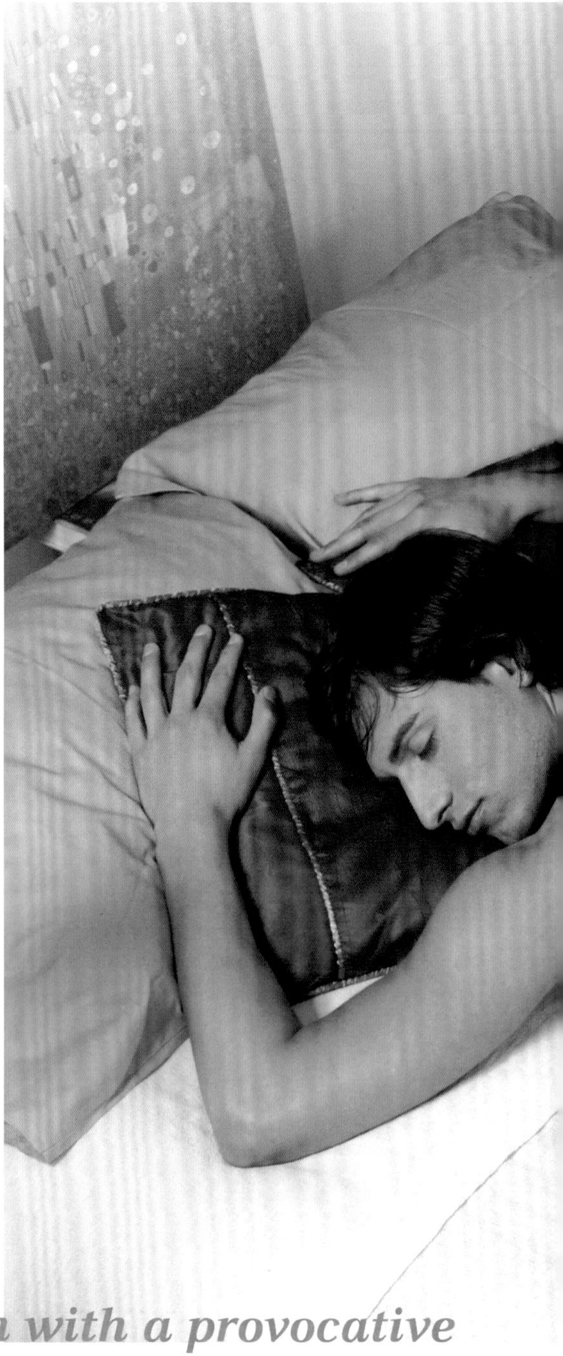

The Grazing Touch

The grazing touch is a form of soft contact, similar to a caress but even lighter. **The thighs and back** are especially suited for using this type of stroke. To learn how to do it, begin on the back, since this is the simplest place for a beginner to maintain control.

Of course, the back can be the site of more intense massage, but using a grazing touch can actually turn out to be more sexually stimulating. We must explain, though, that regardless of the type of touch you choose for erotic massage of the back, you must include **the buttocks** or your partner will experience the massage as incomplete. This is because the butt is the most sensual part of the posterior area of the body and stimulating it produces pleasant chills in the chest, head, and genitals.

In the following sections, we offer some ideas on how to practice the grazing touch.

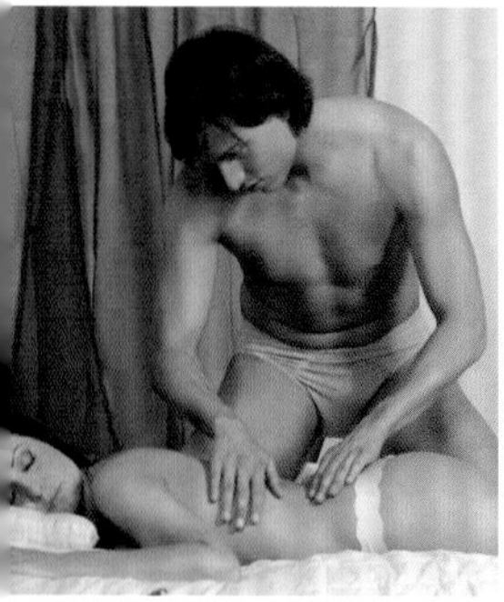

Go all over your lover's skin with a provocative graze of your fingers.

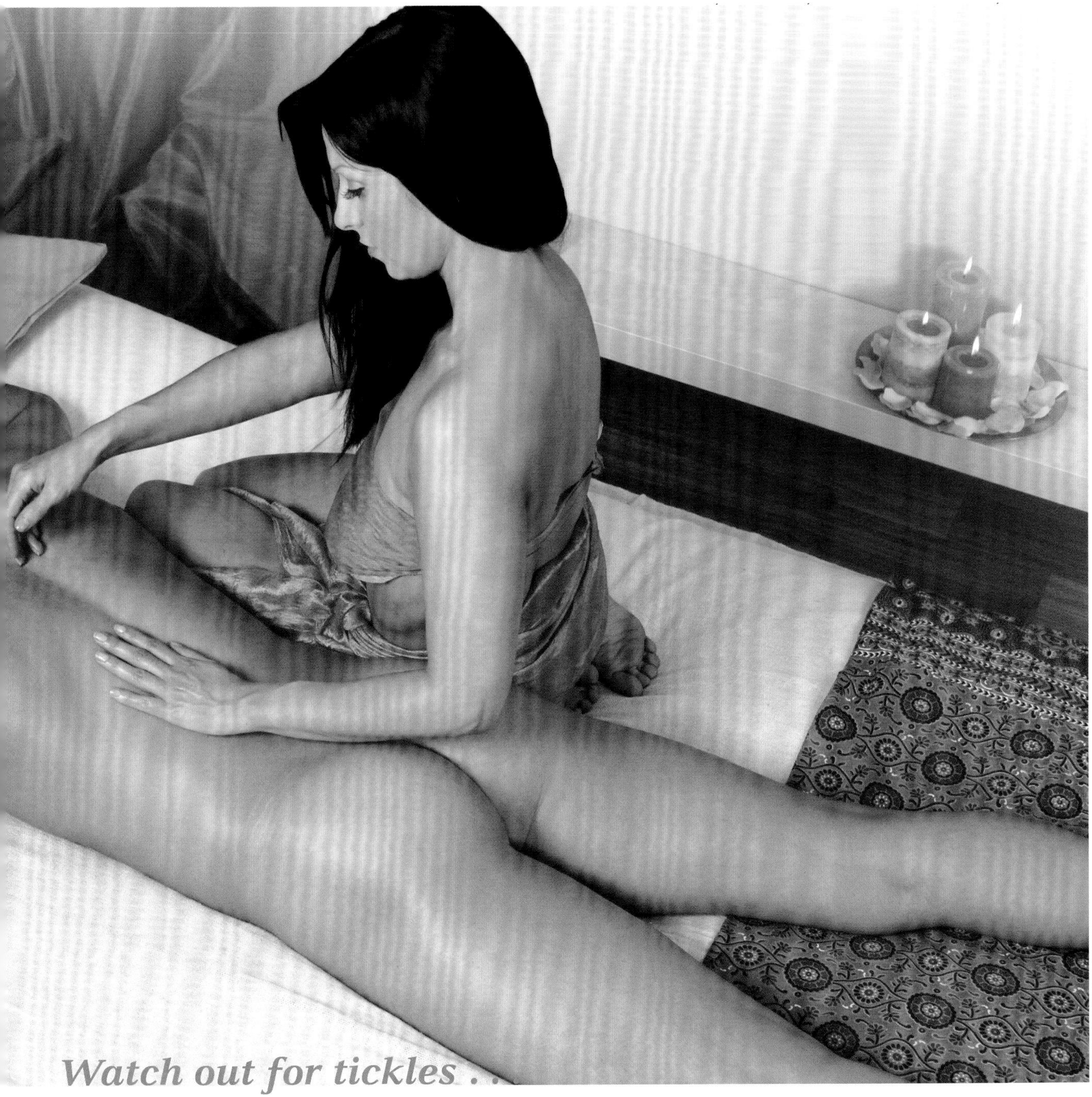

Watch out for tickles . . .

Large Movements

Sit on the right of your partner with him/her face down. Place both your hands parallel on his/her right buttock.

1. Softly slide your hands, one hand following the other, alternating and stroking crosswise outside to inside.

Keep sliding your hands on your partner's back in an upwards direction until you reach the shoulders, using soft and deliberate strokes which barely graze the skin at first, but bit by bit becoming more ample. In this way, your partner will feel the massage is spreading over their whole back.

Change sides and repeat the same sequence on the other half of their body, slowly and tenderly.

Ask him/her how the contact feels to them and if your touch should be more or less intense. If they desire more vigorous pressure, just lean the upper part of your body forward and your hands will automatically deliver greater intensity.

Gliding Touch

Rest your hands, palms down, on each side of the vertebral column with your fingers pointed toward the head.

2. Allow your hands to glide along the entire length of the vertebral column, going over the musculature as your hands ascend upwards. Complete this movement by slowly retracing the same territory with your hands moving apart, inside to outside.

Remember to always watch your partner's reactions. Watch his/her breathing and note any sounds they make. It's important that you know how they're reacting to the massage and if necessary, ask if they like it. Then adjust the intensity of your movements according to your partner's response.

Circular Movements

Place your hands on both shoulders, simultaneously.

3. Glide your hands making gentle circles from the center of the back to the outside, then tracing back again. Start with the barest of grazing then increase the movements bit by bit until the strokes become more firm and intense.

Before rubbing your lover's skin, check your hands.

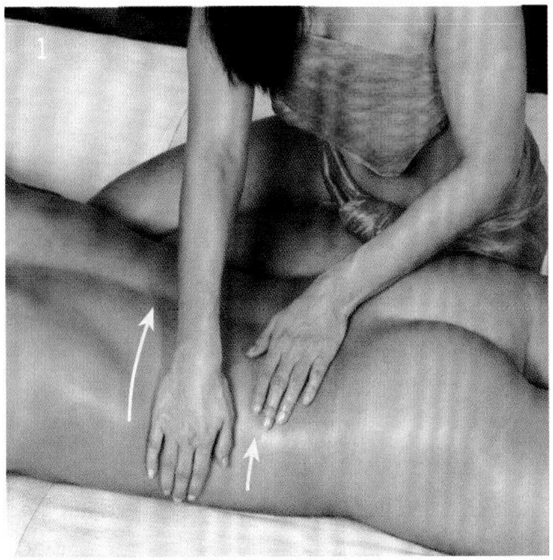
1
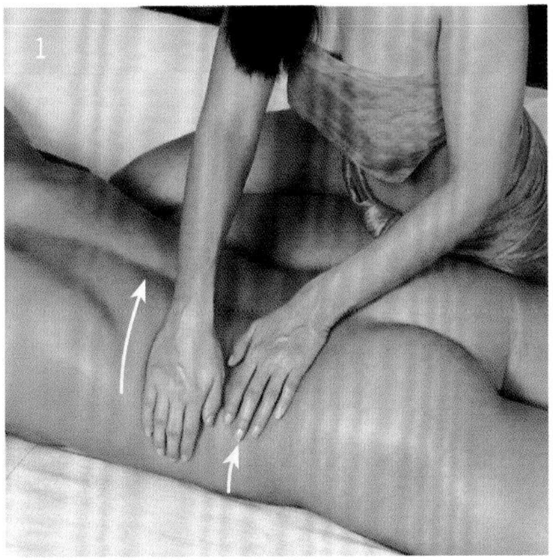
1
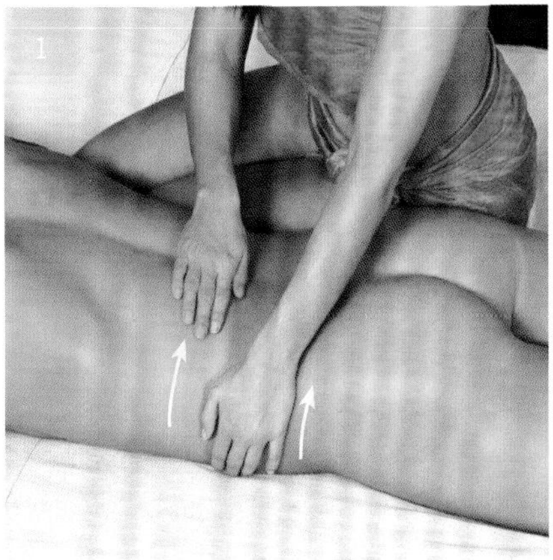
1
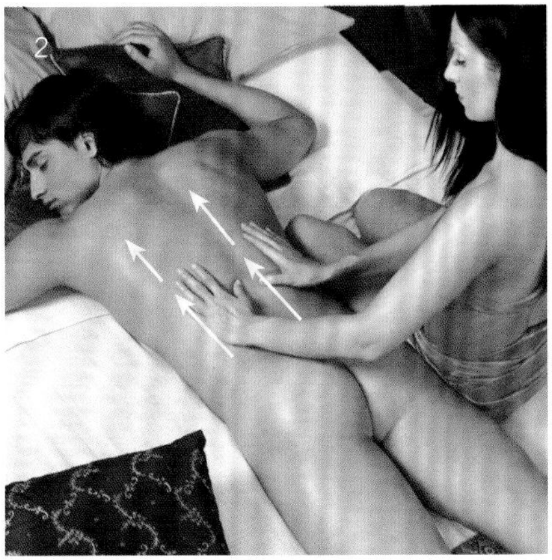
2
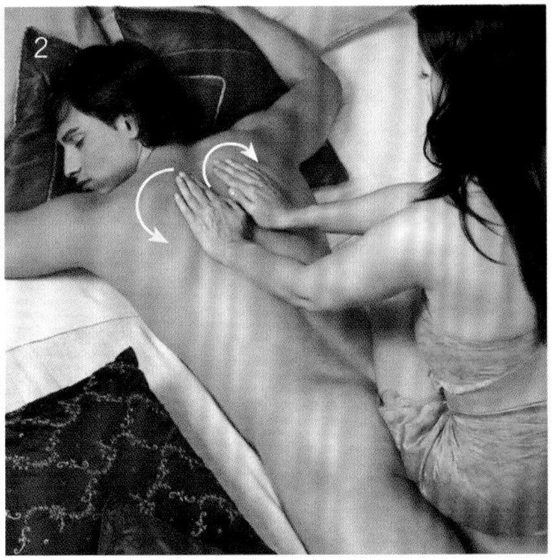
2
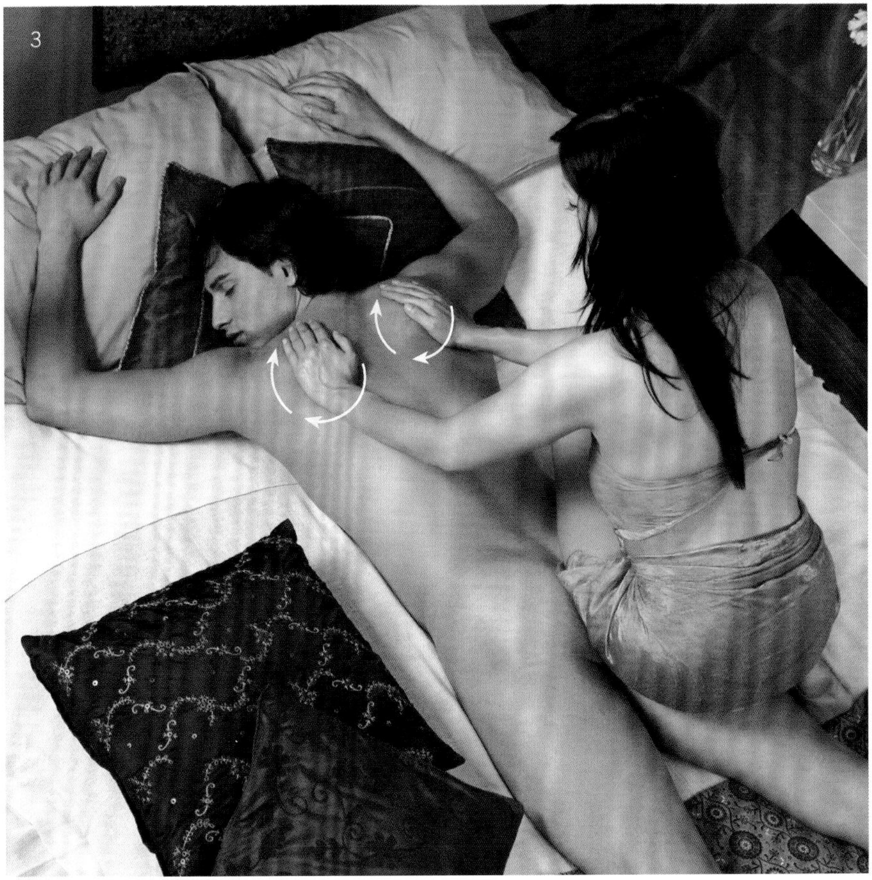
3

The Friction Stroke

This involves rubbing with friction and, in fact, constitutes the basis of couple's massage. The friction stroke **relaxes** tense or cramped muscles and **eases** muscle fatigue. Depending on the amount of pressure applied, this massage will either **stimulate or relax** and always affects the nerve endings of the outer layer of the skin.

It is advisable to start with a light friction that warms and relaxes the muscles before going to a more intense massage. Friction rubbing and caressing are very similar. Both involve **gentle, light sliding over the skin.** Nevertheless, caresses use more deliberate, sensual movement, while with friction rubbing the massage is performed with **more rhythmic and shorter** movements. Friction rubbing is recommended, especially for the arms, thighs, and back.

With Palms of the Hands Flat

1. Kneel next to your partner and give him/her friction rubs on his/her back. Work from the lumbar area upwards, using both hands at the same time.

2. Have your fingertips pointing toward your partner's head. Delicately slide your hands over their back.

Apply even pressure with the palms of your hands kept flat.

Follow the shape of the muscles with your hands and gently outline their contours.

3. Finally, with both hands on his/her shoulders, slide from inside outwards to the arms. Imagine your hands are like ocean waves.

With this type of massage, make sure to apply enough massage oil to the area to be worked.

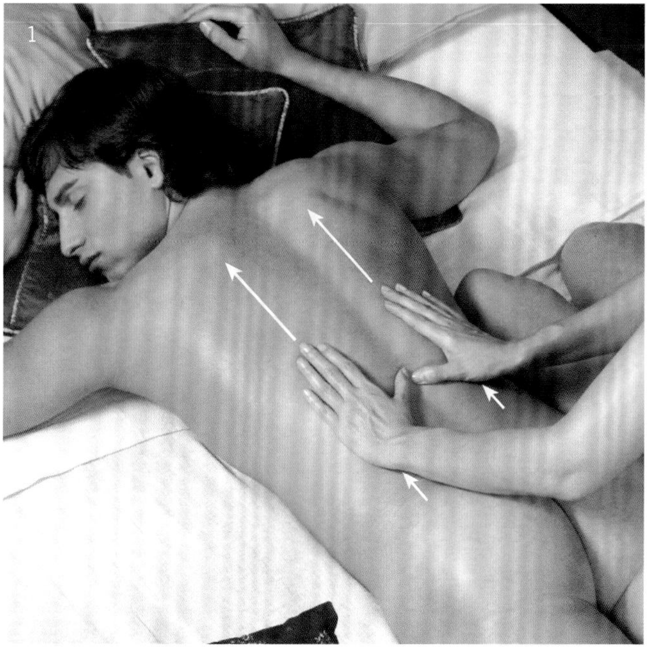
1

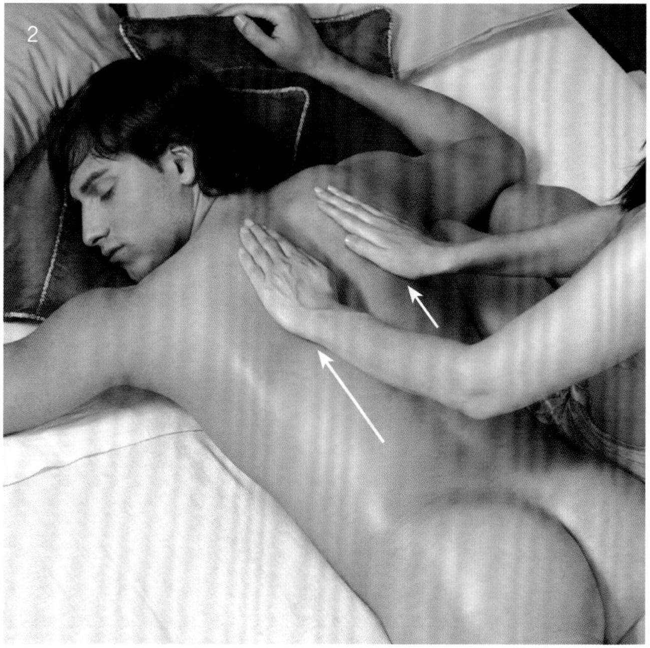
2

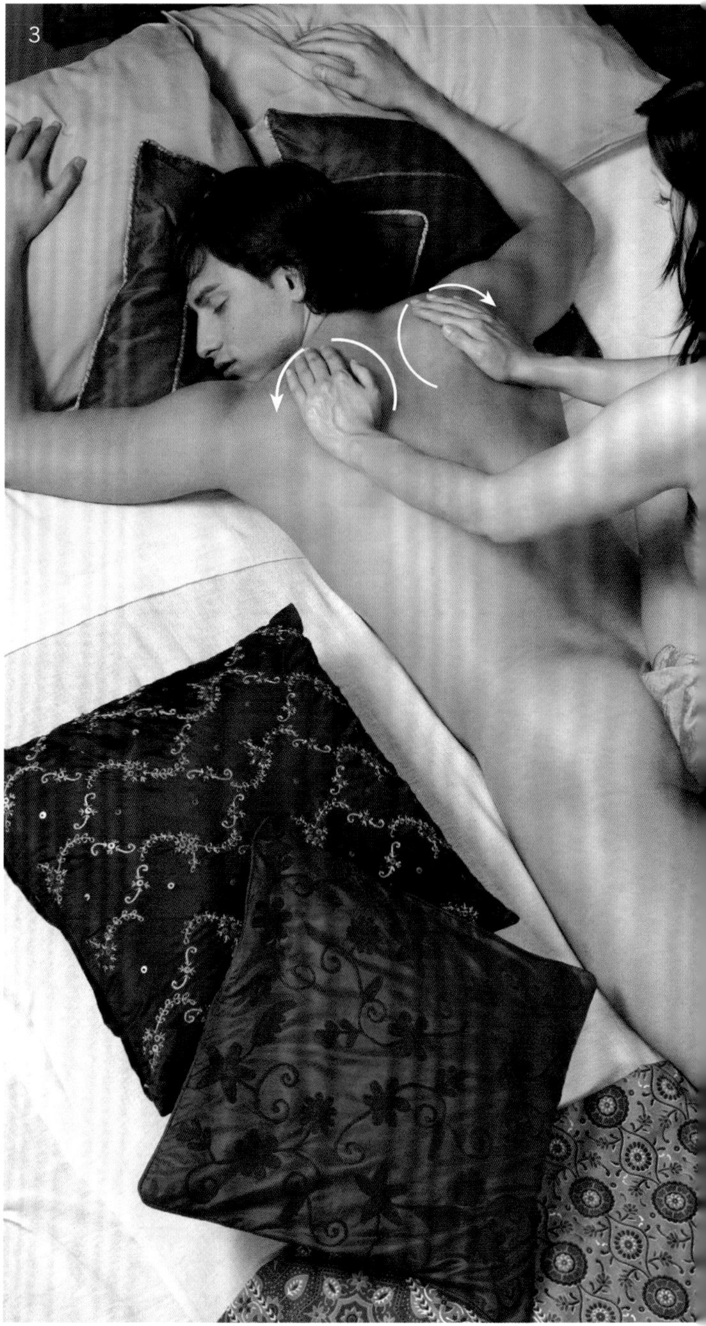
3

Massage with Flexed Hands

The friction stroke with flexed hands is particularly suited for working the arms and legs as shown below:

Sit between your partner's legs or beside him/her with their face down.

1. Place one hand behind the other on your partner's calf just above the ankle.

Sweep your hands exerting light pressure with one hand following the other so that they smooth over the calf up to the back part of the knee.

Ask your partner if they like the pressure. Continue upwards from the knee to the butt, increasing the pressure deliberately and gradually.

2. To finish, start again at the ankle and repeat the sequence as before, only this time increase the pressure.

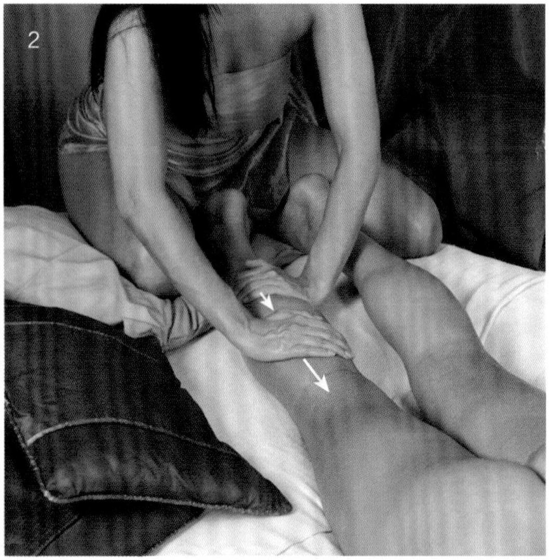

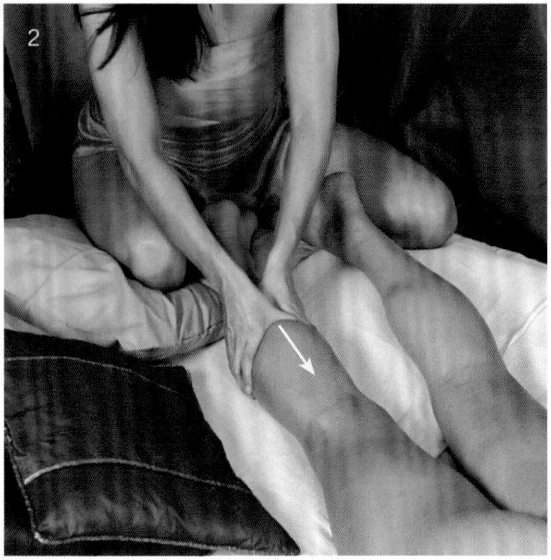

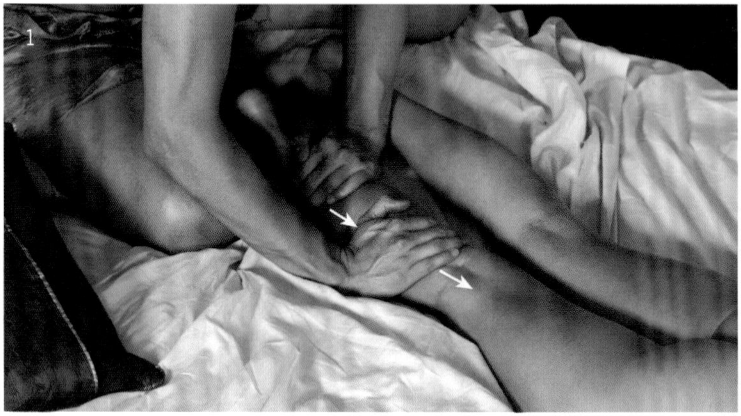

Circular Motions

This technique is a magnificent ending for the massages we have just described. It consists of friction rubs in a "circle 8" pattern that create waves of stimulating sensations.

Do not forget your partner's buttocks since they are the most sensitive part of the body's posterior.

All of these basic techniques will keep appearing in the massages that are detailed throughout this book. They are techniques whose effectiveness has been proved, but this does not mean they are the only ones. In all of the massages we explain you can vary the type of movements and strokes we suggest. The most important thing is to let your imagination go and trust your intuition and capacity to improvise while always being attentive to your partner's reactions and remembering it is him/her we are trying to invigorate and please.

Make circles with your hands on your partner's back.

Make one hand move clockwise and the other counterclockwise.

You will see that your hands tend to overlap and you will end up making "figure 8s" on your partner's back.

Ask your partner what effect the movements are having. Usually they have the sensation that several hands are doing the massage.

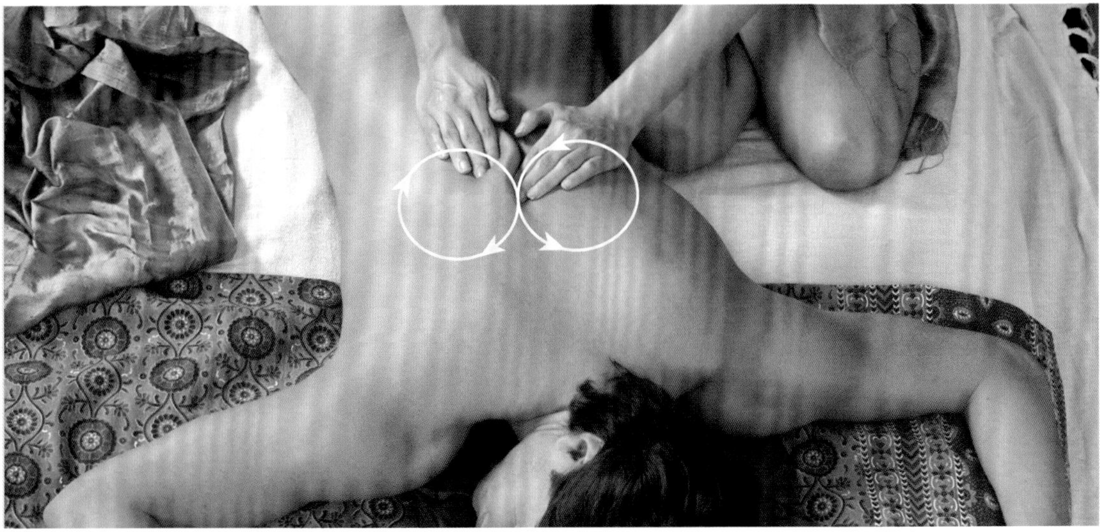

Pressure Stokes

These involve strong and firm movements which can also be done slowly. Pressure is applied mostly with the fleshy pad at the junction of the thumb and the palm of the hand. Pressure strokes stimulate blood flow and this in turn stimulates the genitals.

1. Place your hands on your partner's buttocks, back, or thighs.

2. Draw the fleshy pad of the palm of your hands around this area.

3. Gradually increase the pressure while you rub each of the separate muscles more intensely.

Ask your partner if he/she likes the intensity of the pressure and adjust according to his/her response.

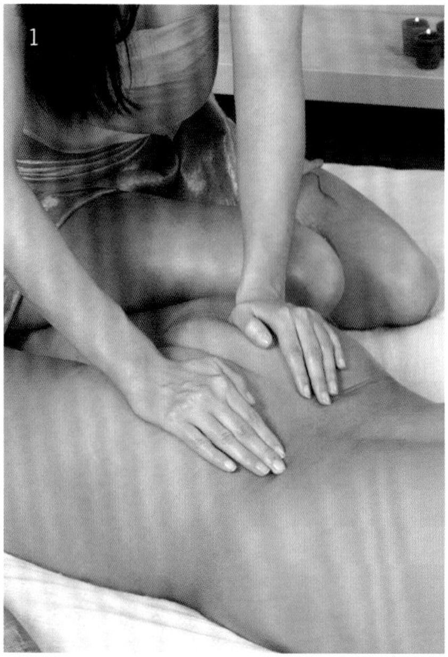

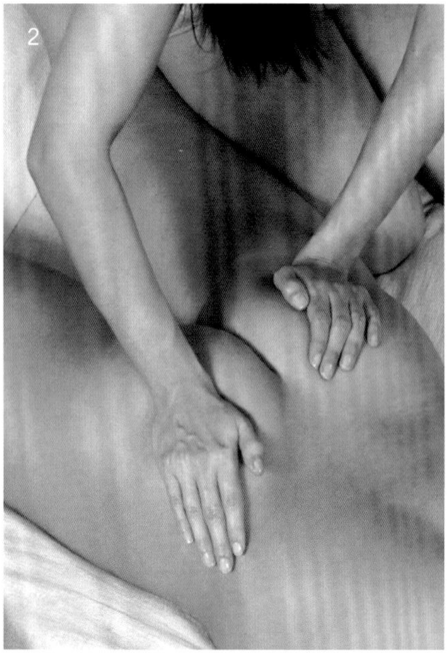

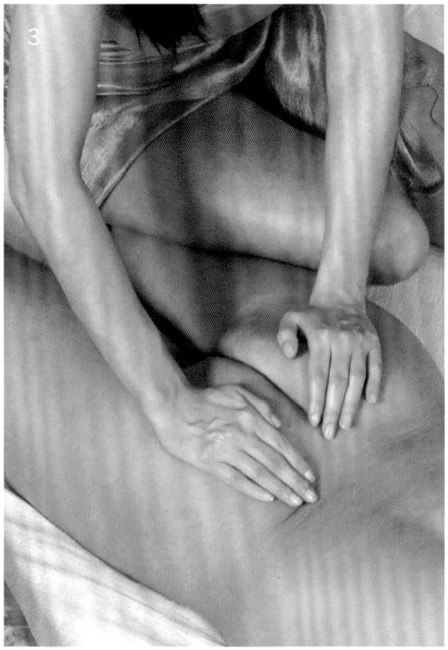

Stimulating your partner's buttocks is one of the most seductive massages there is.

Kneading

This technique is suitable for parts of the body with the most muscle mass such as the buttocks, waist, and shoulders. The movement can be compared to hands kneading dough. This involves deeper rubbing that awakens desire.

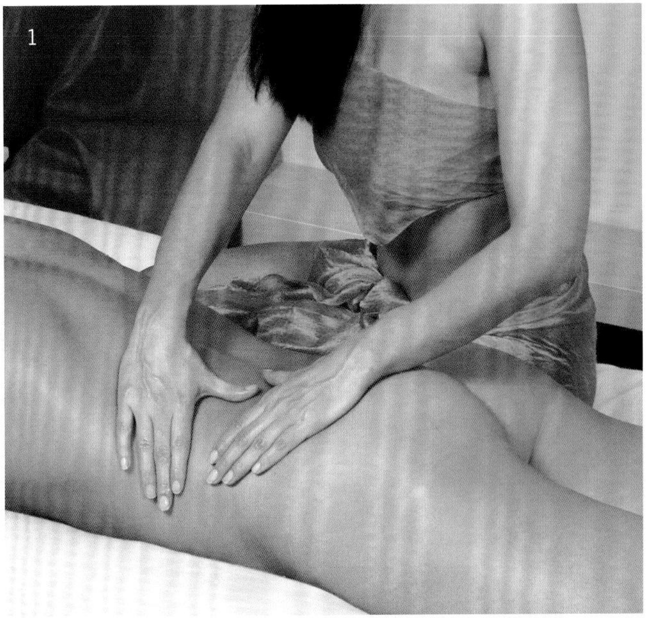

Sit on your partner's right side aligned with his/her waist.

1. Have your hands slide over his/her waist toward their left hip and lean your body over his/hers. Repeat the motion going from the hip to the waist and then back again.

2. Knead the muscle by pinching it gently between your thumb and fingers.

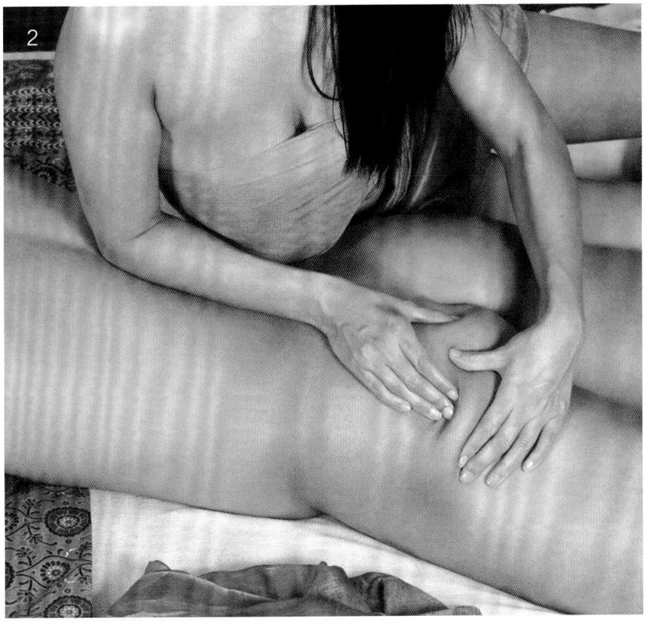

Make sure not to apply excessive pressure and that your partner likes the massage.

Change sides and repeat the same sequence.

The pressure and force of your hands will depend on your partner's preference.

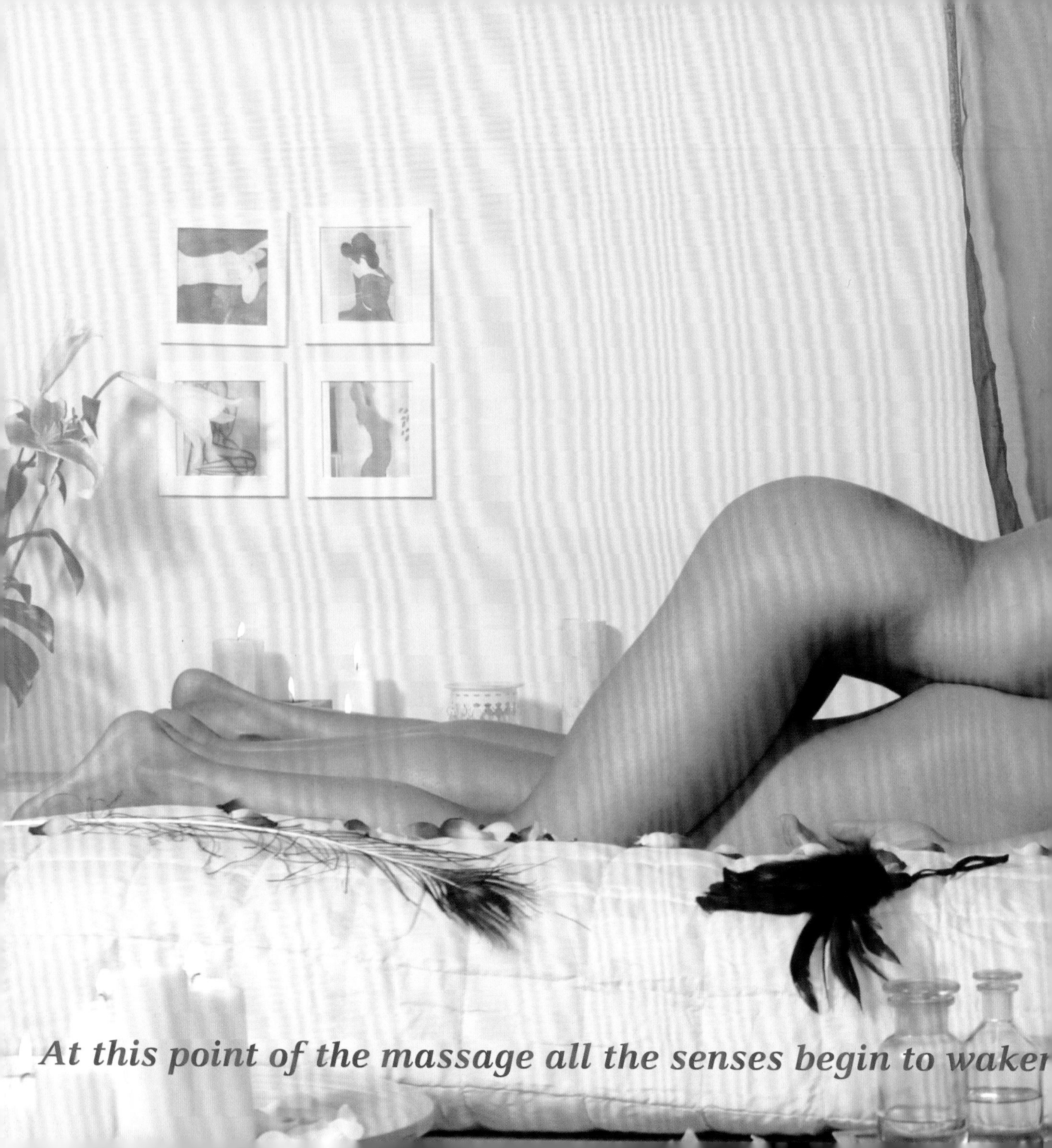

At this point of the massage all the senses begin to wake

Sensual Massages

TURNING UP THE HEAT

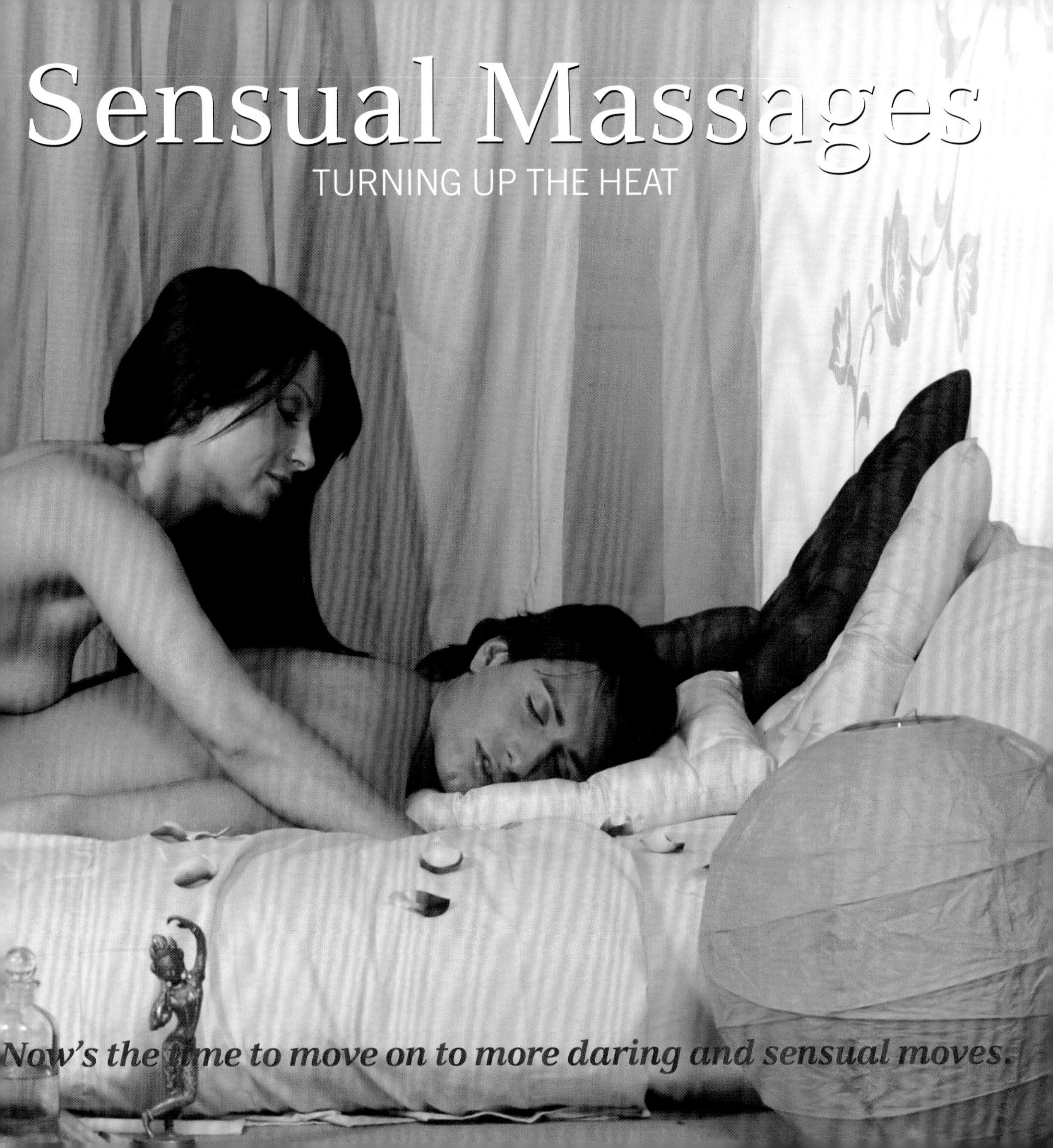

Now's the time to move on to more daring and sensual moves.

The Keys to Success

You now know the basic techniques for a giving a complete, sensual massage. However, for your success to be assured you must be aware of certain guidelines. Following is key advice that guarantees pleasure:

- Make sure to create a **warm and inviting atmosphere** in the room before you begin.
- **Turn off your cell and landline phones.** You do not want anything or anyone to interrupt you.
- Have **oils, towels, pillows, and cushions** nearby and blankets, if you need them.
- The most important thing is to always **maintain contact between your bodies** during the massage. Keep focused on your partner's body at all times and when you change technique or position remember to keep a hand in contact with his/her skin.
- Touch your partner **delicately** and slowly as you show them your tenderness and affection. **Don't hold back** when you improvise. You are not limited to using your hands only and can also massage your partner's skin with your **hair, lips, and tongue** or any other part of your body.
- Encourage your companion to **express his/her desires and fantasies.**
- Pay attention to your partner's nonverbal communication. This means any possible movements or sounds they make, no matter how insignificant they may seem.
- Don't get carried away with the idea of creating too sexy an atmosphere. The most important thing is that both of you **feel comfortable** and that everything flows naturally.
- If your partner suddenly takes the initiative and starts to **stroke or caress you,** let them do it. Don't forget that massages are good for both sexes.

Without Hang-Ups

It's perfectly natural that the first few times we practice couple's massage we might feel ashamed about our own body or our partner's body.

Besides your hands, you can use other parts of your body to do a massage.

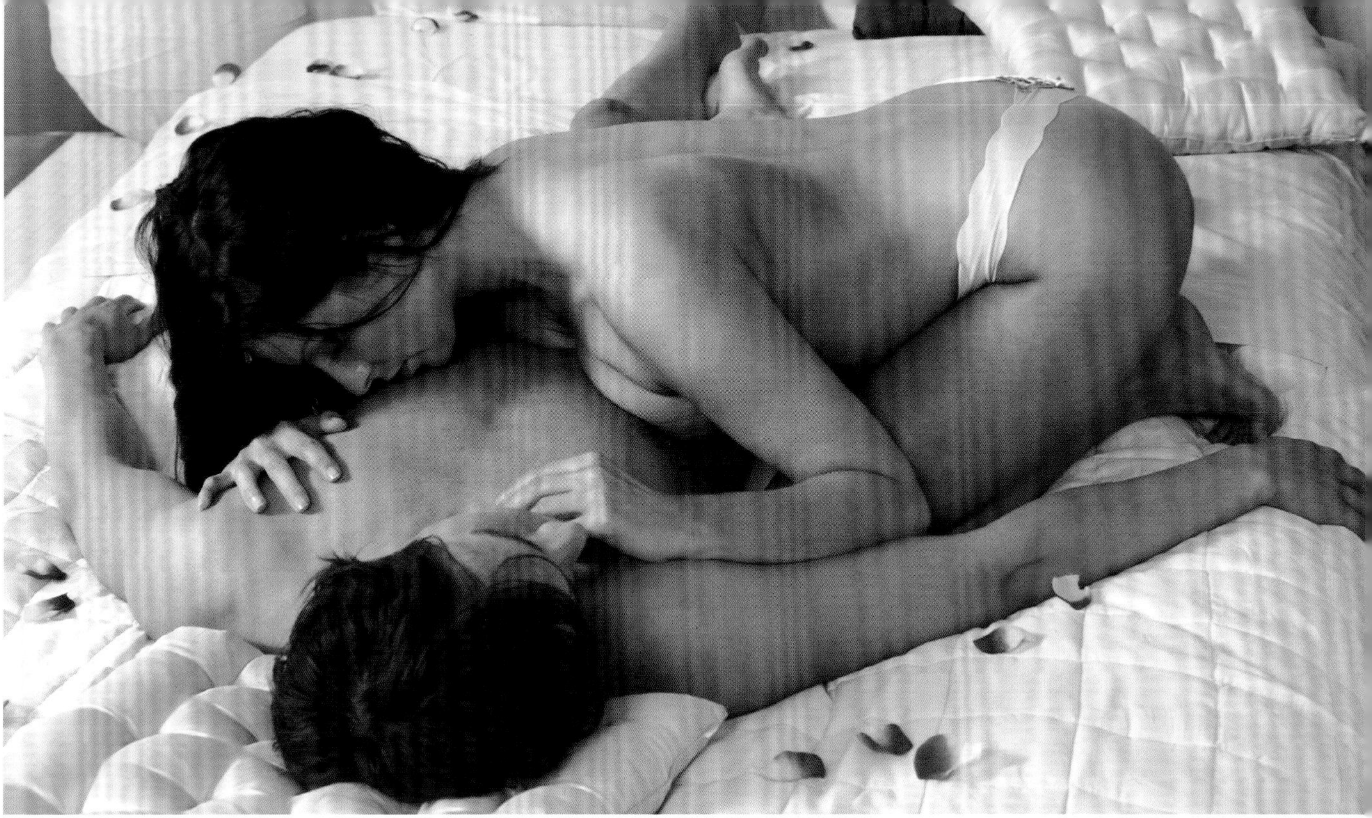

This makes sense if you keep in mind that it is rare to touch or be touched all over the body with such attention and detail as during an erotic massage.

It is also possible that while we are giving the massage we might wonder if we are doing a good job or if our partner is really enjoying it. Perhaps we're afraid we look clumsy or are not pleasing our companion or even, on the other hand, that they are about to reach orgasm and will not want to continue the session after they do. It's also possible that while we're receiving a massage we're afraid that our partner might be bored or tired and isn't enjoying him-/herself.

We need to put all these kinds of worries out of our mind. We must carry on naturally and spontaneously and let what happens take its own course. The essential thing is to get into the feeling and go with the flow.

It is highly recommended that after the massage you both talk about what you experienced and what you would like to try the next time. Also comment on what signals/signs were useful or

Rub your partner's body with your breasts, hair, mouth . . .

would be useful to show what you are experiencing.

It's also natural in the beginning that you or your partner may feel like laughing because you're not used to massage or haven't mastered the techniques, or simply because you're ashamed. This is not something to worry about. In fact, laughing will help both of you to relax and forget about yourselves and release any tensions.

Orgasm isn't the point, but it's nice when it happens.

In the first place it should be clear that the principal objective of erotic massage is not orgasm. It is possible, nevertheless, that sometimes the massage causes it to happen unexpectedly.

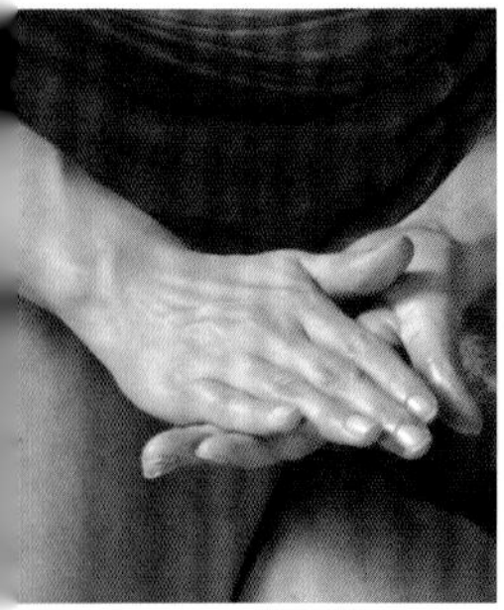

If this should occur while you're receiving a massage let it happen without getting upset. Just relax and enjoy it. When you are the one giving the massage don't worry about your partner getting an orgasm. It can be very enjoyable to both partners if one of them has an orgasm, but it doesn't mean anything if this doesn't happen and the massage can still be enormously pleasing in all respects.

It is possible your partner feels so relaxed that they are not at all aroused. This is nothing to be concerned about. The aim of couple's massage is pleasure in its most widely understood sense and its development depends on many factors, one of which is your partner's mood. Don't push. Enjoy whatever happens without worrying about any preconceived results.

Delaying the Fireworks

Here is a little trick you should try if you want to avoid an imminent orgasm. If the genitals of the man or woman are highly excited, the one giving the massage can divert the energy this way:

- Put your hands on your partner's body so that there is **minimal, light contact.**
- Using a rapid movement let your **hands smooth and sweep the energy** accumulated there to the exterior of the body. It is as if you were pushing the energy out of the body by way of your partner's hands, feet, and head.

Erotic massage should be something fun and natural for lovers.

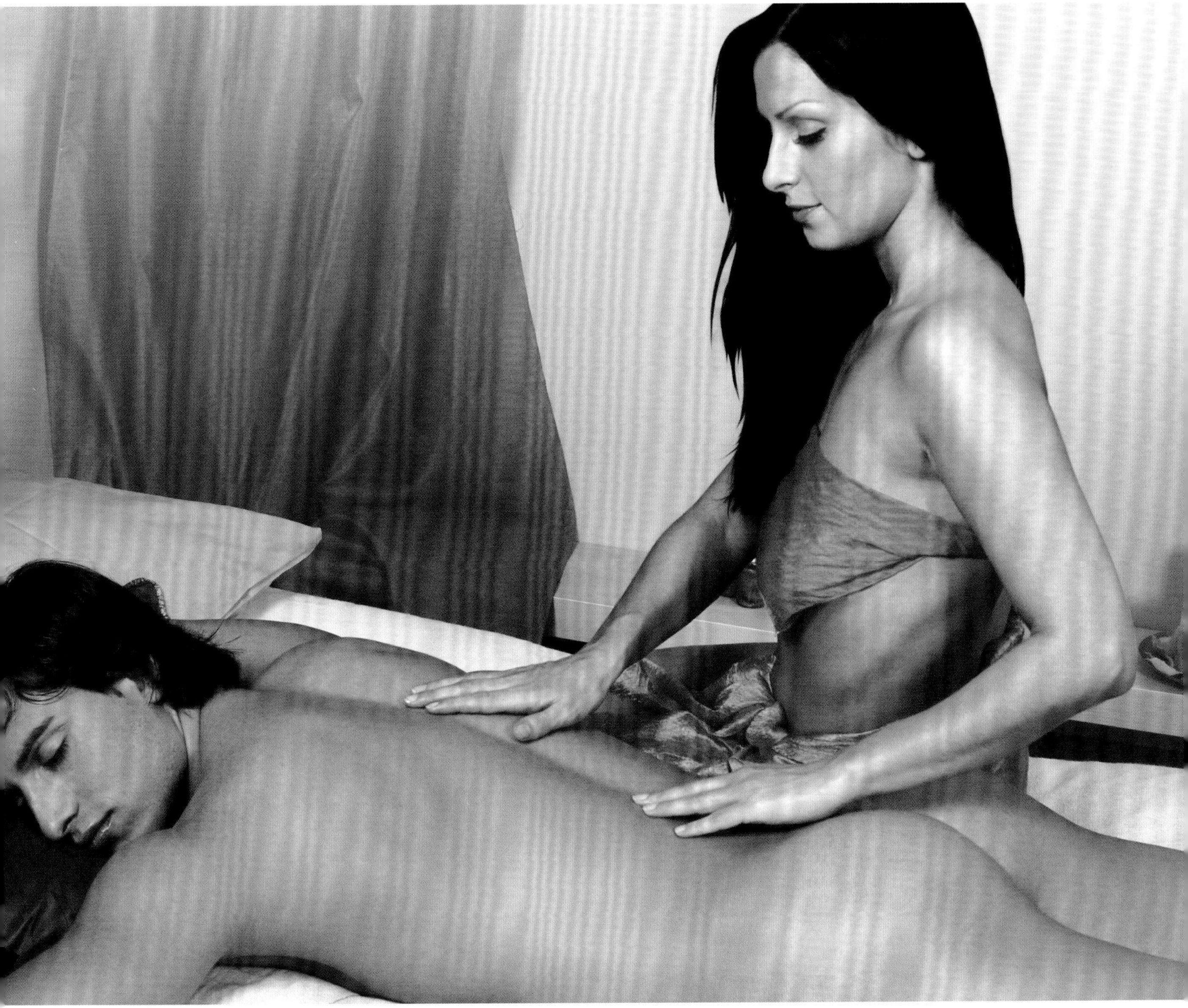

Let your imagination fly, free yourself from tensions, and enjoy.

Foot Massage

Massaging the feet and legs is a good way to either start or finish a full massage session.

Many are unaware that there are important erogenous zones on the feet that rapidly provoke pleasurable sensations. The ankles, for example, with their delicate curves are very nice to caress and rub. Don't doubt for a second that your partner will be excited when you give him or her a seductive foot massage that includes both caressing and kissing.

There are couples that may feel ashamed for including the feet in their sex play, but once they conquer their initial reticence they discover that a sensual massage of the feet can be incredibly relaxing and powerfully stimulating. A good foot massage can unleash chills over the entire body and become a true source of pleasure.

Don't forget to choose massage oils that seduce the senses of both of you. Choose them together. We especially recommend sandalwood oil. Its sensual and delicate aroma mixed with almond oil is particularly suitable for performing a relaxing and erotic massage of your partner's feet.

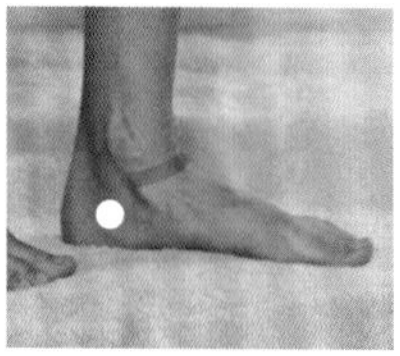

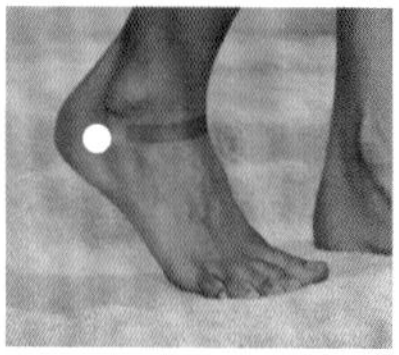

Erogenous Zones of the Feet

Foot reflexology maintains there is a connection between specific areas of the feet and their corresponding organs, systems, or structures of the body.

- For example, on the inside and outside of the heel are reflex points that correspond to the ovaries, testicles, and prostate along with the masculine and feminine genitals (see the images to the left).
- The area that includes the entire heel up to the ankle corresponds to the abdomen. If you apply soft, circular rubbing, the effect is particularly pleasant, seductive, and energizing.
- In the center of the sole of the foot there are three points of sexual stimulation which run in a line from the heel across the arch up to the ball of the foot (see image on right).
- We also observe a fourth point situated apart from this line in the edge of the arch (see picture on right). Make spiral movements rubbing along this line.

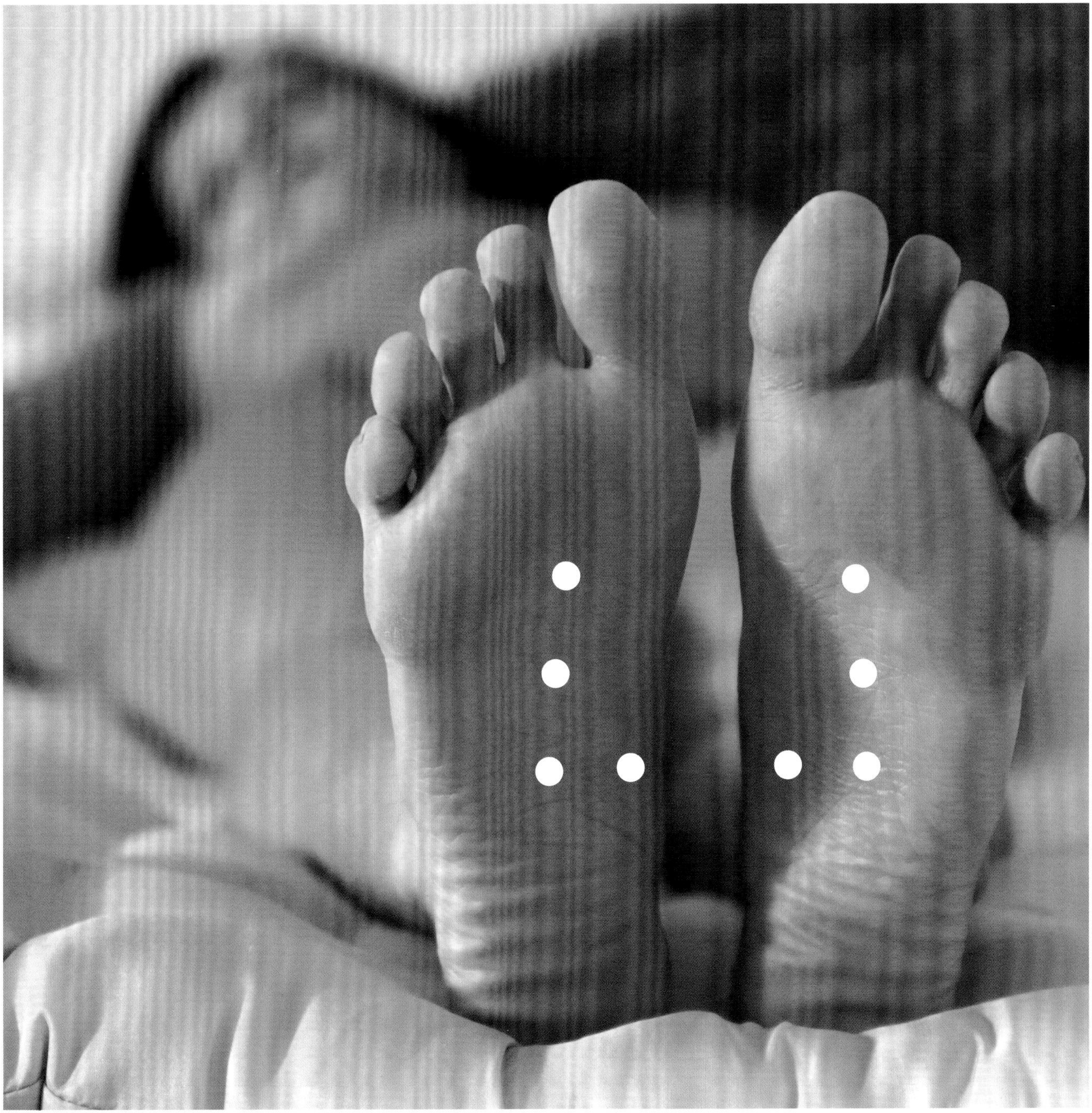

First Sensual Contact

We've divided foot massage into three phases. You can either do the whole foot massage, or stop after the first phase and go on to other parts of the body. It all depends on how you feel at the moment. Take care not to tickle your partner. Tickles on the feet can be really annoying.

Step by Step

Prepare the oil, towels, cushions, and if necessary, a blanket.

Your partner should be stretched out on his/her back. They can be nude, half-undressed, or totally clothed, as they prefer. It's important, though, that their feet remain uncovered.

Place a cushion beneath your partner's knees. The cushions help prevent any bodily discomfort. It is always important to avoid this.

1. Sit before your partner's feet and take them in your hands delicately and tenderly.

Put massage oil in your hands and rub them together to warm the oil and evenly spread it.

2. Begin by taking the right foot in both your hands and use your thumb to apply clockwise circular movements around the ankle on both the inside and outside.

Repeat the same motions on your partner's left foot.

Next, put the tips of the three middle fingers of each hand on the exterior of the joints of both feet.

Apply circular friction to the ankles. Make five circles in one direction, then make five circles in the opposite direction.

3. Then use the tips of your fingers to slowly trace "figure 8s" on the outside of the ankles of both feet.

Ask your partner if they like the friction and if you should increase or decrease the pressure.

Play with the "figure 8" movement, changing the size of the figures.

Give your partner enough time to experience the energy flow spreading throughout their body.

With this massage it's important to watch your partner's reactions.

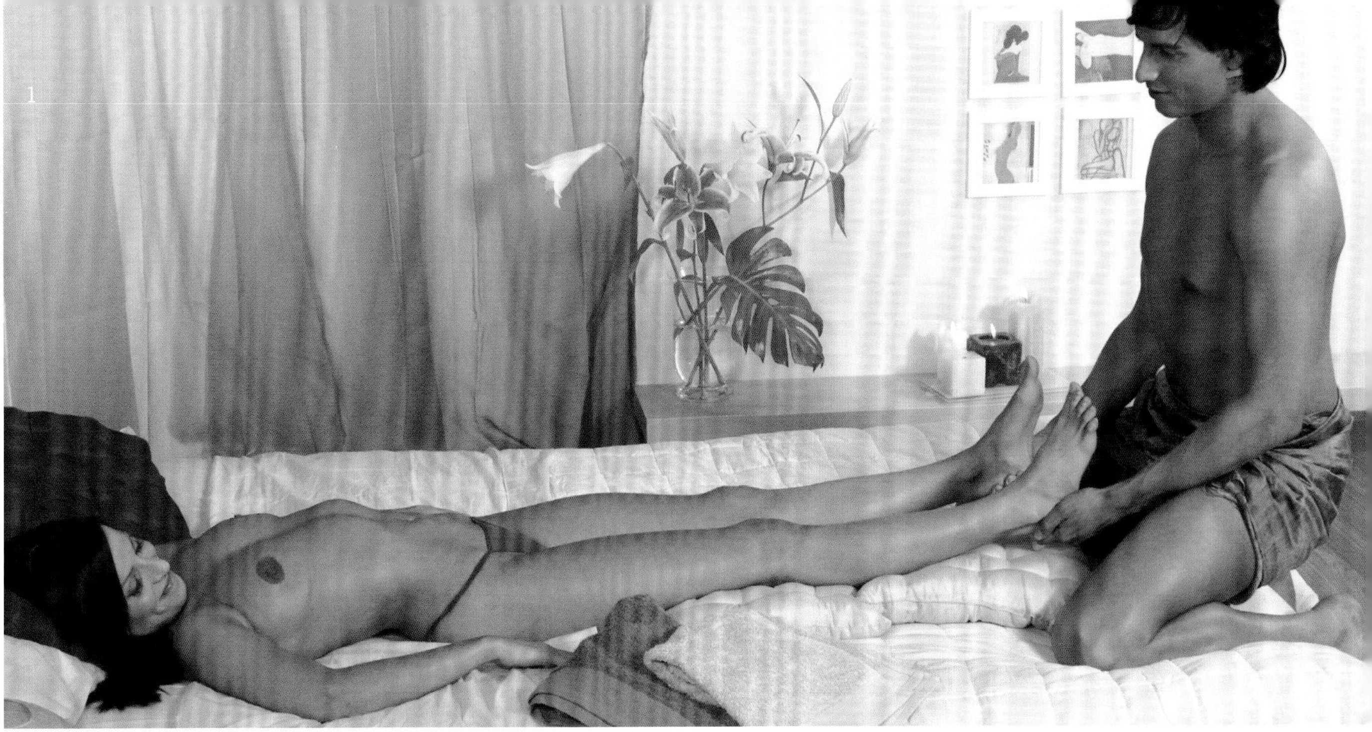
1

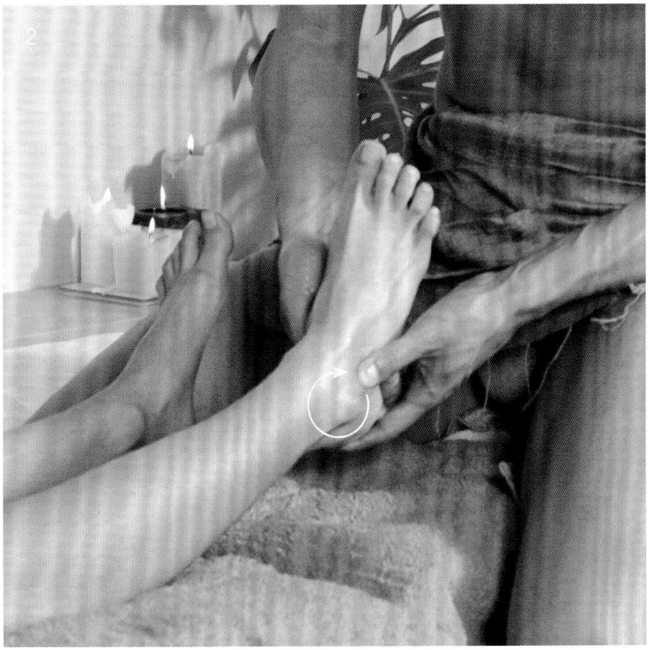
2

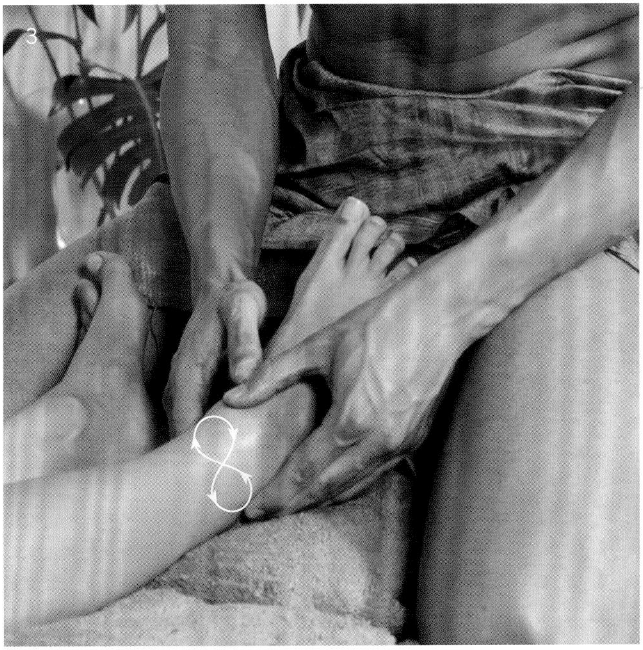
3

Press and Glide

We now begin to deeply work the muscles of each foot. Using a generous quantity of massage oil, it is time to apply intense pressure and stimulation.

1. Take your partner's foot with both hands and anoint it with oil. Pay special attention to the instep and sole of each foot.
2. Rub with both hands stretched and wide open from the tips of the toes to the calves. Make one hand follow the other in succession.
3. Do this several times. Make the friction continuous, dynamic, and flowing.
4. Keep your partner's foot right between your hands. Slide your hands toward the tips of his/her toes. Repeat this several times.
5. Take your partner's foot with both of your hands around the instep and rub with the fleshy pads of your palms. Move slowly outward and downwards. Use the fingertips of both your hands to apply light pressure to the sole of the foot with a consistent rhythm of pressing.

Do the same motion in the opposite direction up to the joint where the foot joins the calf.

Repeat this sequence a couple of more times and remember to always pay attention to your partner's reactions. This way you can vary the pressure as they like.

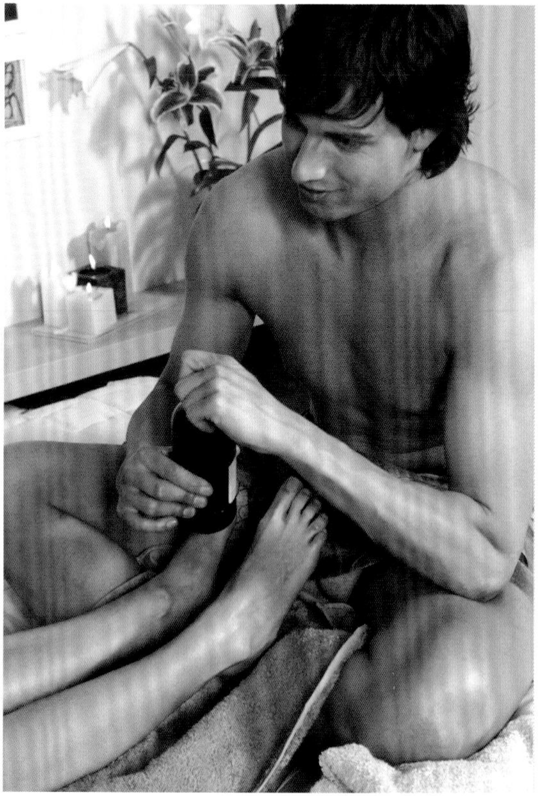

With this massage you must maintain constant, intense pressure.

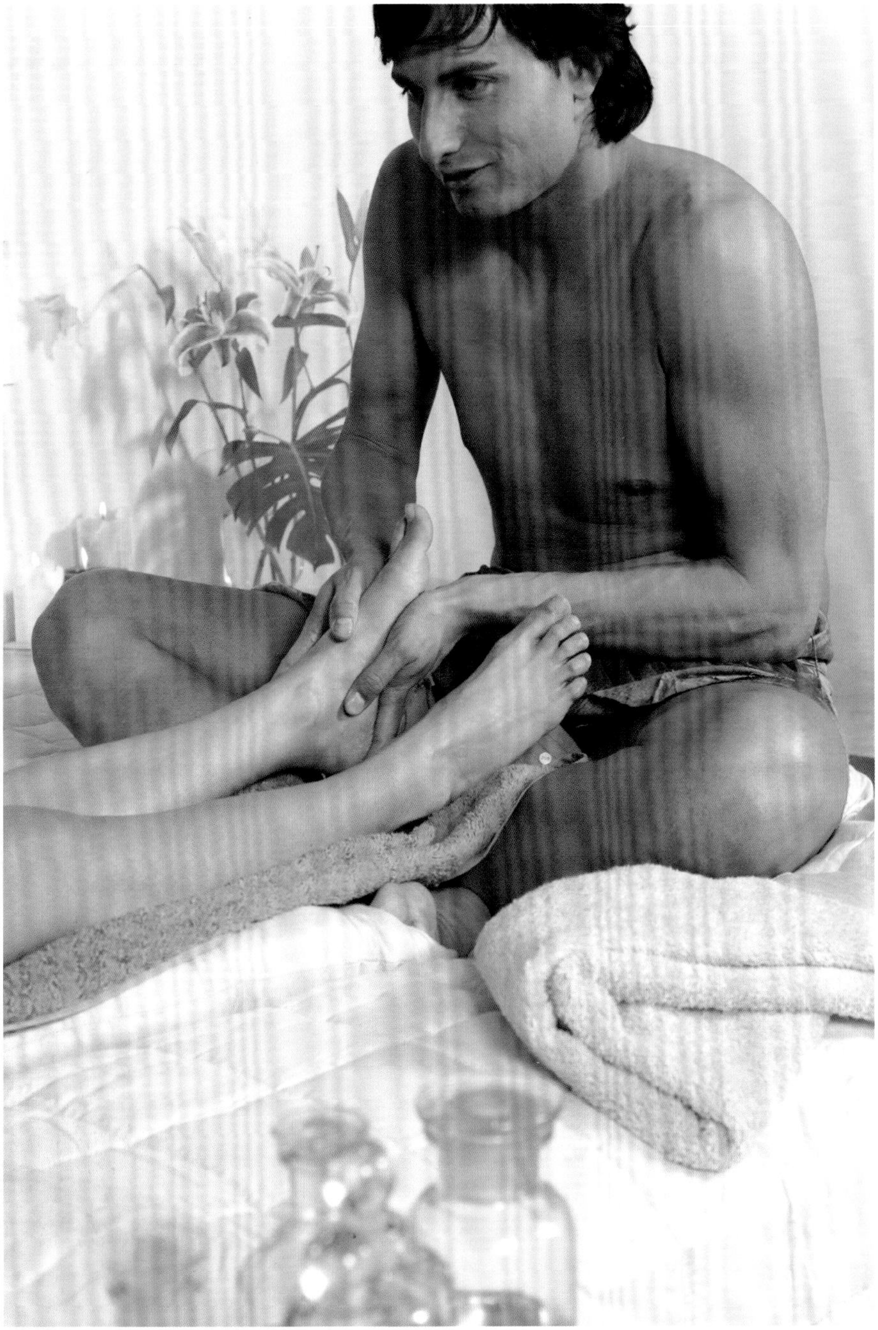

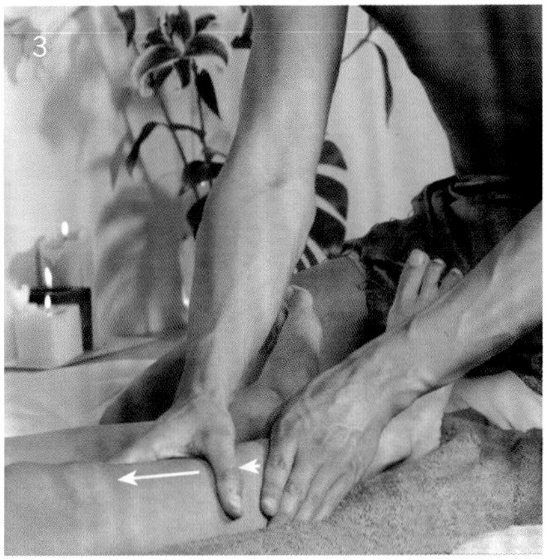

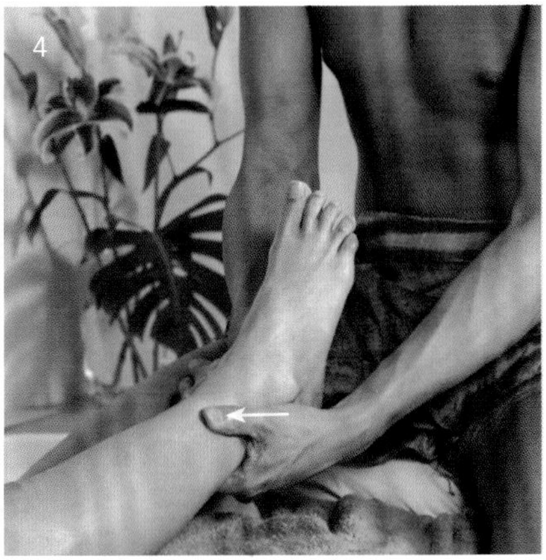

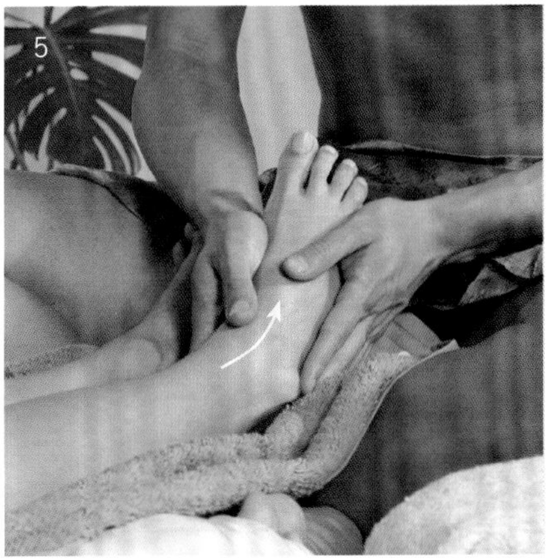

This way, the effect will be more pleasurable.

Stimulate the Key Points

6. Next, continue with pressure on the upper part of the instep with both your thumbs, rubbing in opposite directions. This is where the foot joins the leg and it constitutes an important point of reflex stimulation for the groin area.

7. Make "figure 8s" on the inside and outside of the ankles and all around with wide and gentle circular movements.

8. Grasp your partner's foot with your right hand and use the thumb of your left hand to draw small circles on the sole of the foot, lengthwise. Use gentle pressure and linger on the pressure points we described earlier.

9. Now pay attention to the toes. Rub each one in a circular motion using your thumb, index, and middle fingers. Feel free to kiss his/her toes; the sensation of your lips is sure to be very sensual. Remember to use your tongue to explore and moisten every little cranny.

Now let your partner's right foot rest. Cover it so it keeps warm and repeat the same sequence with their left foot.

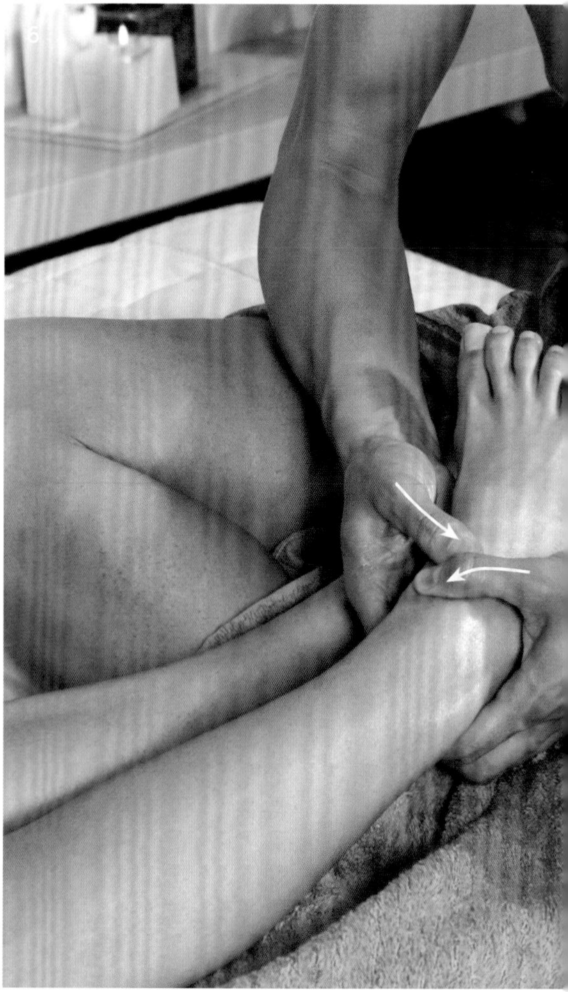

Deeply stimulate your partner's feet and turn on their desir

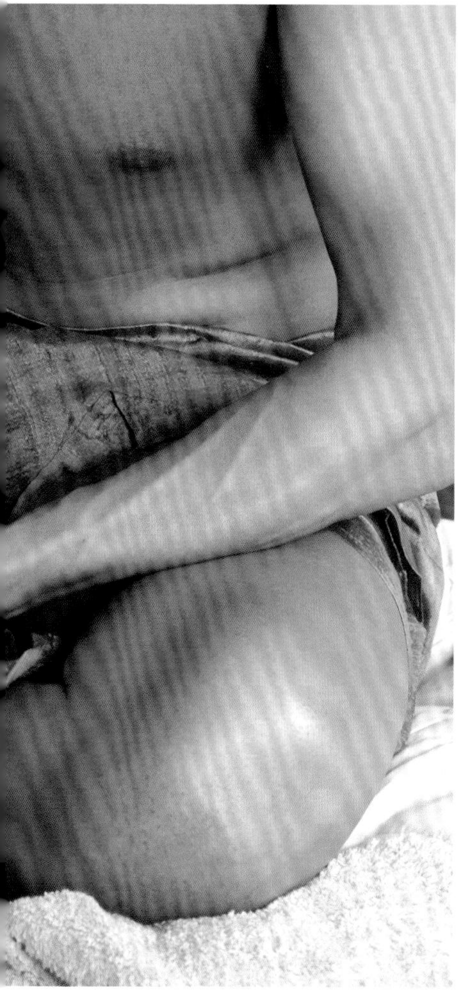

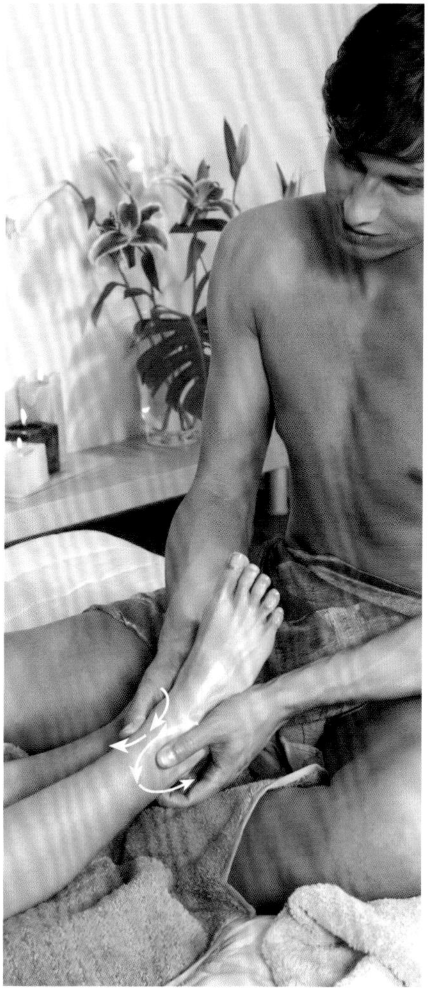

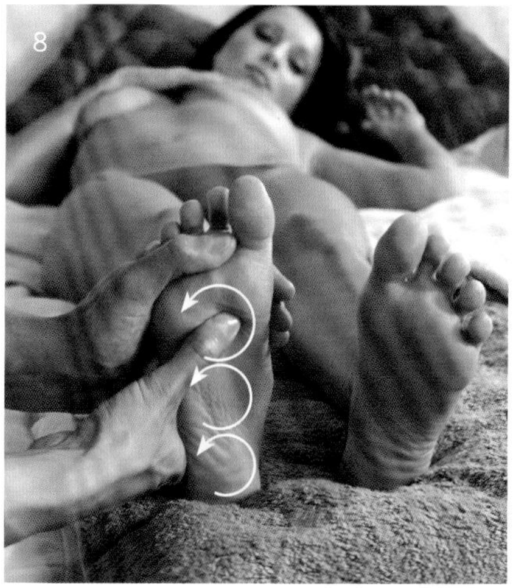

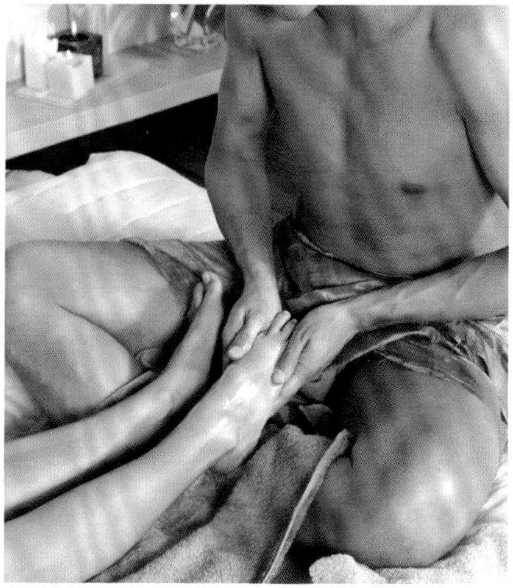

Do this firmly but gently and maintain a good rhythm.

A Relaxing Finish

With both feet uncovered, apply a liberal coating of massage oil and completely anoint them.

1. Go back to the ankle and make "figure 8s."

2. To finish, take each foot by the heel and pull it without jolting your partner. To make the movement even more relaxing, gently shake the leg you are working on.

3. As a final touch, rub the toes of your partner with your lips and kiss them tenderly, or go around them with your tongue.

To Be Continued…

Although erotic massage of the feet constitutes a complete massage in itself, it is certainly difficult to leave things at that after just having experienced such thrilling and pleasant sensations. This type of massage is often a prelude to other, more sensual massages . . .

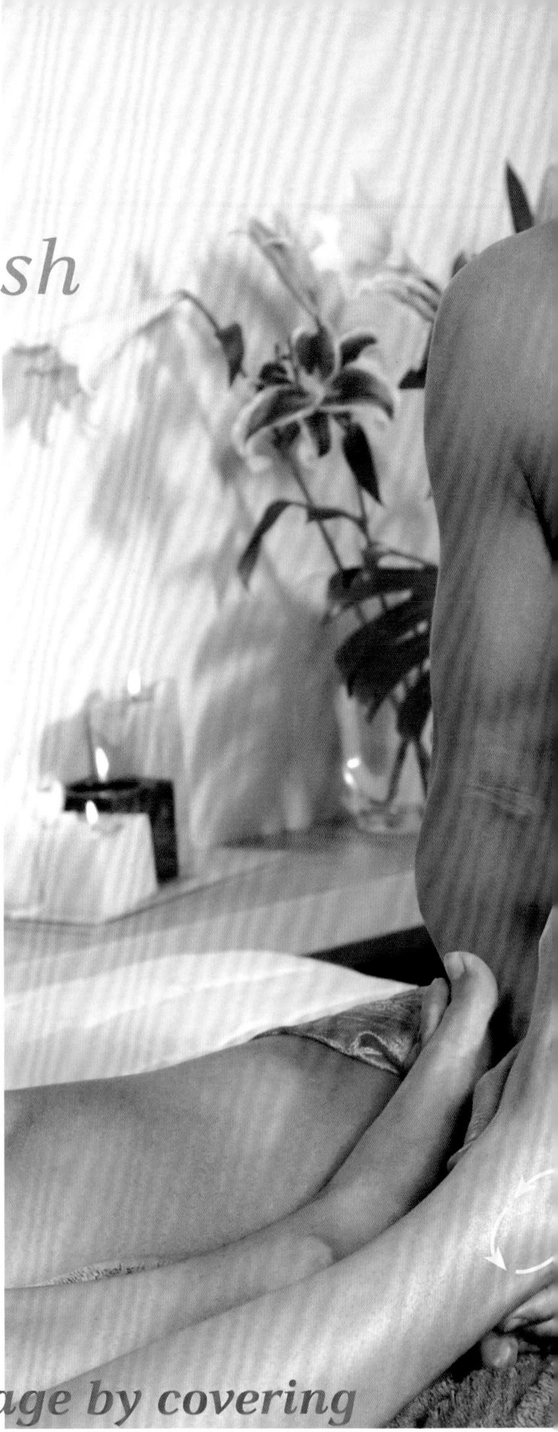

You can finish this erotic massage by covering your partner's feet with kisses.

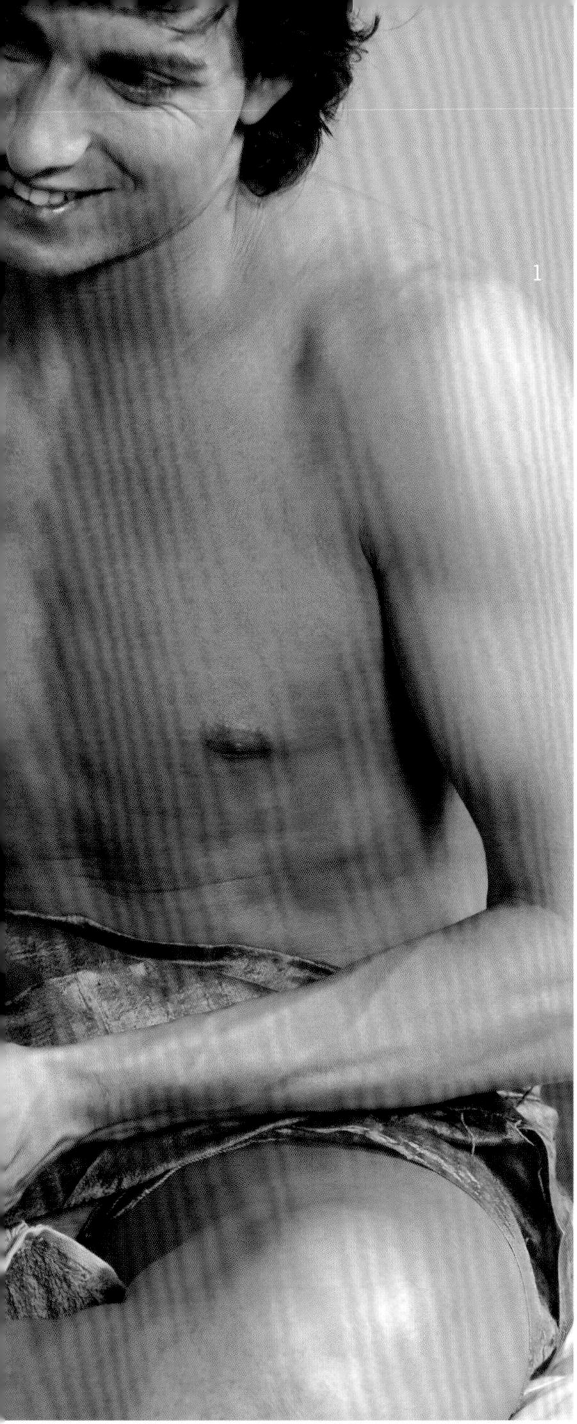

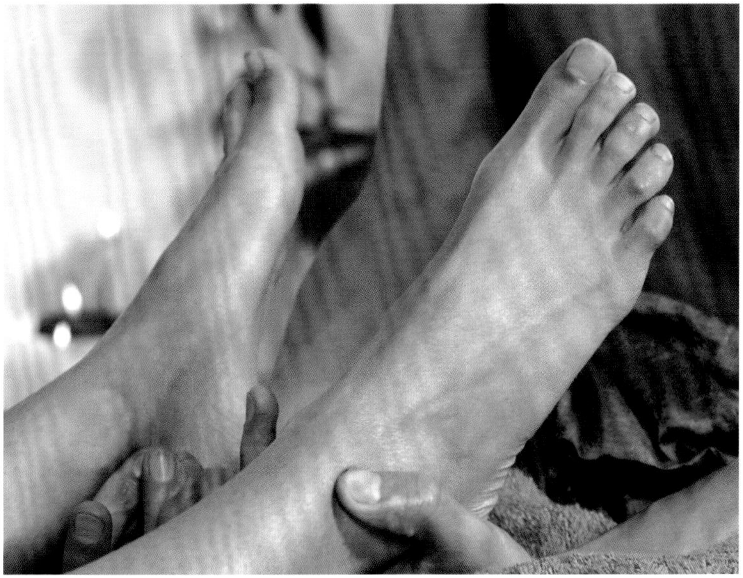

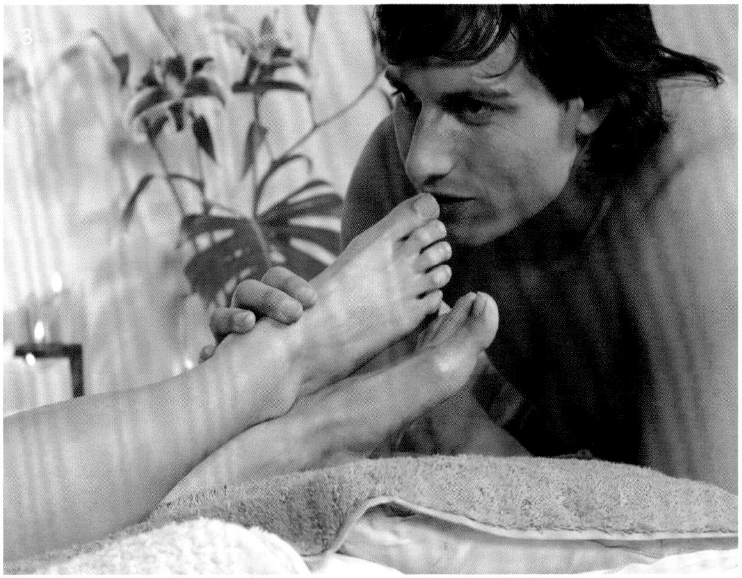

The Back and Lumbar Area

The back is the perfect area to begin practicing couple's massage for all those people who are timid about or ashamed of their own bodies. When face down, the person receiving the massage feels much more protected and can relax while they enjoy the pleasant sensations the massage gives them.

In the back we find nerve plexuses, which are connected with all parts of the body. Remember, as we explained earlier, both men and women have numerous points of sexual stimulation that provide exquisite sensual pleasure when stimulated with delicate stroking or pressure.

Erotic massage of the back is different from classic back massage. You start at the neck and end at the gluteals; the object is to be more stimulating than relaxing.

You can use any of the techniques we've seen so far to massage the back and lumbar area. As with all erotic massage, remember that it is essential to vary your techniques and try different things. With practice, we discover what types of strokes are more sensual as well as little tricks or ideas that work best on our particular partner.

The first thing you need to do a back massage is a comfortable place with a solid support for stretching out. A bed that is too soft will not work. It is better to put warm blankets, sheets, or towels on the floor and use that instead. Don't forget to choose massage oil blends that you both enjoy.

Preparing Your Massage Oil

A Fresh, Soothing Aroma
4 tablespoons of almond oil
2 drops of sandalwood essence
2 drops of Ylang Ylang
3 drops of orange sanguine essence

A Long-Lasting Fragrance
2 tablespoons of almond oil
1 tablespoon of rosehip oil
2 drops of jasmine essence
2 drops of rosewood essence
3 drops of red mandarin essence

Back massages are ideal for shy lovers.

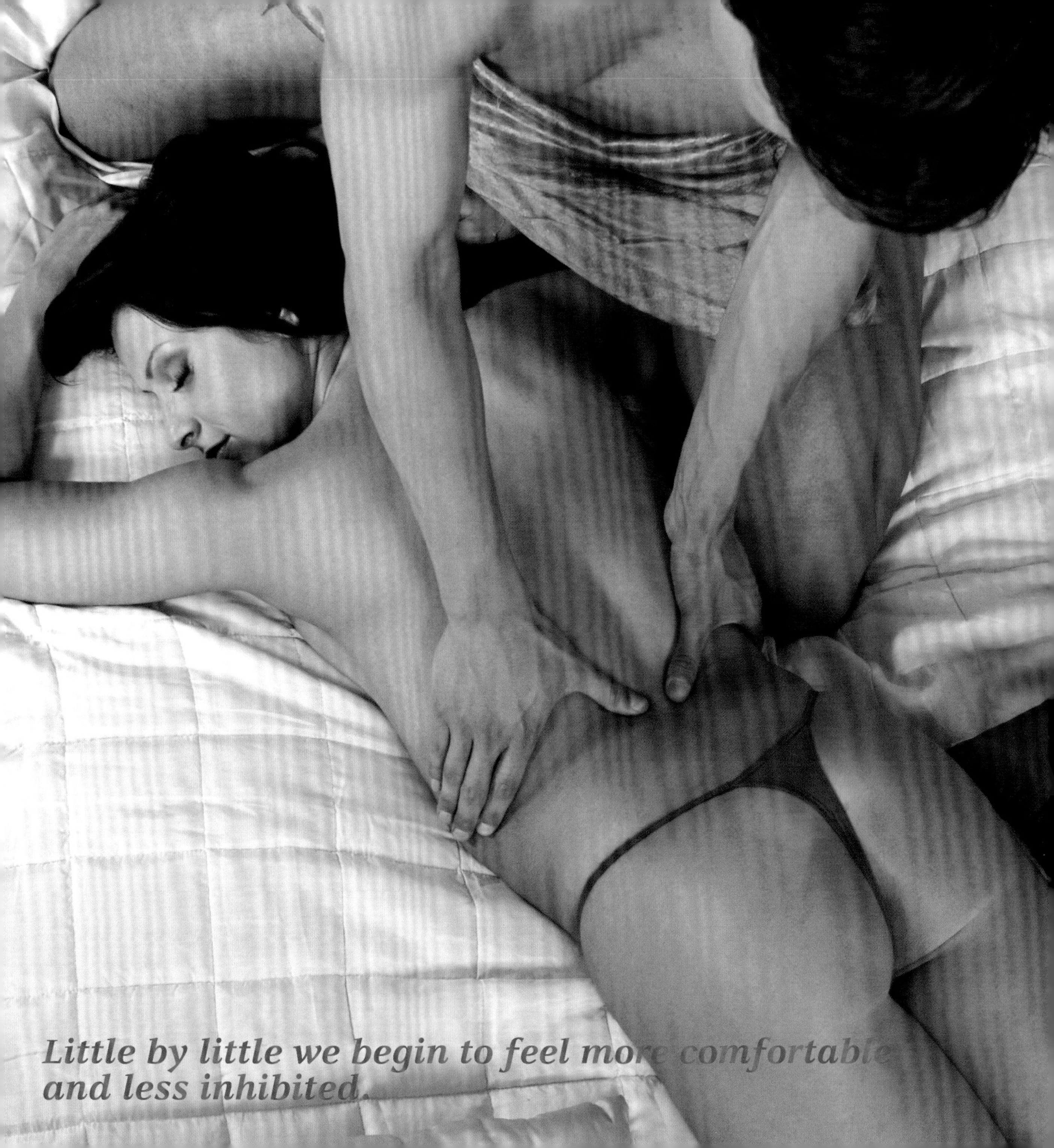

Little by little we begin to feel more comfortable and less inhibited.

A Stimulating Back Massage

Prepare the massage oil mix you have already chosen with your partner.

Put cushions underneath your partner's ankles, chest, and forehead. The support must be firm, and your partner must feel comfortable and relaxed.

Cover your lover with a towel, sheet, or cloth from the bottom of their buttocks and over their legs. The back and gluteals remain uncovered.

1. Use both hands to anoint your partner's back with massage oil. Slide it on using your palms and don't forget to cover the entire area from the neck to the top of the buttocks.

Follow the contour of his/her back with movements that are as slow and rhythmic as possible.

At any time, bring your hands close to your partner so he/she can breathe in the pleasant aroma of the oil. This will help them to relax. Though you are the one who is giving the massage, you can also enjoy the seductive fragrance that wafts through the air.

Take this opportunity to explore and become familiar with the skin and muscles of your partner's back.

2. Next, place your hands on the area at the base of the neck and run your fingertips in the direction of your partner's butt.

Then massage the whole back from top to bottom, applying friction on both sides of the spinal column. With a hand on each side, go down and gently press until you reach the top of the rump.

3. Separate and extend the fingers of both hands and rub both sides of the area where the back and buttocks meet, rubbing both hands in opposite directions.

Then run your hands upwards, keeping both hands apart on the outside flanks of the back from the rump to the neck and do this gently, without pressing.

Each time you do this sequence, replenish your hands with the aromatic oil blend and don't forget to rub your hands together to warm it. This way you can glide your hands or trace curves on your partner's skin without causing any unpleasant tugging.

With your hands stretched out make circles on your partner's shoulder blades.

Make the same circular motions along the spine downward until you reach the butt.

Repeat these movements at various times over the back, varying the pressure. You can also vary the rhythm by going faster or slower.

When doing this the first few times, don't forget to ask your partner if they like the pressure and rhythm you are using. With experience, you and your fingers will acquire the necessary touch for delivering the ideal intensity at any moment.

This time, sit on the left side of your partner and place your hands on the right side of their back with the hands parallel on the lumbar vertebras.

Continuing, gently and delicately apply friction from the lumbar area to the upper middle part of the back with one hand following the other in succession. Run the palms of your hands upwards as far as the shoulder blades. Then go back to where you started and slowly repeat the same movements.

Change sides and do the same sequence on the opposite side.

Re-apply oil so that your partner's skin stays smooth and flexible.

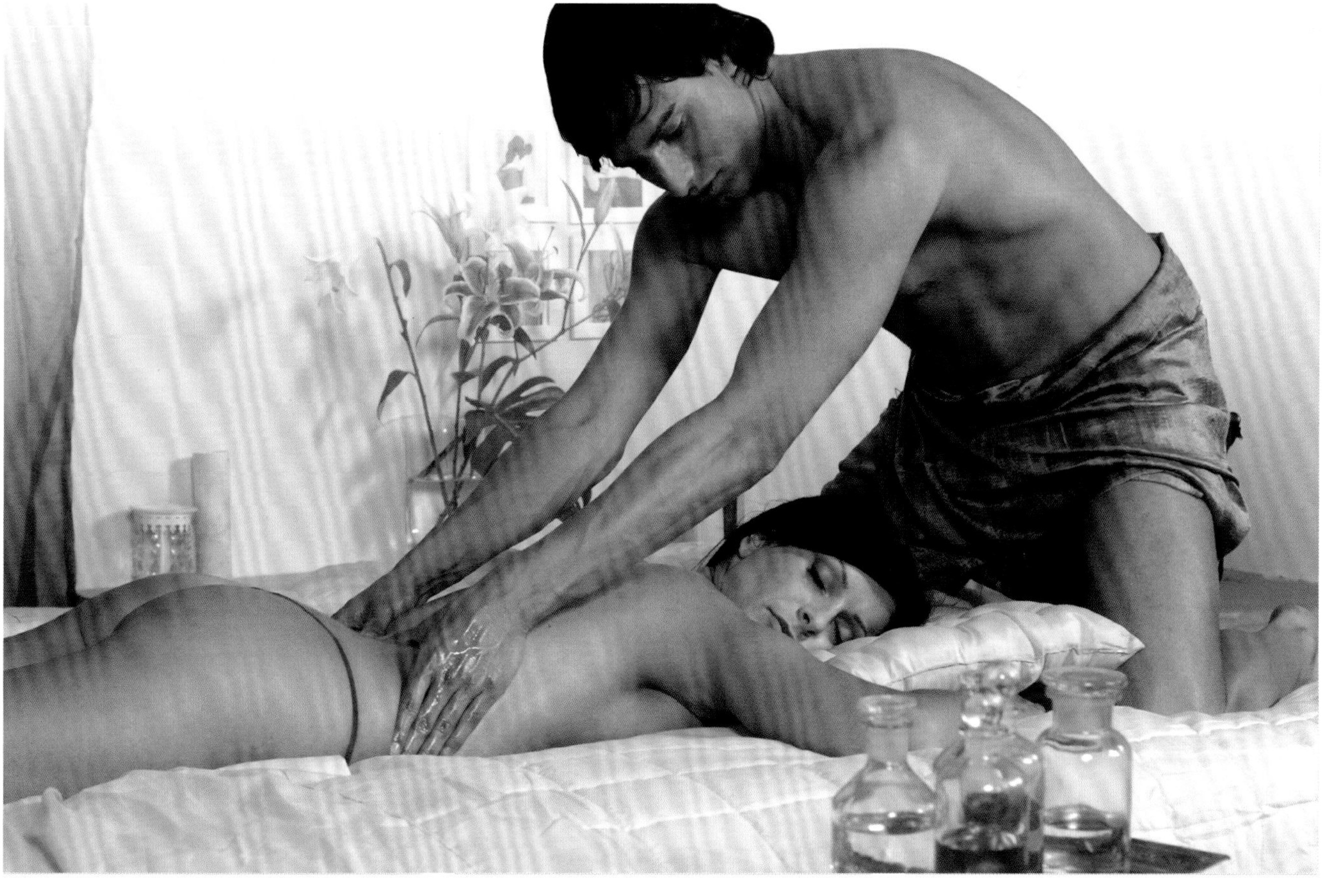

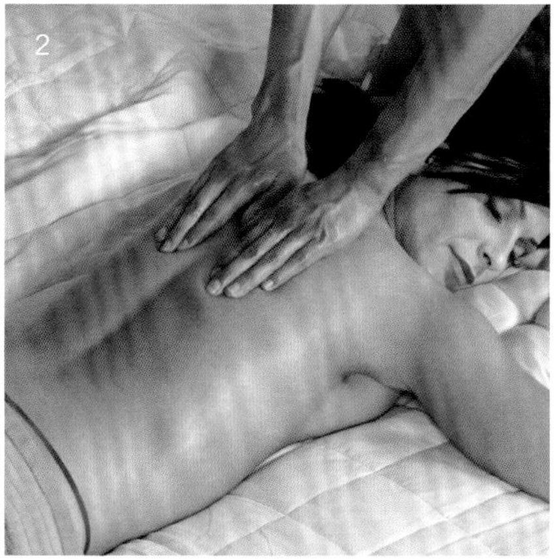
2

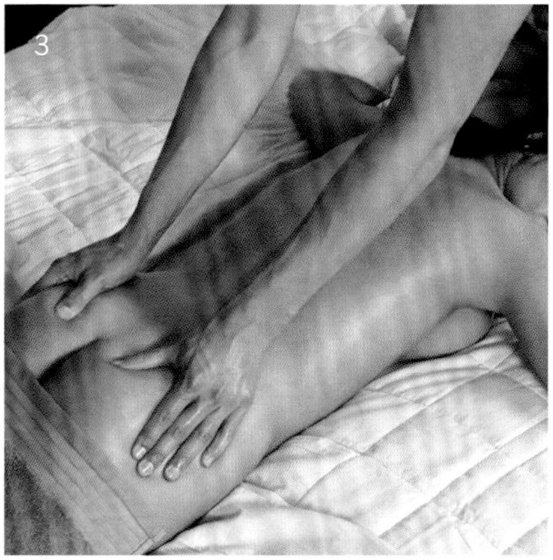
3

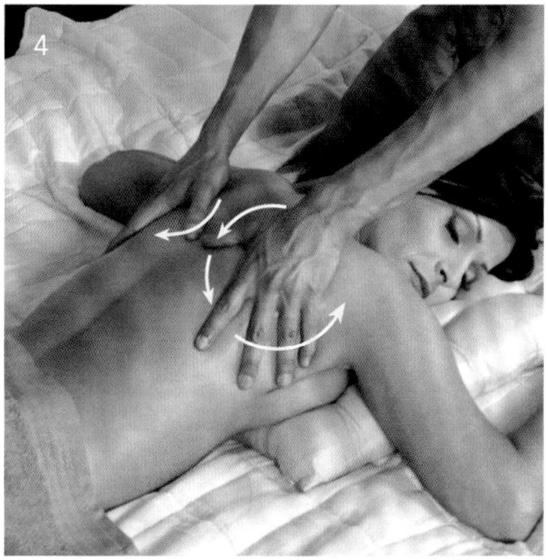
4

A Back Massage for Him

On the back of a man as on the back of a woman, we find various points of sexual stimulation.

In the man, these points are located approximately 3 inches (8 cm) below the zone of the navel, at the end of and on each side of the sacrum. In the woman, on the other hand, these points are located 3 inches (8 cm) above the coccyx (you can see the diagrams of the erogenous zones and points in the chapter "With Great Pleasure").

Step by Step

Begin by sitting on your partner's buttocks. This will give the massage, right from the start, a powerful erotic charge. If, however, it is not comfortable for him to support your body weight, you can sit next to him at the level of his hips.

1. Place your hands on both sides of your partner's spinal column on his sacrum.

2. Use your fingertips to massage, gliding softly and making circles, moving outwards. Gradually slow down your movements.

Not only is it probable that your partner will enjoy the massage, but it is also likely he will become more excited as things go along. If you notice he is getting too excited and you still want to continue the massage, apply soft friction rubbing over his entire back maintaining a constant rhythm. Do this first on one side and then the other.

3. Next, make circular movements using your thumb or fingertips on his lumbar area and specifically at the point which is level with his navel. Proceed upwards along the spinal column, gently tracing circles.

If you really want to excite him, make these circles on his buttocks.

Glide the palms of your hands across the area of the lumbar vertebrae, linking the right and left sides with "figure 8s."

4. Continuing, go up his back gradually making "figure 8s" until you reach the shoulder blades and continue with his arms, making wide figures.

Top off the massage by gently caressing your partner's entire back. He will find this simply irresistible.

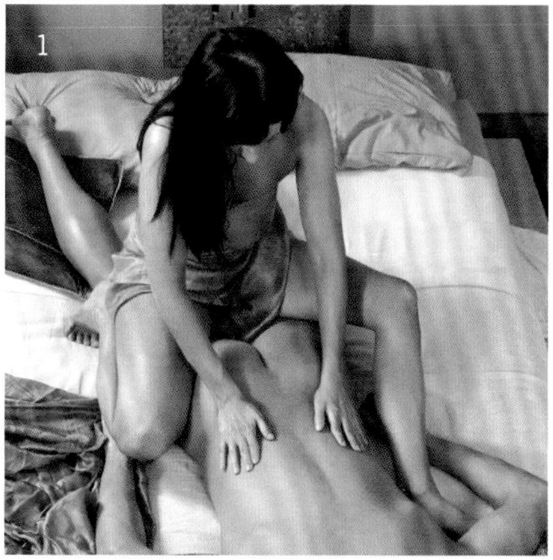
1

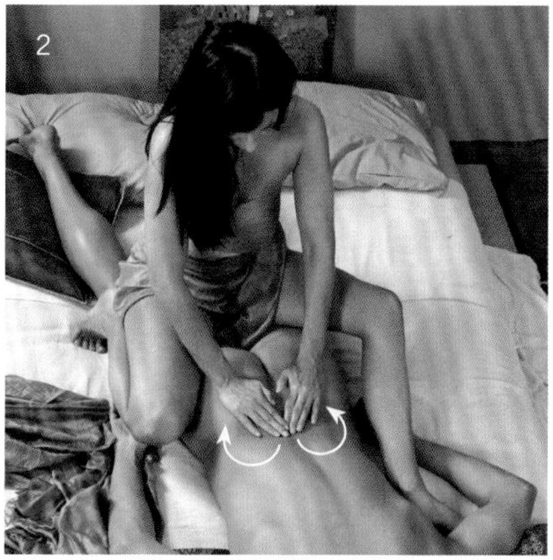
2

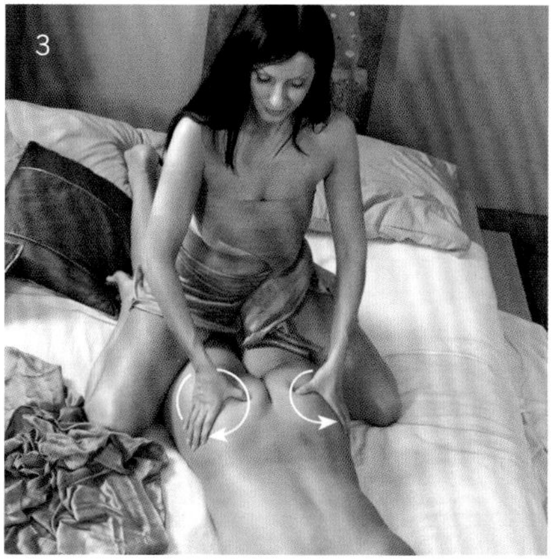
3

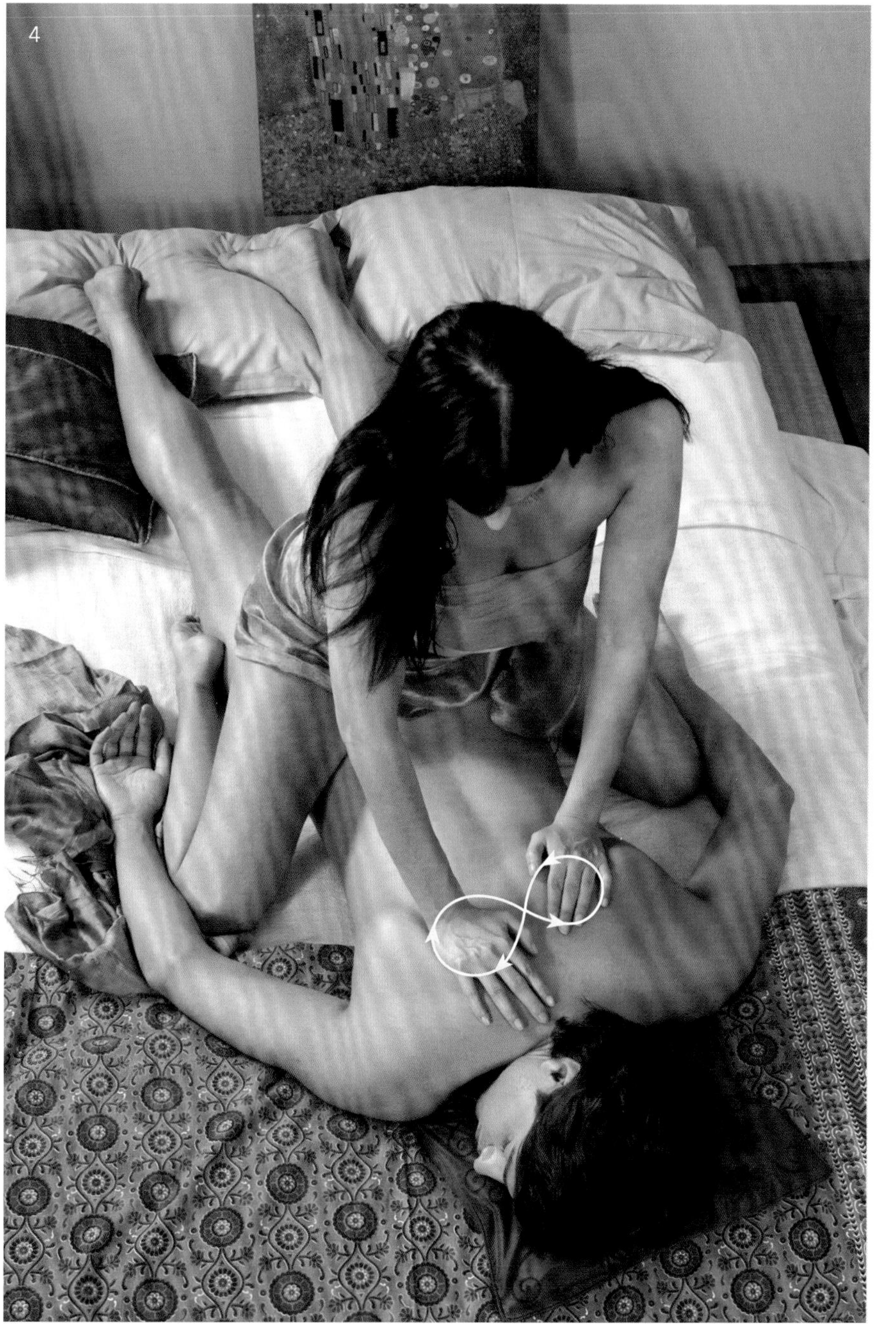
4

A Back Massage for Her

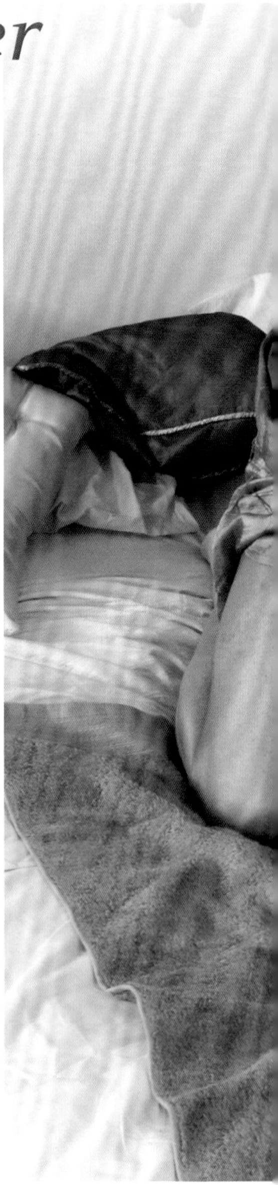

Try sitting on her gluteals. If she is not comfortable with this, then sit beside her at the level of her hips.

1. Place the palms of your hands totally flat on both sides of her spine on the lumbar area.

2. You should know that a magical point of sexual stimulation lies about 2 inches (5 cm) above her coccyx. Stimulate this area by making small and gentle circles with your thumbs.

To continue, stimulate the points along both sides of her spine as described in the chapter "With Great Pleasure."

Begin massaging the area level with the coccyx by making small circles. Proceed upwards until you reach her waist.

Pay attention to her reactions. Make sure she is enjoying your massage.

3. Next, place your fingers about 1 inch (2.5 cm) away from each side of her spine and continue making small and gentle circular movements from below upwards until you reach her waist.

Repeat this sequence of moves until it causes her muscles to quiver.

Just as was explained in the previous section (A Back Massage for Him), apply "figure 8s" using the palms of your hands. Begin at the lumbar zone and make sure you run the figures over both sides of the back.

Go upwards gradually until you reach her shoulder blades and shoulders. Then go on to her arms, making sure to massage both of them simultaneously.

Women have an especially erogenous point on their back.

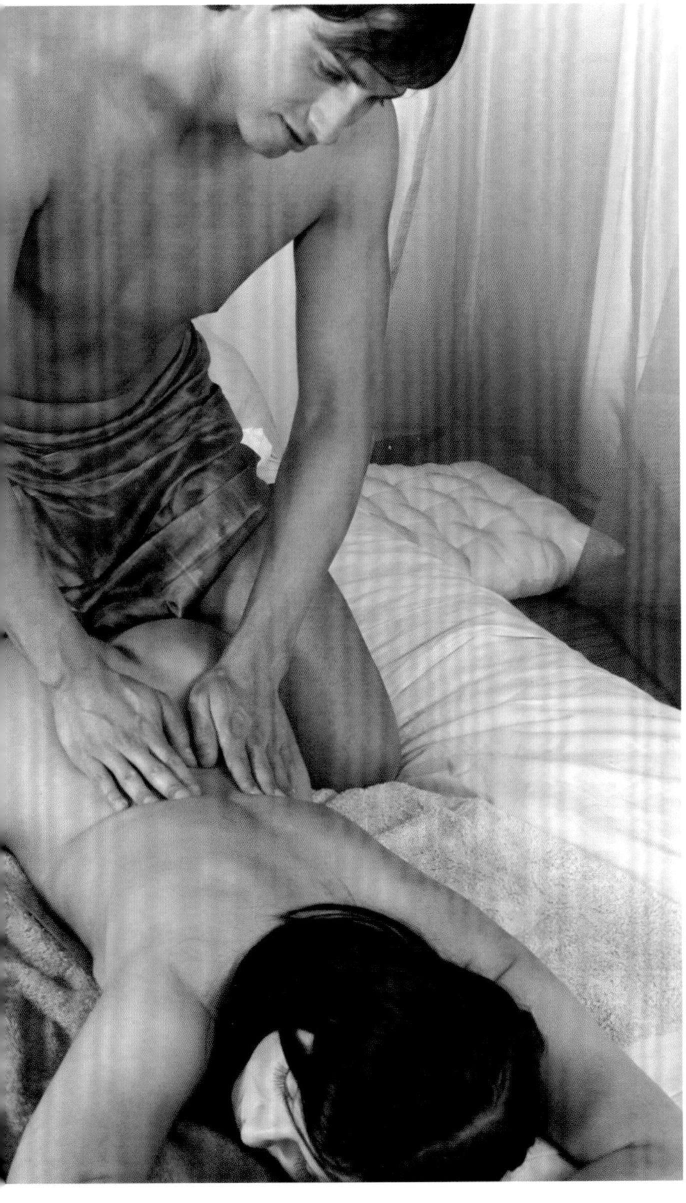

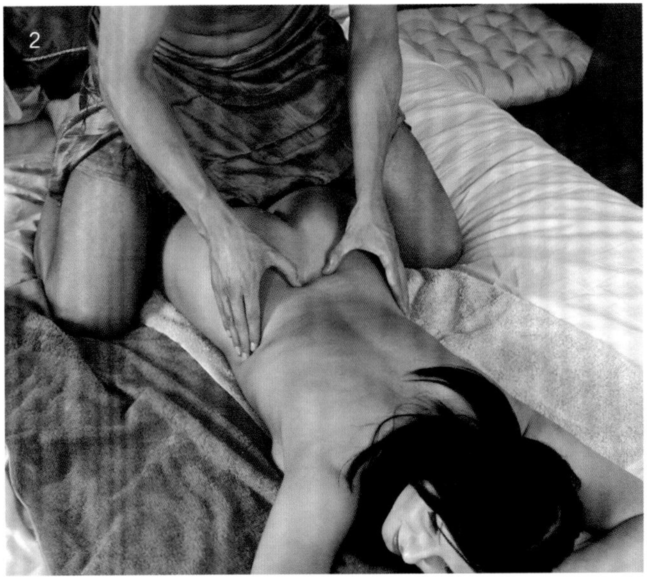
2

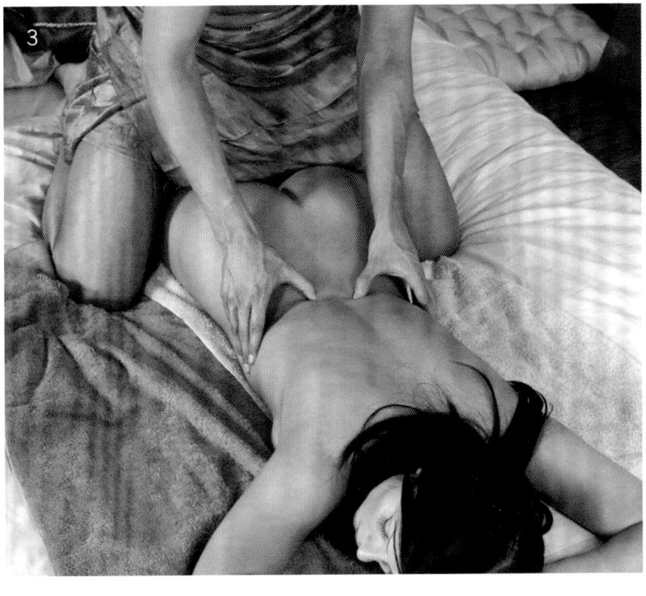
3

Buttocks and Legs

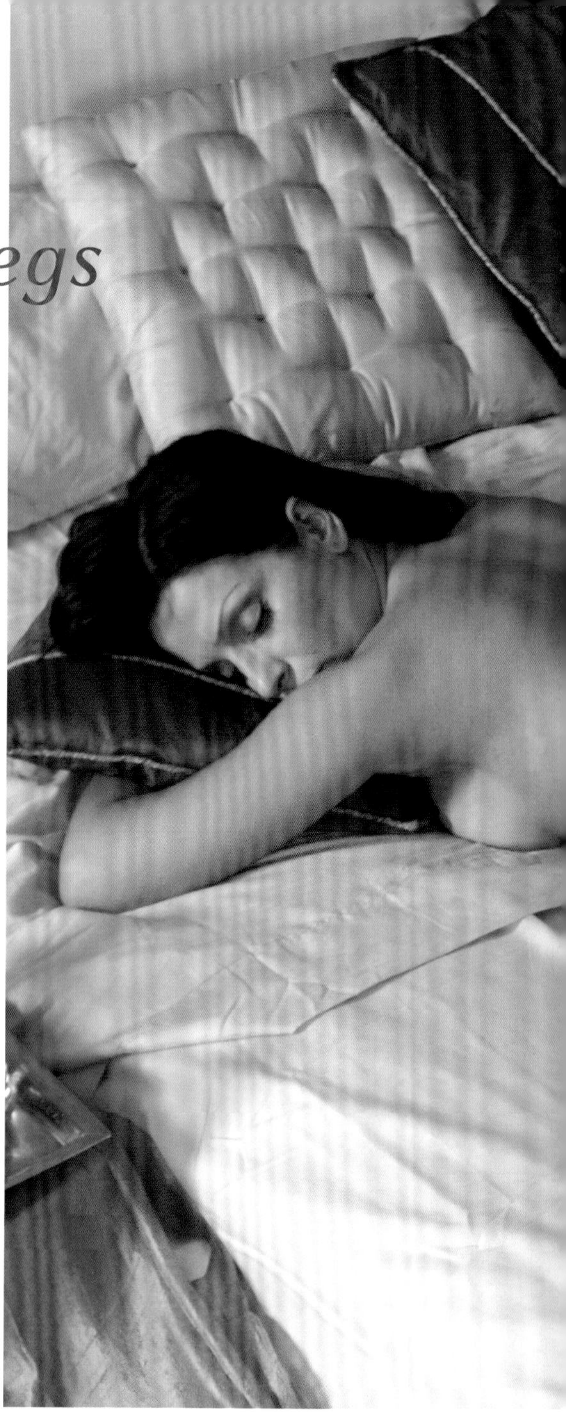

The buttocks and legs are **extremely sensual areas of the body** whose curves and folds are especially erotic and enjoyable to touch. The gluteal muscles are very tender and fleshy and are just waiting to be massaged and squeezed.

You partner will be delighted with a good sensual massage here and it will alleviate any tensions that might interfere with the sexual act.

From Less to More

It is best to **start with gentle caressing** on the inside of the thighs. This will be highly pleasurable. You can do this with your fingertips, or even your lips. **Later** go on to the **buttocks and upper part of the thighs.** In these areas we recommend a more vigorous massage. **Kneading and friction rubbing,** which we have explained before, are ideal for this. Little "chops," pinches, or slaps work well to stimulate these areas. Nevertheless, make sure you start very gently.

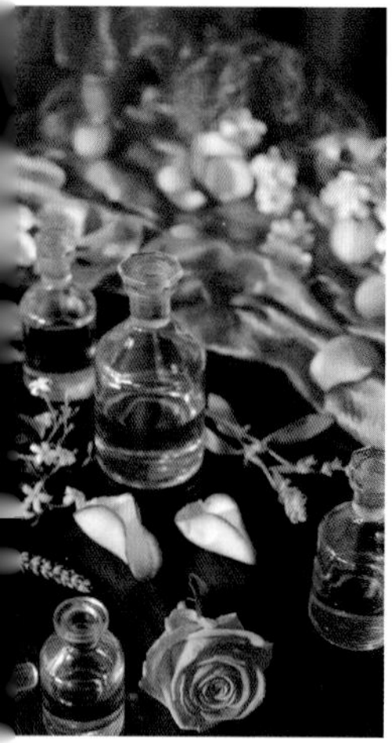

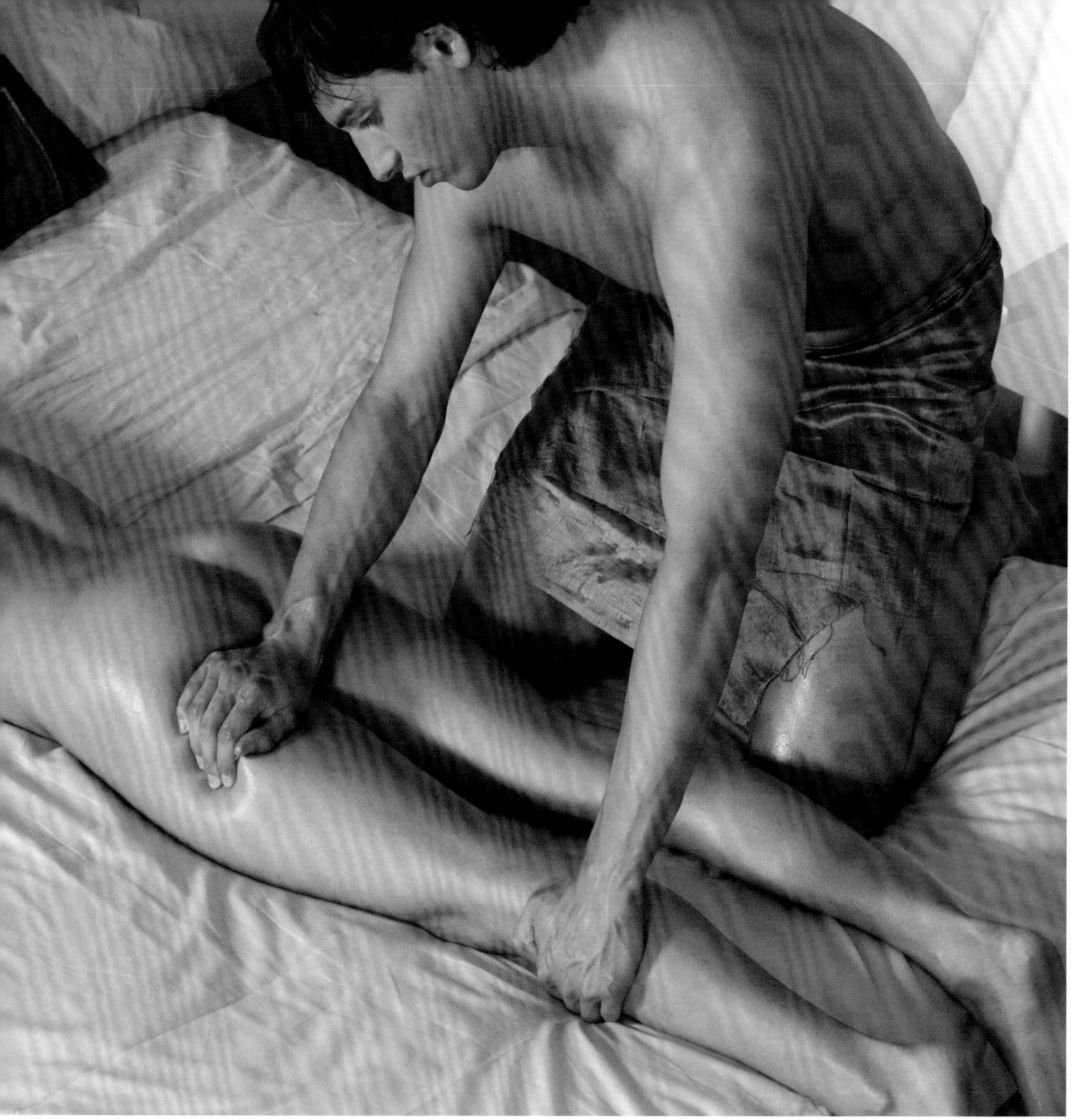

Step by Step Butt and Legs

With your partner face down, sit next to his/her left leg.

Place your hands just above the ankle of their right leg with your fingertips pointing toward their buttocks.

1. Glide your hands over your partner's calves, crossing over them, the knees, and the thighs until you reach the buttocks.
2. Rub the buttocks, imitating the motion of a fan, going from the center of the rump and moving outwards.
3. Next, place your hands on each side of your partner's leg and rub it up and down. Do this several times.
4. Continue by using the pads of your palms to go from the rear of the knee up the thigh and to the butt. When you reach his/her rump, massage it from inside outwards.

As always, ask your partner if he/she is OK with the pressure you are applying and make any adjustments they want.

Draw your hands along the side of your partner's leg, upward and downward. Do this several times. You will see how this completely relaxes him/her.

Later, put your hands above the ankles, one behind the other. Apply rubbing friction with the palms of your hands cupped and go over the leg up to the coccyx.

Bend your body slightly forward to increase the pressure and repeat the previous sequence.

Continue by following all of the previous instructions and massage the other buttock and leg.

Finally, knead and caress the two buttocks in detail, moving in opposite directions. You will enjoy the pleasure your partner is getting from this.

5. For a final touch, stimulate the sexual pressure points of the gluteals. You will find them in the illustration in the chapter "With Great Pleasure."

For More Excitement . . .

If you really want to give your partner a special thrill, completely massage the **buttocks and lower part of the back,** applying different pressures and intensity. **You can also use your forearm** and give your partner a sweet sensation like that of smooth velvet. This will be especially pleasing to him/her. You can also put your forearms, or even your fists, on both buttocks and move them in soft circles on their skin.

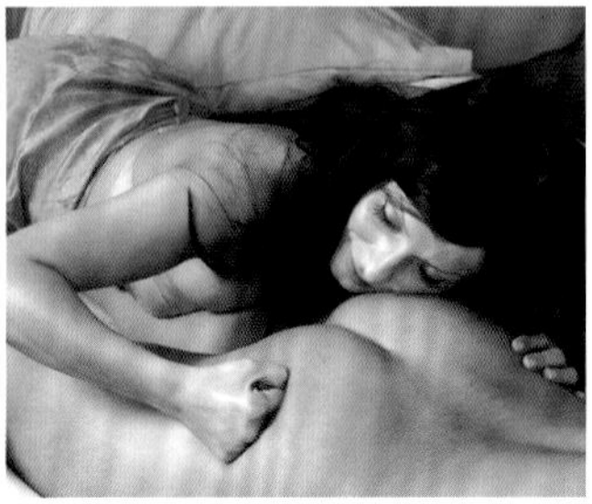

The pressure used for this massage is different for men and women.

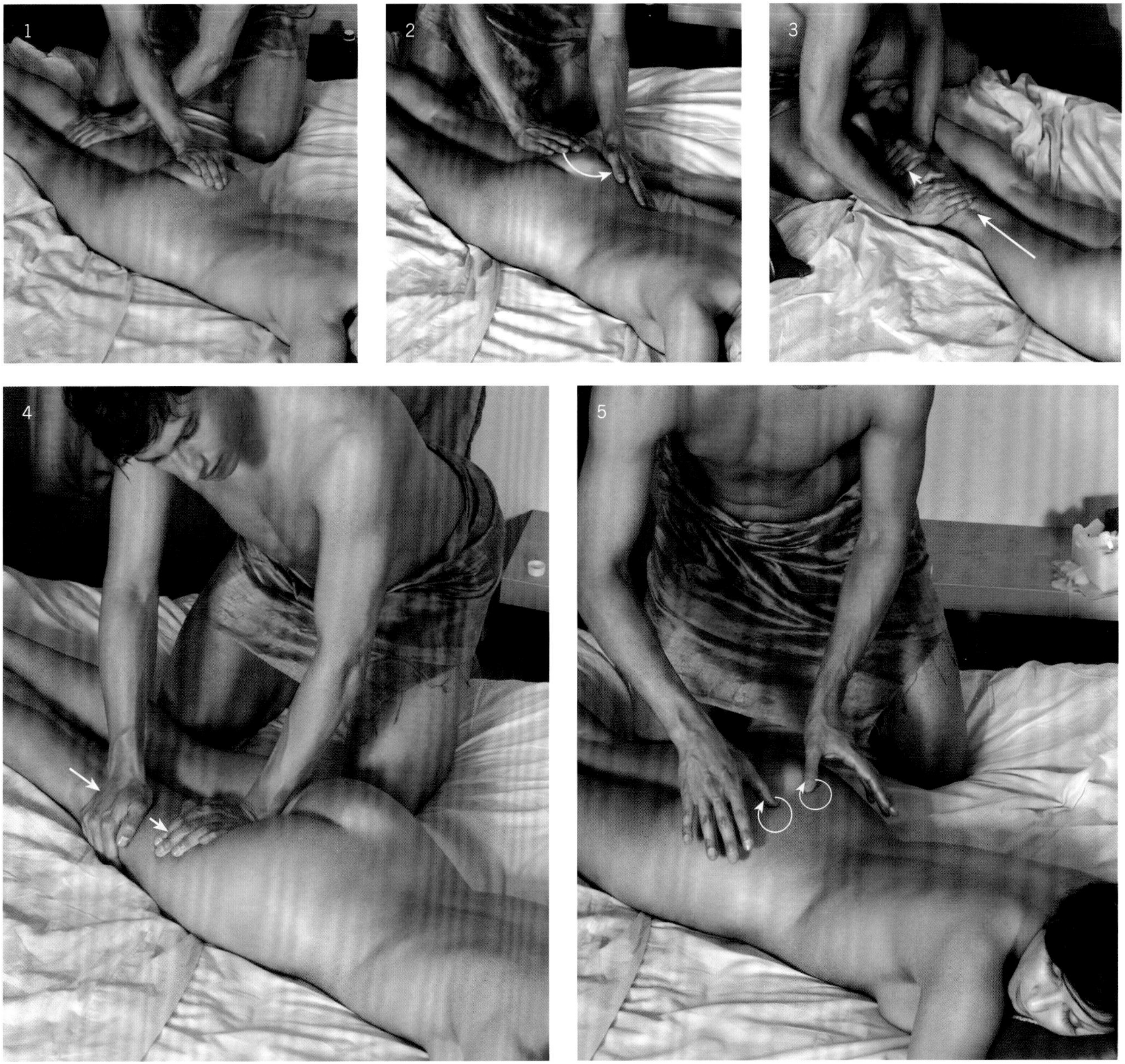

Men are excited by strong pressure and women by a softer touch.

Hands and Arms

From the viewpoint of sensual massage, hands and arms are simply marvelous instruments that provide **pleasure and communicate sensually.** They are the main tools we use to caress, connect with our partner, and strengthen our relationship.

We use our hands a lot in our daily life. We use them less, however, for sensual communication, as "tools for caressing."

Whoever does a massage should pay special attention to these parts of their partner's body. Even when doing massages of the chest and abdomen, it is a good idea to start off with the hands and arms since there is no better way to begin connecting with your partner.

To Begin

A good time to massage the hands and arms of your partner is right after a back massage.

- Start by carefully helping your partner to sit up. It's possible, especially with the ladies, that your partner will feel a bit chilly since their body is so relaxed after the massage. Cover them gently. Have them lie on their back and cover their chest and genital areas with soft towels or blankets so they stay warm.
- Begin rubbing their hands. Then take your partner's hands in your own and kiss the fingers, one by one, until the two of you feel an intense sense of closeness.

Fragrant Friends

One-half glass almond oil

3 drops rosewood essence
1 drop neroli oil
3 drops bergamot oil

A Fresh Aroma of Vanilla

1 tablespoon of almond oil
2 tablespoons oil of macadamia nuts
1-3 drops of essence of benzoin
2 drops of rose oil
1 drop of neroli

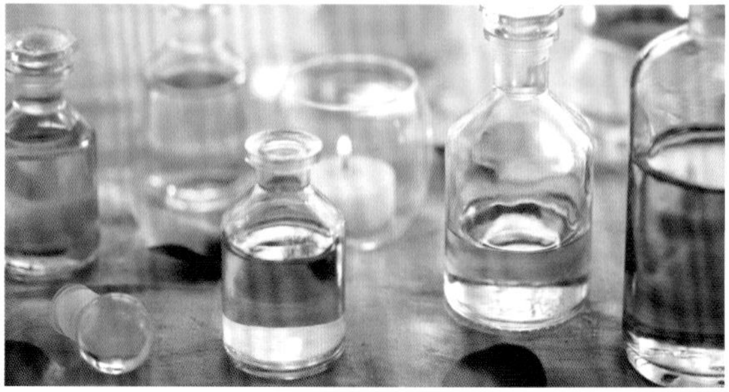

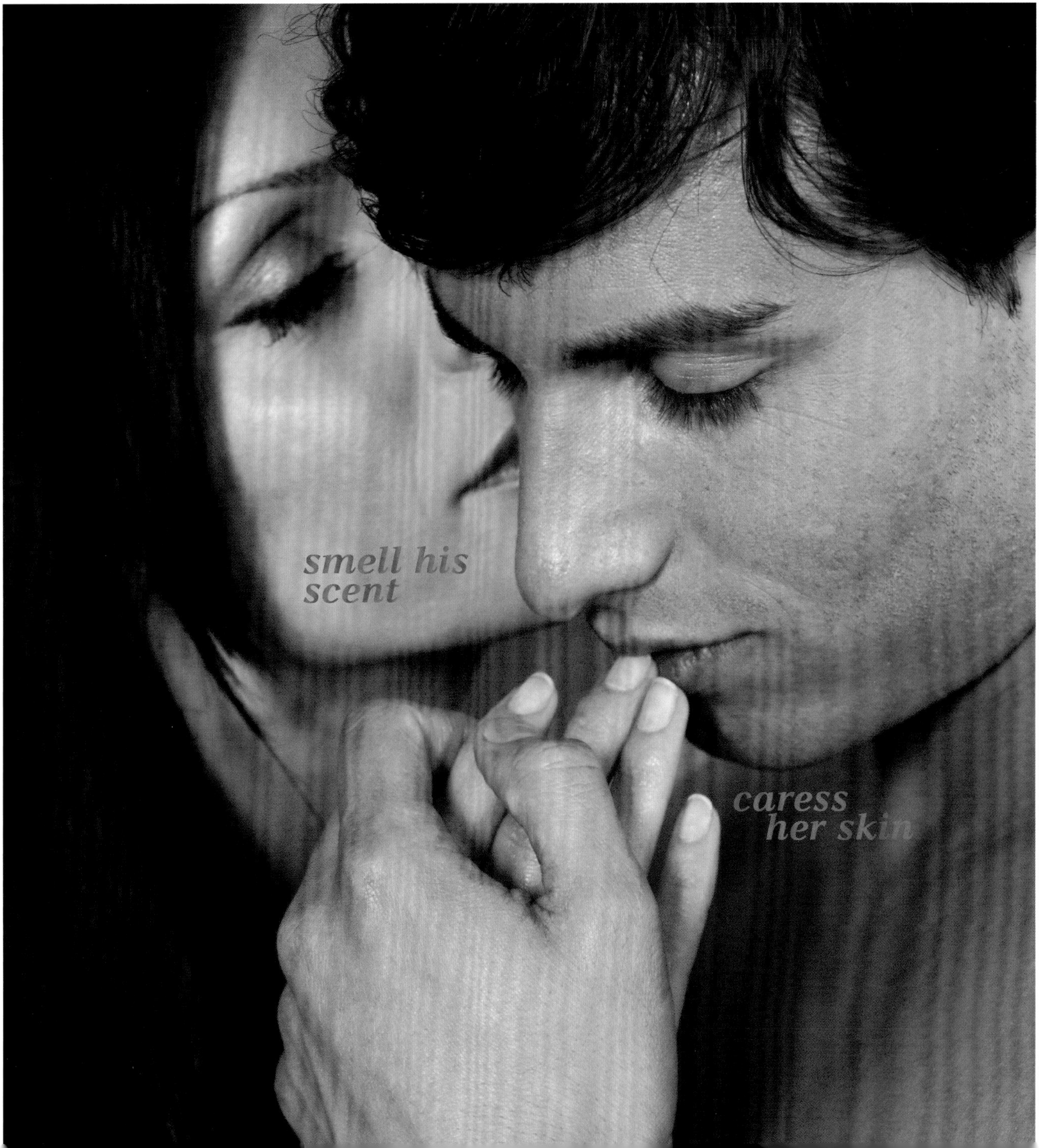
smell his scent
caress her skin

Step by Step Hands and Arms

Sit on the right side of your partner.

Pour a bit of massage oil on your hands. Take your partner's right hand and hold it in your hands for a few moments.

1. Continue to hold your partner's right hand with your left hand and place your right hand on his/her wrist with the fingers pointing at their shoulder.

2. Go over the arm very slowly with your fingers fully extended, from the wrist to the elbow and then from there to the shoulder.

Apply the same movement downwards from the shoulder to the wrist, but this time along the back side of the arm.

Repeat this movement several times softly and don't forget to re-apply oil when necessary, especially if the arm is hairy. Don't forget to ask your partner if the pressure you are applying is OK.

3. Continue by placing both hands on your partner's forearm and perform friction massage with cupped hands. Begin at the wrist and proceed upwards up to the shoulder. Make sure to apply consistent pressure.

Glide your hands from your partner's shoulder down to their wrist. This time, do it softly without any pressure. Repeat this movement several times.

Again, take your partner's hand in yours and place it so that the palm faces up and turn it gently.

4. Press and rub the muscular areas of your partner's hand with your thumbs.

Continue by gliding your index finger on the insides of your partner's fingers slowly and gently, up and down, as far as the palm of their hand so that you have gone over all the area between their fingers.

If you like, you can do the same thing with your tongue. Slide your tongue along the inside of your partner's fingers and kiss his/her fingertips gently and delicately.

Then gently caress the palm and top of their hand with your fingertips and the edge of your nails.

To finish, go back and apply gentle movements from your partner's shoulder down to their hand. When you get to the hand, let your partner see how your movements are slowing down and maintain contact with his fingers to the last moment.

Before you remove your whole hand, keep contact with just one finger. This way you will preserve the intimacy and bonding that has been built up between the two of you. It is a wonderful moment that deserves remembering.

Now sit on the other side of your partner and repeat the above sequence on their left arm and hand.

The posterior part of the arm and forearm is especially sensitive.

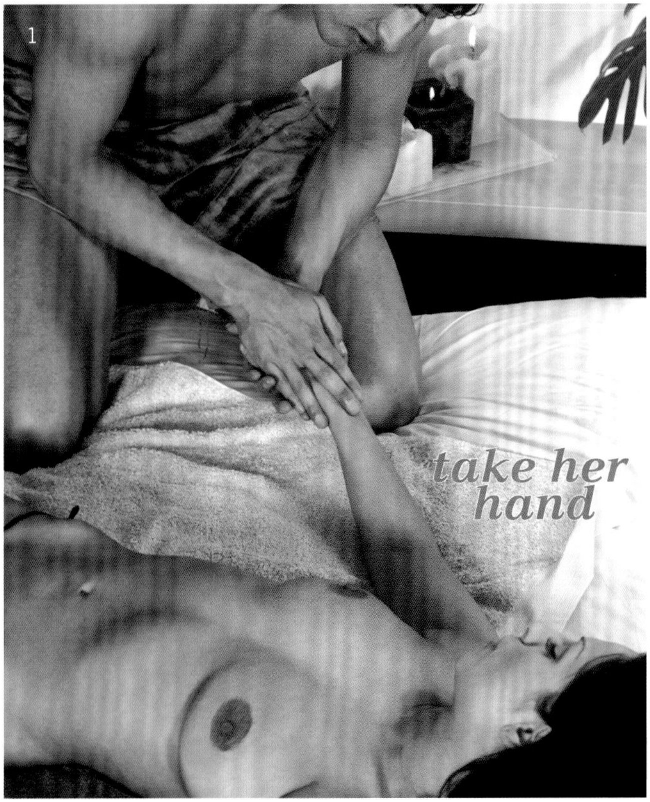

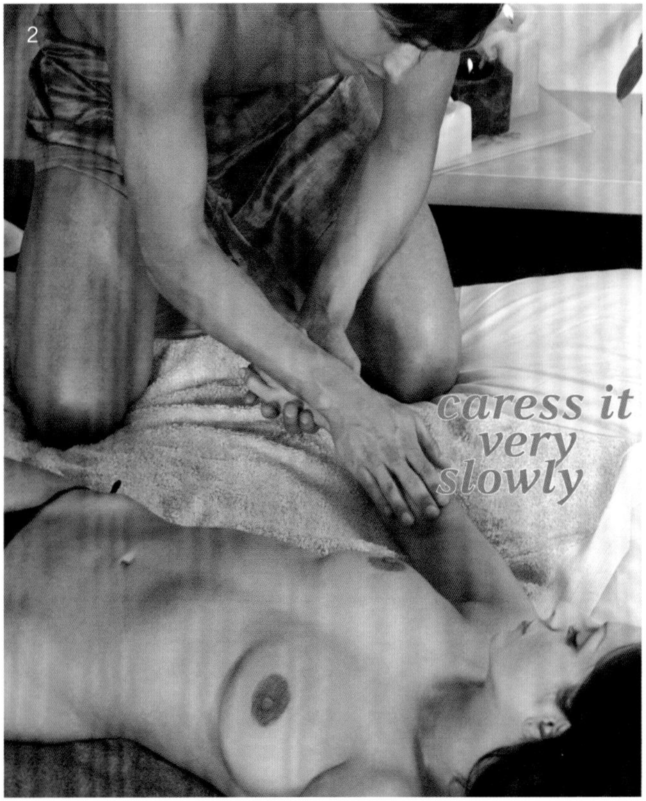

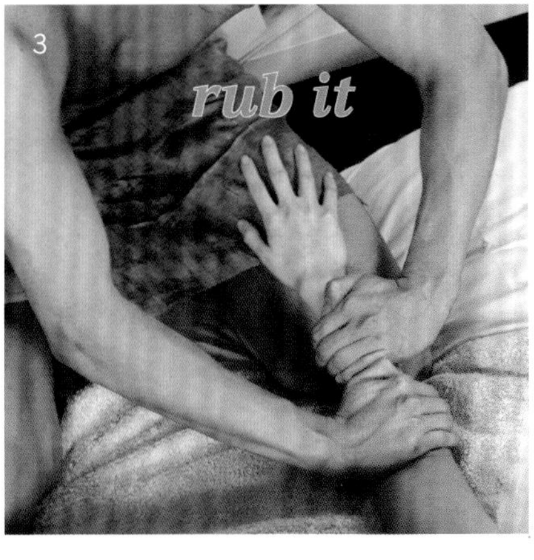

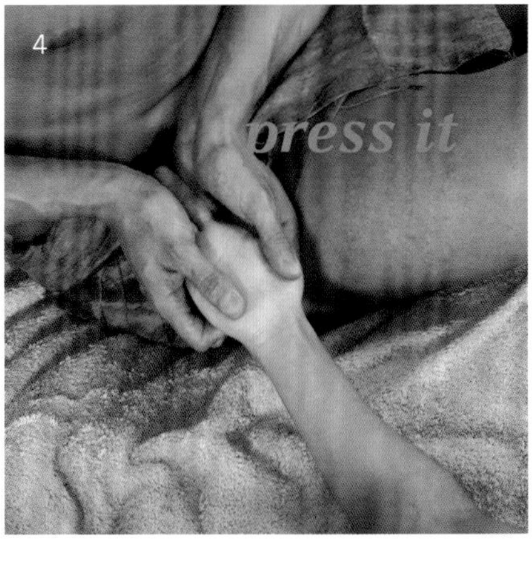

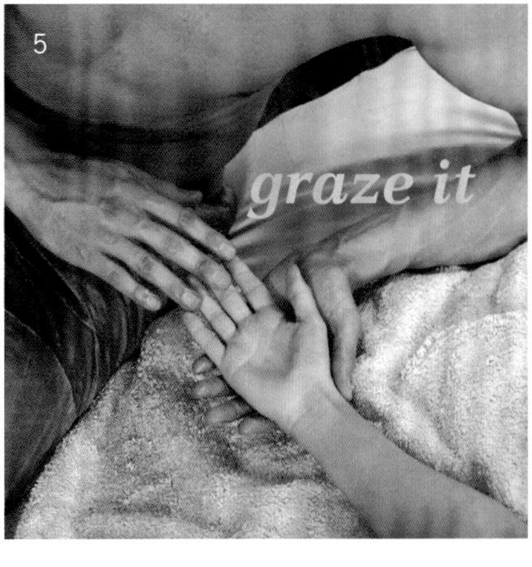

Caress the whole area and go over it with your fingers and mouth . . .

Chest and Abdomen

The chest and abdomen are the most sensitive areas of our body. Whoever receives a massage here feels especially vulnerable since they are totally exposed, offering the other person their fragility.

It is also usual to feel more uneasy when you are lying nude face up than when you are face down. For this reason it is very important that when we massage the front part of our partner's body we are **particularly gentle** and do everything we can to make sure they are comfortable and can relax.

When we massage the chest and abdomen we must **create a bond of sexuality and intimacy** with our partner. If this doesn't happen it means something has gone wrong.

Preparation

As we've already said, massaging the chest and abdomen when they are totally nude involves a very sensitive zone of the body and we have to be very careful, even in the summer, to **make sure the room** stays at a **suitable temperature (warm in the winter, cool in the summer).** Remember, it is impossible to enjoy a massage if you are shivering from cold or sweating from the heat.

If it's winter, before you begin you can **put blankets or towels on a radiator to warm them up a bit.** If you want to do something extremely sensual, wrap your partner in warm towels perfumed with orange blossom or rose water. This will turn on the two of you as nothing else will.

If it's summer, cushions and sheets should be fresh and not too rough.

Fragrant Massages

A Light and Sexy Perfume

one-half glass of almond oil
1 drop of rosewood oil
1 drop of jasmine oil
2 drops rose geranium oil
3 drops verbena or bergamot oil

An Aphrodisiac Fragrance

one-half glass of almond oil
2 drops vetiver oil
2 drops Ylang Ylang
3 drops sanguine orange essence, orange essence, or oil of litsea cubeba

If you wish to make a more refined perfume, add a drop of osmanthus essence (keep in mind this is quite expensive).

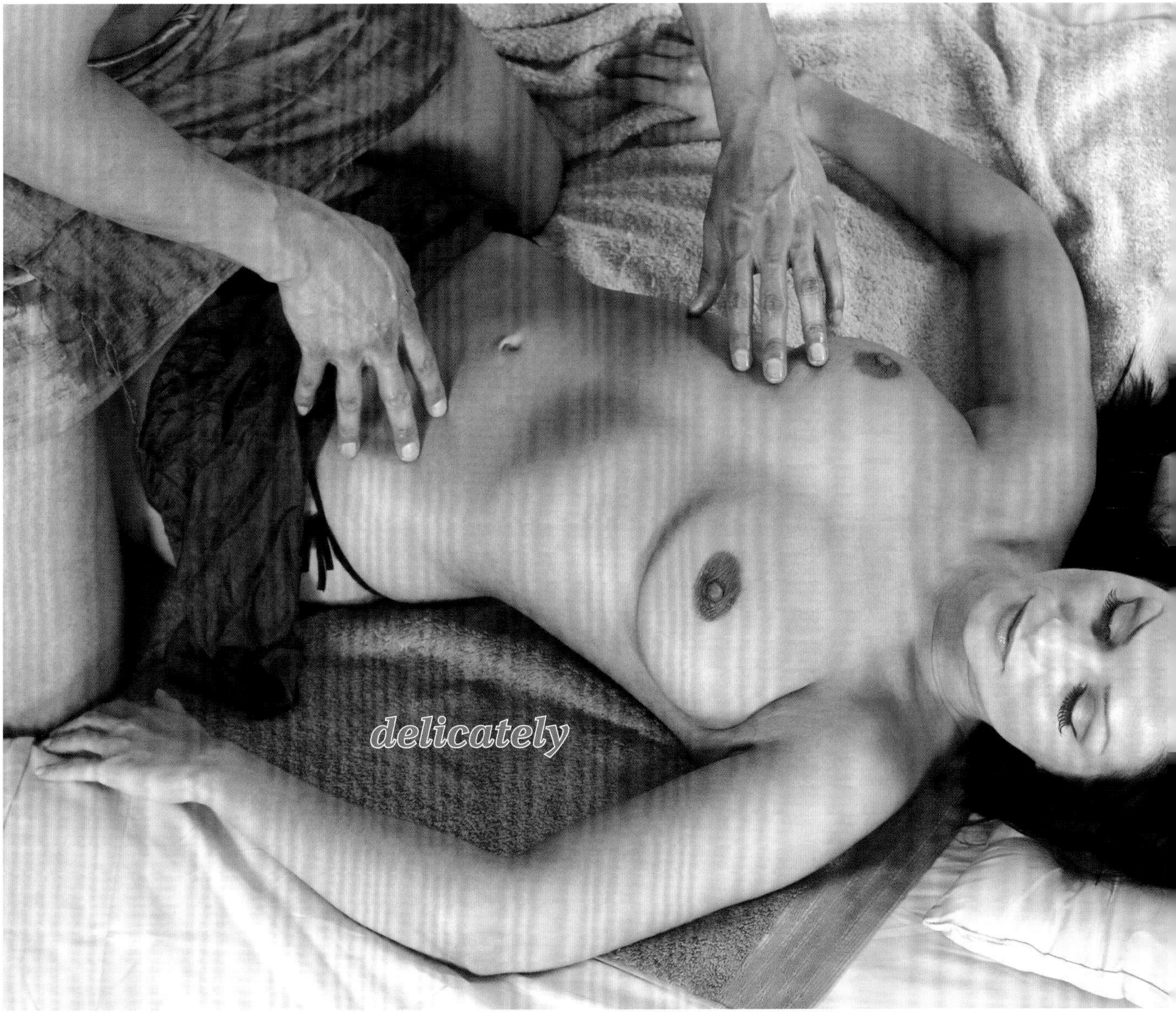
delicately

Step by Step Chest and Abdomen

Kneel behind your partner's head. Put oil on your hands and rub them together until it's warm.

1. Put your hands on your partner's chest with your fingertips pointed toward their feet.

Both hands should be at the side of his/her neck with the pads of your palms lightly touching right below the collarbone and the thumbs grazing the center.

2. Glide your hands gently forward up to the pubic bone or until you can't lean forward any more.

Make sure to use enough oil, especially if the chest is very hairy.

Keep in mind the pressure you apply on the chest should be vigorous, while on the abdomen you should apply softer pressure each time you go there.

Remember to ask your partner if they like the intensity of the massage and change pressure as they prefer.

Continue to go over their frontal area downward until you reach the pubic bone. Once you're there, slide your hands outward, separating them from each other in the direction of the hips.

Draw your hands up along the sides of your partner's body in the direction of his/her head. Do this slowly but firmly until you reach their armpits.

3. Now place your hands below your partner's armpits and continue to slide the palms of your hand and wrists forward, forming a semicircle until you reach the top center of his/her chest. When you finish the semicircle continue with your fingertips pointing toward your partner's feet.

Repeat this sequence several times uninterrupted with wide and slow movements.

Find a regular rhythm and remember to ask your partner if they like what you're doing.

Make sure your hands closely follow the contours of your partner's body while you run them over him/her.

4. To finish, slightly raise your partner's head, supporting it from the back of the neck and put a cushion underneath it.

If you sit behind your partner the massage will be more seductive.

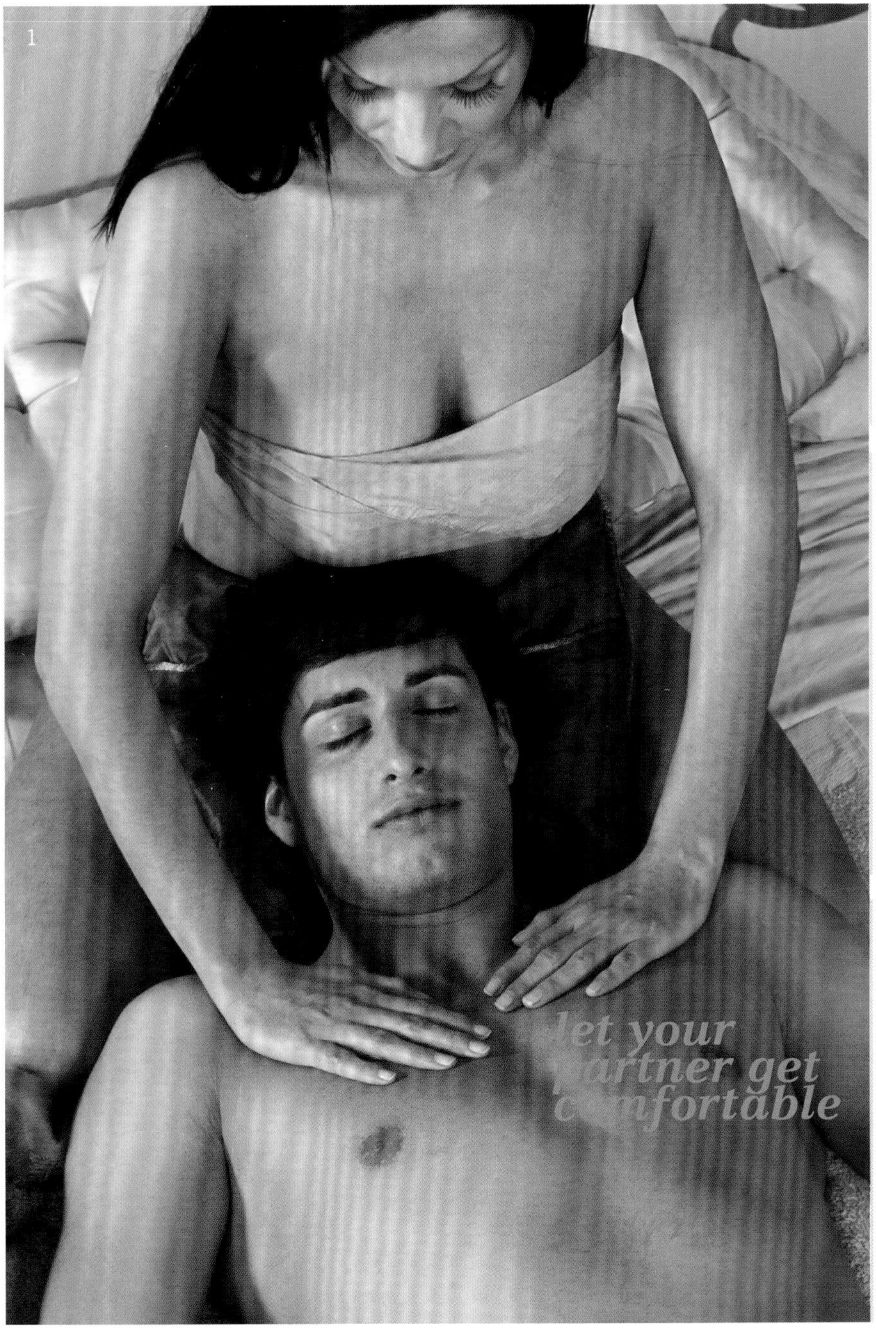
1
let your partner get comfortable

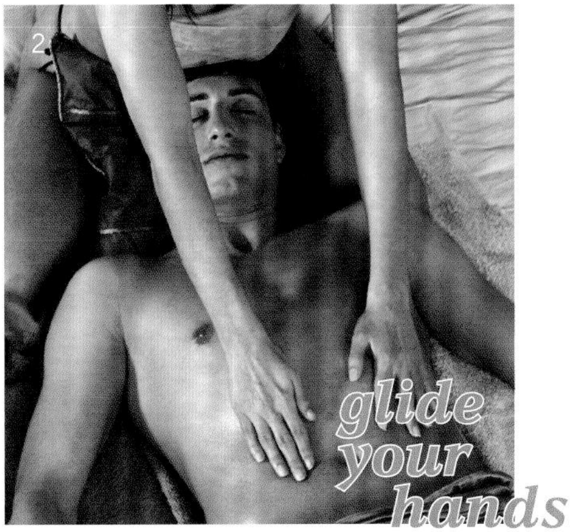
2
glide your hands

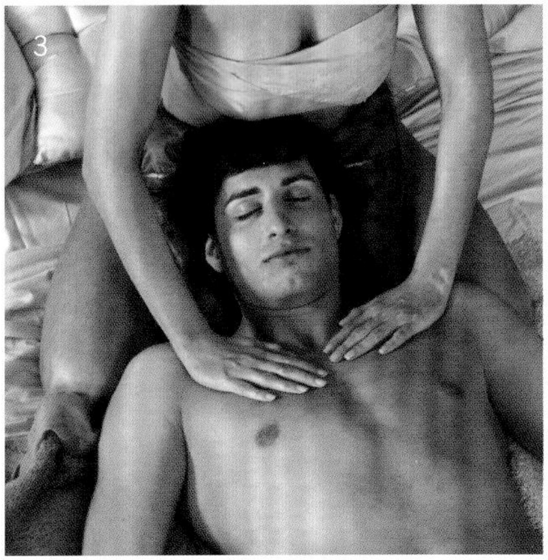
3

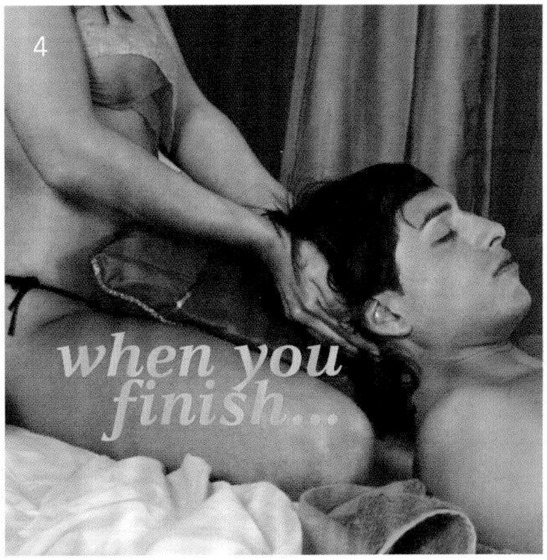
4
when you finish...

A More Sensual Chest Massage

It is best to begin with the manipulations we first suggested and then go on to a deeper, more sensual massage whose effect is highly stimulating and exciting for both the man and woman.

Step by Step

Sit on your partner's right side or on top of him/her (without putting your weight on them, as in the photo).

1. Place your hands on your partner's breast and make small circles with your right hand going clockwise and your left counterclockwise.

From time to time make these circular movements so that your partner's breasts move toward each other.

2. Make three circular movements outwards so that your partner's breasts separate.

You can also make "figure 8s" around your partner's breasts, softly. Ask your partner if they like the intensity of the pressure.

3. Imagine that your partner's breasts are two wheels with the nipples at the hub. Have your hands glide gently around his/her breast just as if you were making the spokes of the wheel move.

Gently pinch the skin, letting it move between the tips of your index finger and thumb. Increase the sensuality of this technique by constantly varying pressure and intensity.

You will certainly notice your partner's nipples getting hard, which will excite both of you.

Lastly, kiss your partner's breasts and delicately graze the skin of the nipples with your fingertips. You can also use feathers or a soft brush (more details in the next chapter).

This is a very pleasant and exciting massage for both.

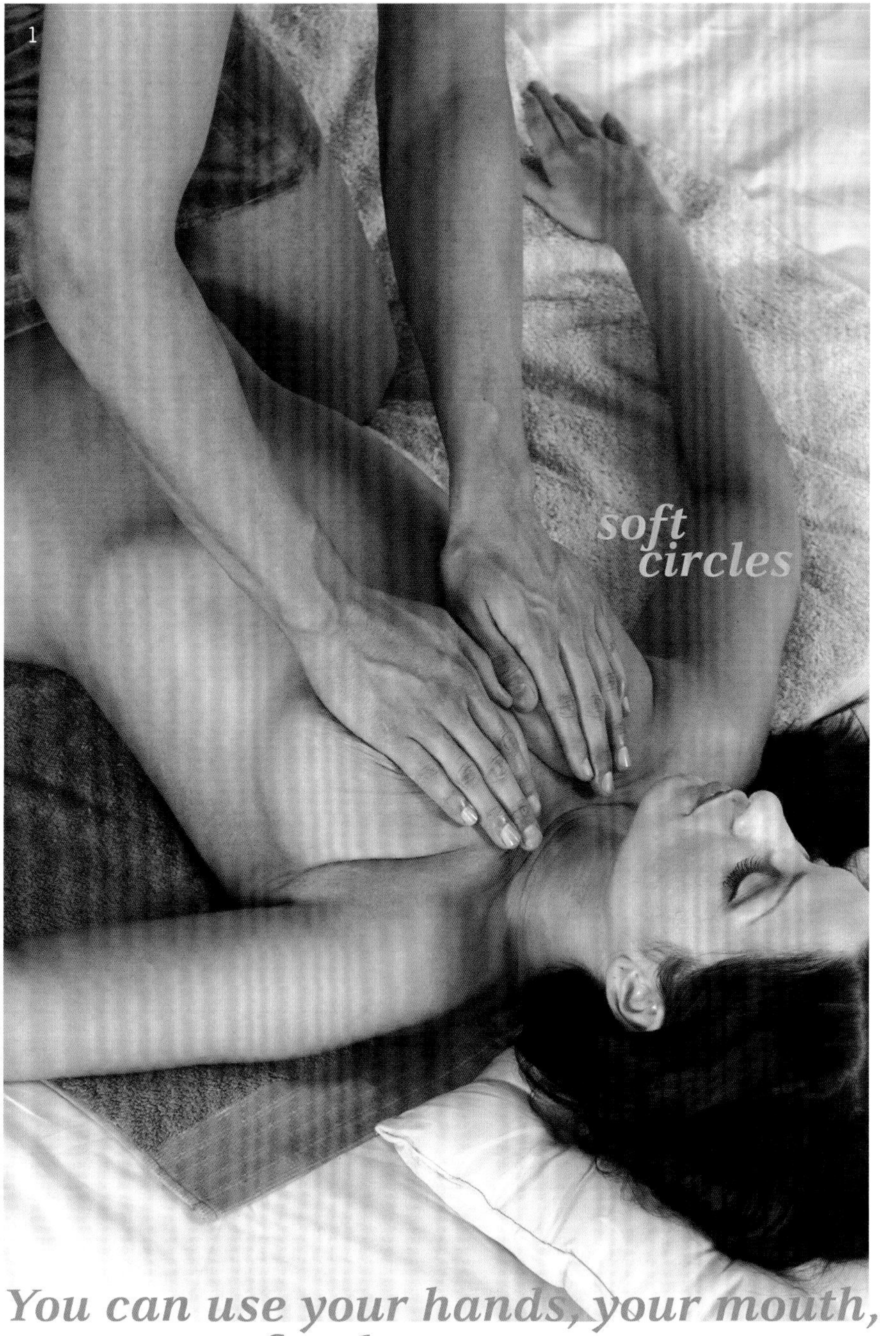

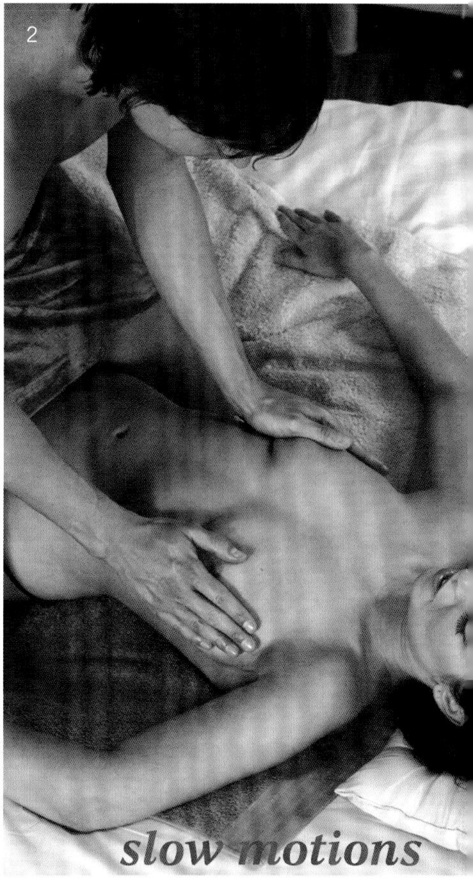

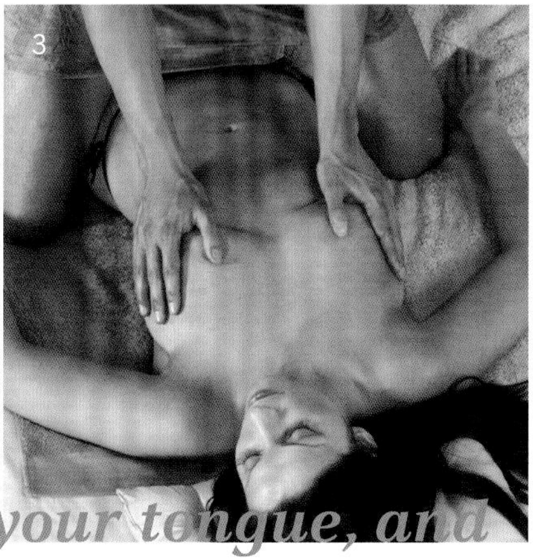

You can use your hands, your mouth, your tongue, and even some feathers.

A More Sensual Belly Massage

Sit close to your partner's right side, or on top of him/her (without putting your weight on them). Before putting the oil on your partner, rub your hands together to make sure they are warm.

Place your hands on your partner's abdomen with the fingertips pointing toward their face.

1. Make small circles with your fingertips moving from the center of their belly to the chest.

2. Now place your hands on both sides of their chest. Slide the palms of your hands all the way downwards and then back up to their waist.

Move your hands over to the lower part of your partner's abdomen and massage it with gentle circles. Go from the center to the sides and then back again.

3. Remember there is a stimulation point for the vagina one palm width above the pubic bone. You can massage all around this point, using your fingertips to make small, gentle circles or use delicate rubbing.

4. On a man, the points of sexual excitation are located in the area below the navel. Stimulate them with gentle friction (this will be pleasant for her too).

Gently massage the inner part of the groin using small, sliding circles. Slow down the rhythm with each pass and make the circles more deliberately.

It's usual that this kind of massage results in heightened sexual excitation. Your partner's pleasure will be obvious. Just don't forget to ask if the intensity suits them.

5. Apply light, rhythmic grazing or soft friction all over your partner's belly. You can change places with your partner, with the one having received the massage going on to give it themselves.

Keep making small circles and add kisses and caresses. If you want to try something new, spread a little bit of whipped cream or honey around your partner's navel (you will find more seductive suggestions in the following chapter).

6. End the massage by caressing your partner's body all over.

The massage should turn into love play without you or your partner noticing, in a totally natural flow. No one is immune to the magic of touch.

Being close to the genitals makes a belly massage very exciting.

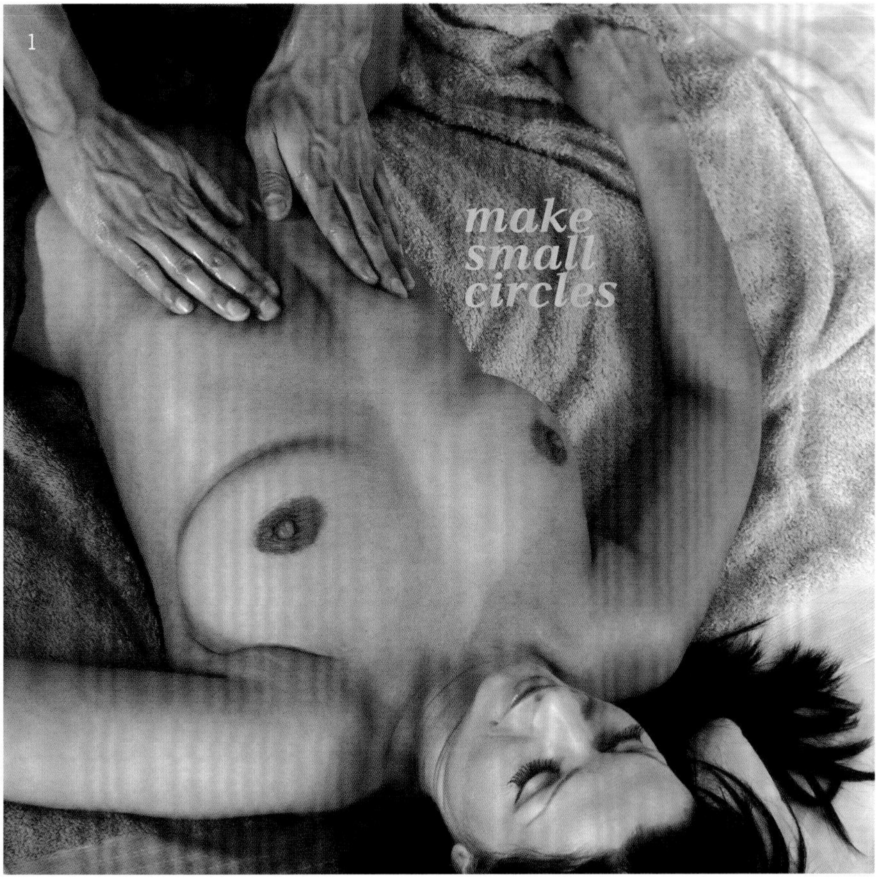
1
make
small
circles

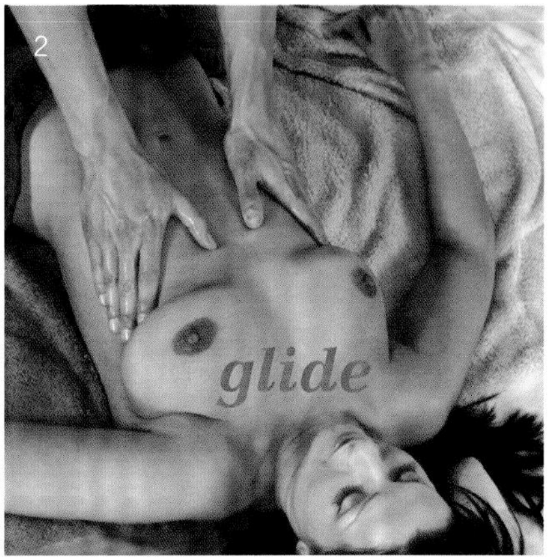
2
glide

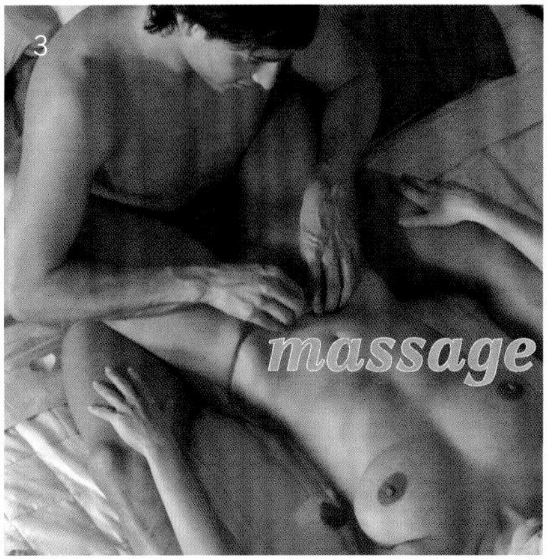
3
massage

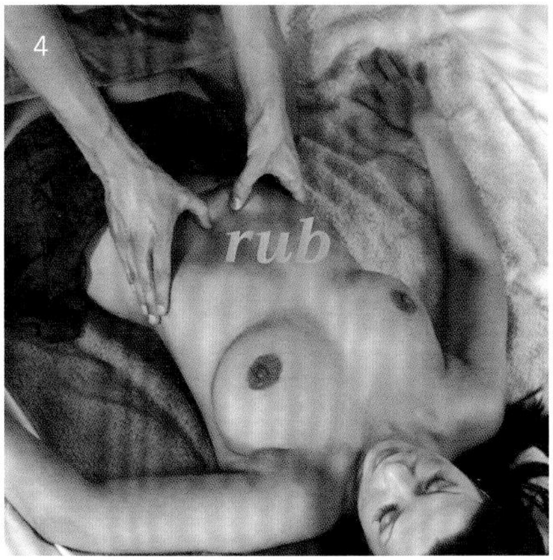
4
rub

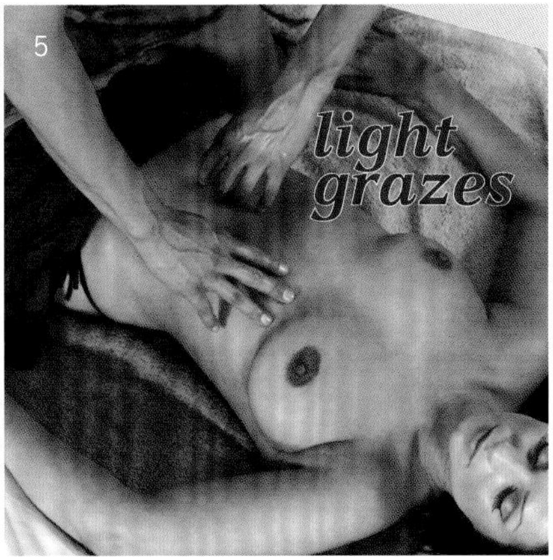
5
light
grazes

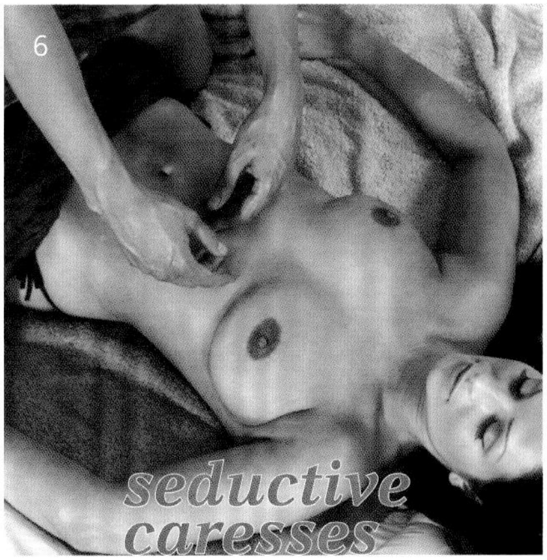
6
seductive
caresses

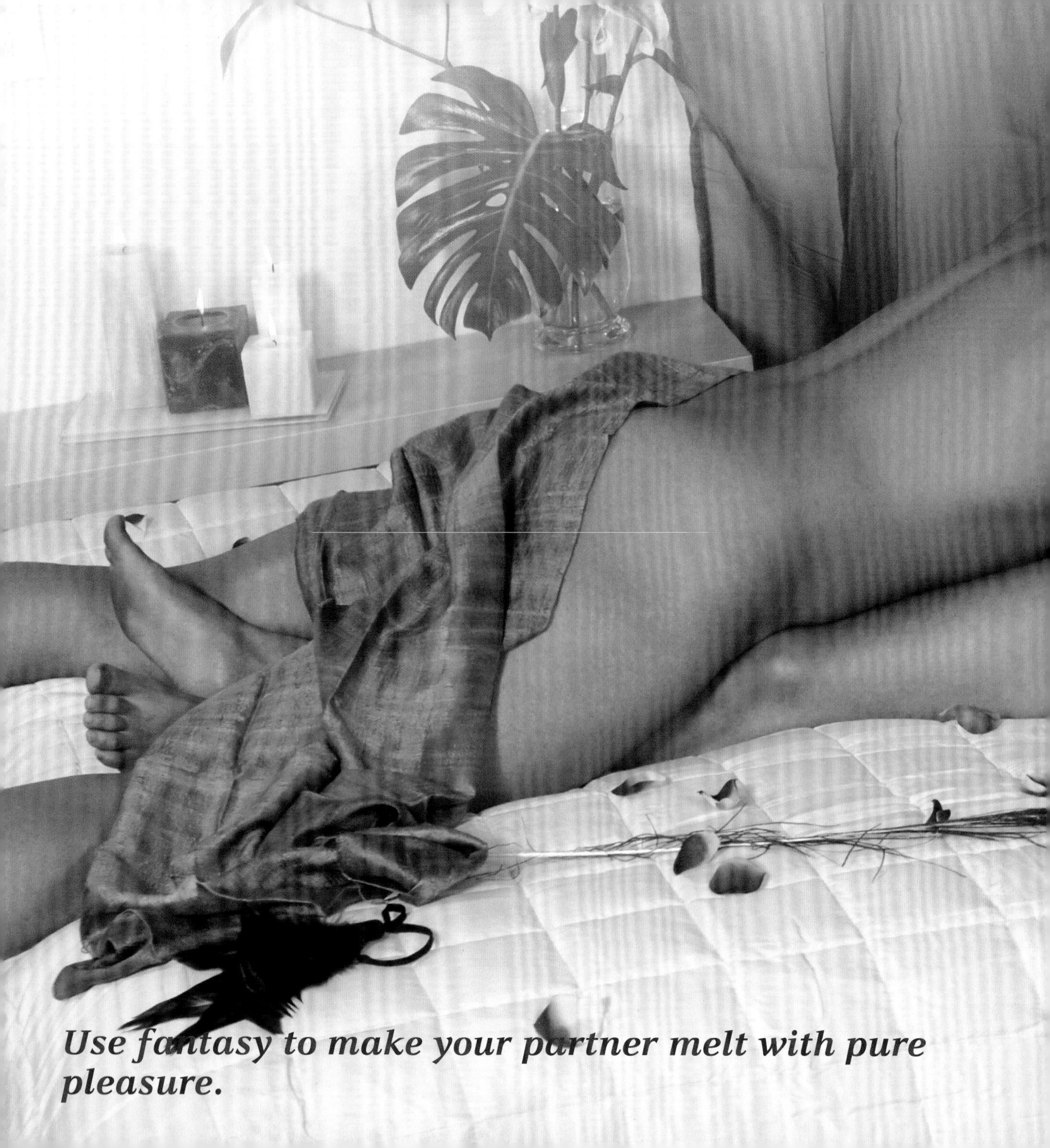

Use fantasy to make your partner melt with pure pleasure.

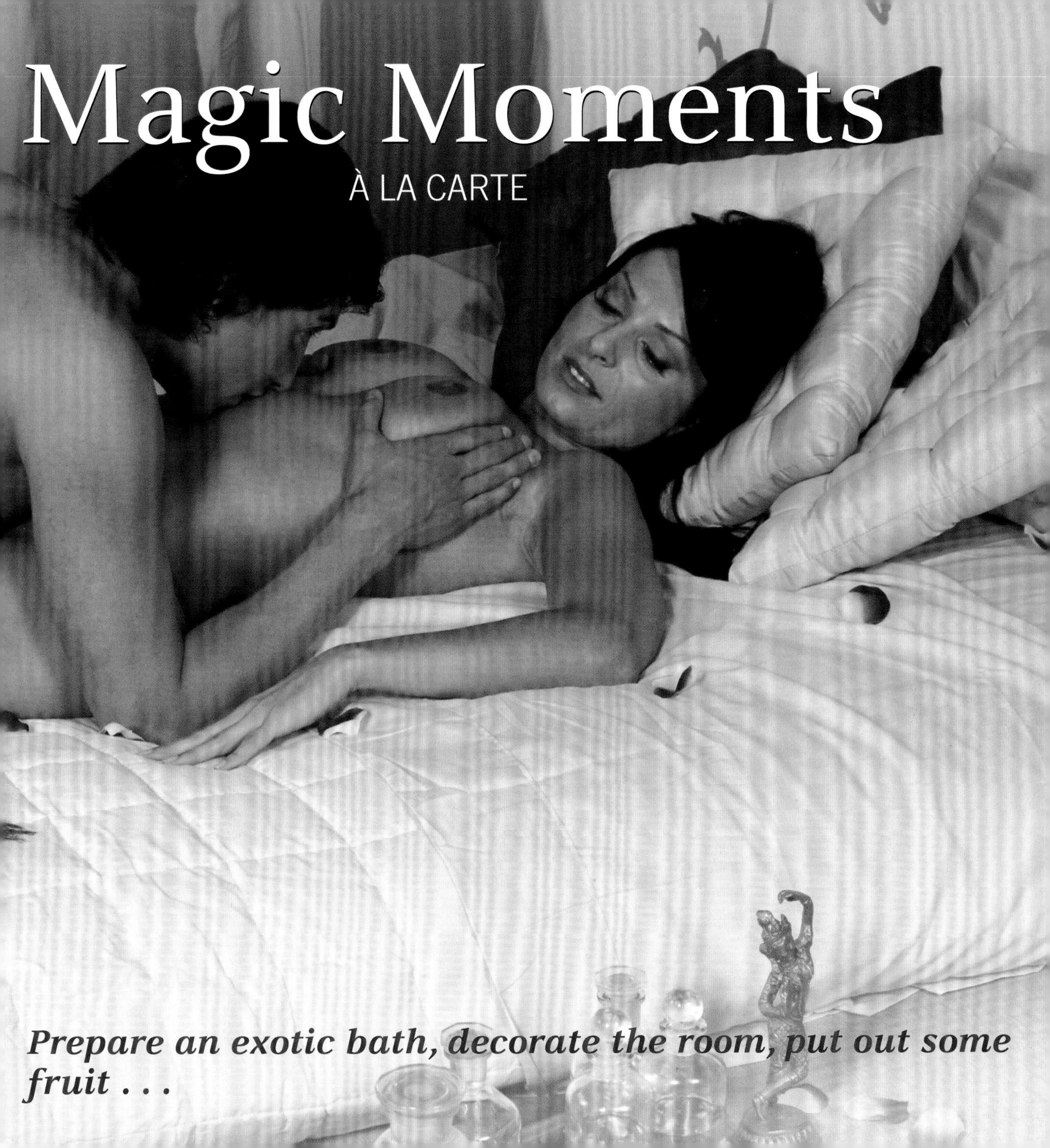

Magic Moments

À LA CARTE

Prepare an exotic bath, decorate the room, put out some fruit . . .

Love's Oasis

In the last few years spa hotels have proliferated, especially those that focus on health and beauty, inspired by Eastern therapies where you can get pampered with baths and massages.

These centers offer a wonderful opportunity to get away from home for a few days and escape with our partner to a special place where we can relax and forget about everything else.

Though it's true we can't always allow ourselves these escapes, there is, nevertheless, something else always available. We can decide to take a whole day to rest and relax (or even a whole weekend) without leaving home, at a much more affordable price.

So enough with the day dreaming and get to work planning and organizing this special day! It is better if the two of you do the preparations together. You can, for example, buy and cook **something sumptuous**. This can be something that helps raise the sexual heat and passion between the two of you. Later, **decorate the bedroom with suggestive props**.

Make yourselves an **aromatic bath** as an appetizer and continue with an erotic massage to awaken your sexual hunger. You don't have to reach too high a state of excitation or go for orgasm. You can keep it on the level of **flirtatious, sensual play**. Just let yourselves get into it totally.

Make it a point to try the different techniques that you've learned in this book. Alternate who gives and who receives the massage for a given session and discover your preferences. In time, a new understanding and confidence with sensuality will arise between the two of you. Follow this faithfully and do everything to give it enough time, even though everyday life, with all its demands, will not make it easy.

At least once a month, if you can't manage once a week, you should practice this very special erotic communion which is intended to bring you closer and make you crazy for each other. Resolve to enjoy the voluptuous pleasure of seducing your lover with a love feast personally designed by you. This is the perfect way to nourish the relationship with your partner.

Surprise your partner by preparing a special evening for just the two of you.

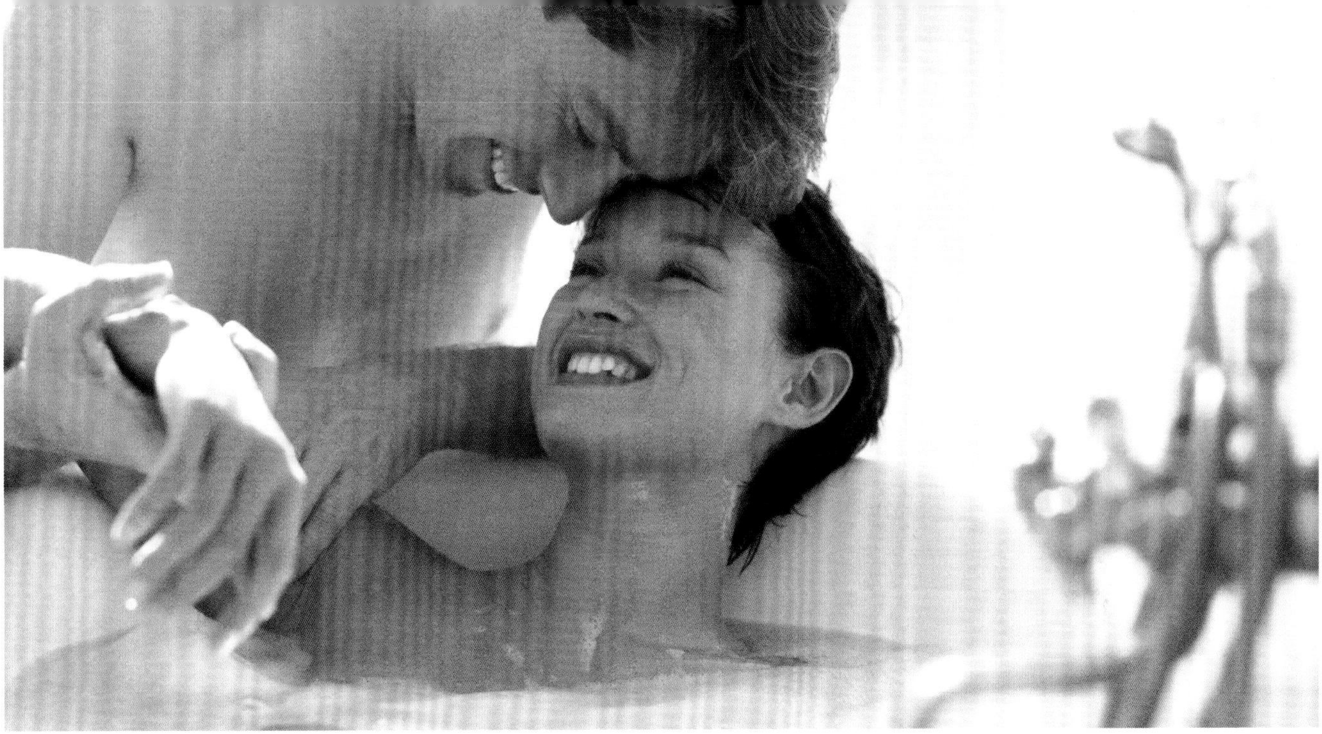

Beyond Fear and Hang-Ups

It's possible that if you've never practiced erotic massage before you feel insecure about your skill as a masseur/ masseuse and are concerned that, in spite of your determination, your hands will fail you when it comes time to deliver.

Put all of this out of your mind. Know that if you let your feelings and intuition guide you nothing bad can come of it. The most important ingredient of a successful massage is **being in sync** with your partner. Remember, also, that your partner can always instruct you on how they want you to touch them.

With time, you will gain confidence. Go ahead and stimulate your partner's erogenous areas and massage them freely. Whatever you do, your partner will react positively. It can be very exciting to see how you are gradually gaining in your ability to give them pleasure. Your efforts will result in your partner's body becoming more responsive to your touch. Even a brief massage, if it is done in a properly supportive environment, can turn out to be an unexpectedly sublime experience.

Organizing it will be fun and the result will be worth the wait . . .

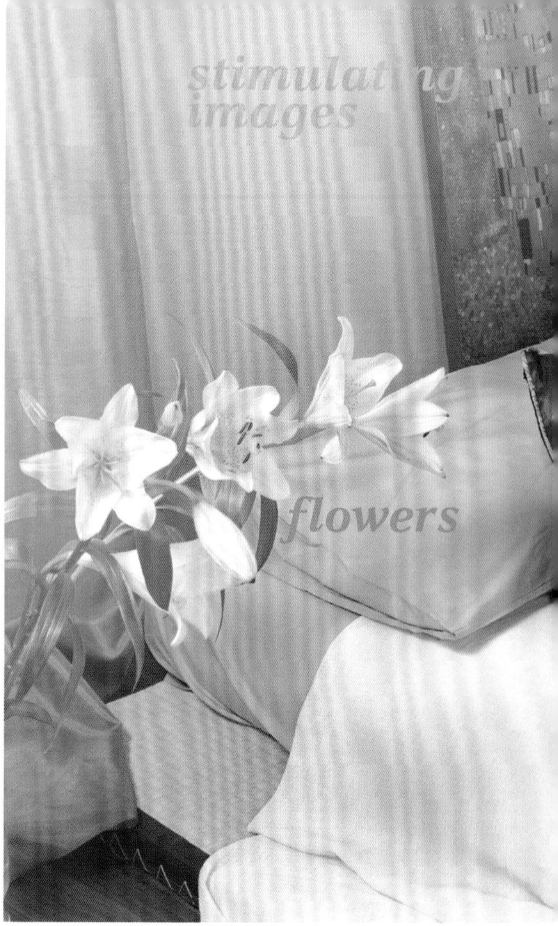

The Bedroom

The bedroom, or whatever space you choose for your sensual encounters, should be a genuine oasis of comfort and should be big enough so that you can recline with full ease (it doesn't necessarily have to include a bed). Of course, the bathroom should be arrayed in an inviting manner as well.

A colorful, fragrant boudoir intensifies sensual pleasure. And you don't have to go crazy to make this happen. It's enough to choose your favorite sheets, include an aromatic oil heater, place a jar of flowers nearby, and display some of your treasured photos or an erotic image that turns on the two of you. Use beautiful scarves or shawls to cover those things in the room which recall the mundane or practical, such as the laundry basket, the telephone, or your laptop. You can also arrange silk pillows on the bed or on the carpet and avail of soft blankets and silk handkerchiefs.

fragrances and colors intensify sensual pleasure

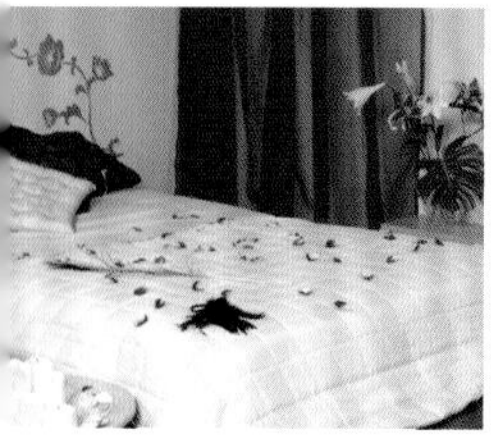

Lighting and Colors

Color, as well as lighting, has a direct effect on our mood. You must take this into account when you go about choosing things to decorate the bedroom. Red and orange are the most sensual colors and have a particularly stimulating effect.

Awaken your senses with surroundings that are sensual and charged with erotic energy.

the color orange is profoundly linked to eroticism

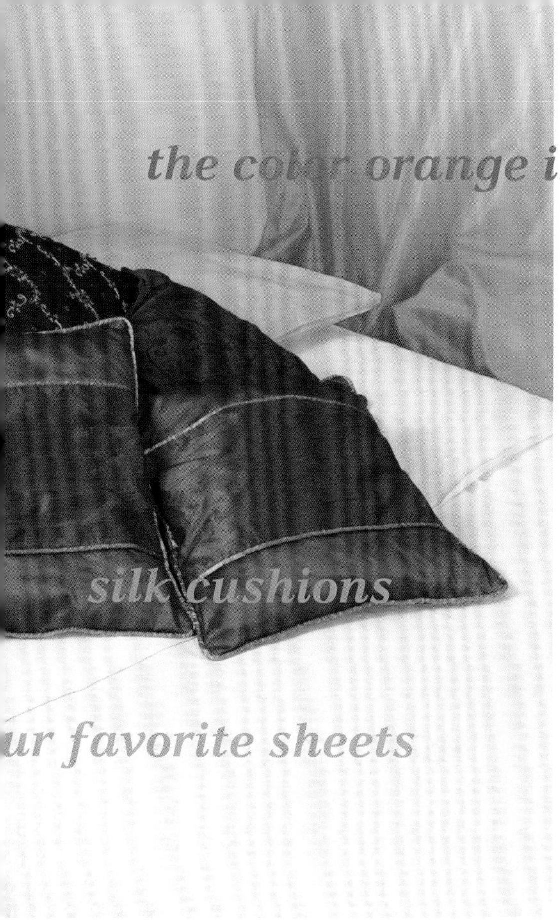

Red expresses the force of life and is the most vital color of the chromatic palette. It is associated with passion, eroticism, energy, enthusiasm, and ardor. It is the color of blood and causes our heart rate and blood pressure to increase. It also stimulates our nervous system. In color therapy red is identified with the ovaries and testicles. Red creates an atmosphere full of life, eroticism, and sensuality.

Orange is associated with a positive state of mind and the setting of the southern sun. It has an anti-depressive effect and being equally strong and intense as red, it should not be used if you are stressed out since it increases nervous stimulation. Orange is also strongly linked to eroticism. In anatomy it is associated with the adrenal glands and, in the case of women, with the uterus.

Yellow is associated with sincerity, joy, and charisma. It has a stimulating effect on the mental faculties and can help with depression since it tends to bring to light one's unconscious issues. Yellow has a curative effect on a number of organs, especially the pancreas, and improves metabolism and benefits the region around the solar plexus.

Lighting, as much as color, is fundamental. You can make it more or less intense or more or less direct according to how it makes you feel about your body. As a rule, candlelight or a dim lamp is the most sensual option. There is nothing more inviting than a dimly lit bed.

Experiment with the colors, fragrances, and textures of your space.

Pleasures of the Palate

Food and sex are a wonderful combination.

You can start with a **romantic candlelit supper** including delicious little mouthfuls and powerful, aphrodisiac cocktails. In this chapter you will find some inviting suggestions.

A tray of fruit next to the bed (strawberries, grapes, cherries, figs, bananas) works fine as well as **a bottle of champagne in an ice bucket (the ice cubes will be available for other stimulating pleasures . . .)**. You can feed each other decadently or nibble on the fruit using your partner's belly as a plate. Just let your fantasy fly! You can also attempt a **tasty belly massage with strawberries or honey**, or begin with the "Venus massage" that you will find later on for massaging the chest.

A Scent for Every Occasion

Fresh citrus overtones such as bergamot, tangerine, orange mandarin, orange, and lemon.

Erotic floral fragrances such as jasmine, mimosa, rose, rose geranium, tuberose, osmanthus, and Ylang Ylang.

Exotic spice overtones such as cardamom, cilantro seed, cloves, black pepper, green pepper, and cinnamon bark.

Invigorating, stimulating herbs such as verbena, mint, and patchouli.

Relaxing herbs such as agarwood or sandalwood.

Sensual woods such as agarwood or sandalwood.

Wood tonics such as cedar and rosewood.

Soothing balms such as oil of benzoin, storax, and incense.

Sensual extracts such as honey, cacao, or vanilla.

Your Choices of Aromas

We've already talked about how it's worth the trouble to make your own blends of aromas and to try new things. Just avoid using too many fragrances at the same time.

The quality of the oils you choose is important too. The best ones to use as bases for your blends are jojoba, almond oil, macadamia oil, oil of evening

A platter full of exotic fruits accompanied by a chilled bottle of champagne

feed your lover with sumptuous little bites

primrose, and sesame oil. They should be 100% vegetable oil and totally natural. They are sold in natural health food stores and some pharmacies. These products are not cheap, but your skin will appreciate the extra expense you've paid. The essential oils (you'll use just a few drops of these to enrich your blends with delicious fragrances) also should be 100% natural, since only those that are 100% natural have beneficial effects on your organism, including your body and mind.

It is important to know that a 3-ounce bottle (100 ml) should contain between 0.5% and 1.0% of the blend. That is to say, for every 3 ounces of oil base you should add between 10 and 20 drops of essence (100 drops = 1 tablespoon; 1 ml = 20 drops).

The examples of blends that appear in this book have proven to be successful before. When you gain experience you will also be able to improvise and create oil blends that align with your personal tastes.

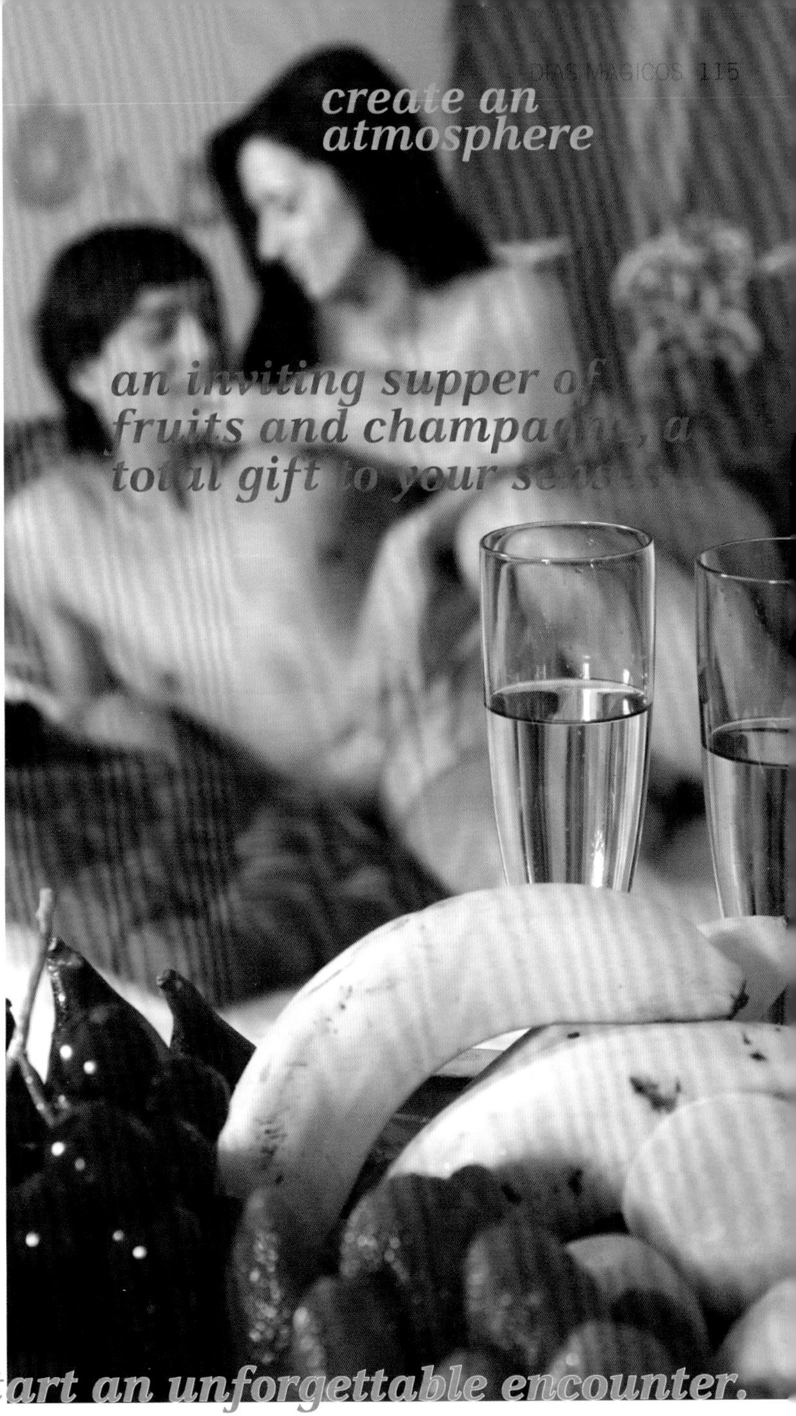

create an atmosphere

an inviting supper of fruits and champagne, a total gift to your senses can be the best way to start an unforgettable encounter.

Getting Ready for a Special Day

This day you have chosen as homage to love is a day that belongs to both of you. It is a good idea to change roles and make sure it isn't always the same person giving the massage. To give and receive alternately will end up being a lot more pleasant for the two of you.

You can start off with a **sensual bath** together while you are deciding who is going to give the massage first. Best is a **gentle massage** all over your partner's body.

Be Prepared!

For the Room:
- Silk cushions or soft blankets and scarves
- Warmed towels and sheets (also bathrobe or dressing gown)
- Flowers, photos, and pleasant items to look at
- A tray with fruit and things to nosh
- Soft music
- Erotic poems to read aloud
- Candles and an oil heater, 100% natural essences

For the Bath:
- Candles
- Bathrobe or warmed towels
- Bath oil or whipped cream and honey
- 100% natural essential oils

For the Massage:
- Silk gloves
- Feathers
- Brushes (fine and large)
- Silk scarves
- Aceite sensual para masajes.

The Bathroom

In ancient cultures aromatic baths and products for bodily hygiene were extensively used.

For men as well as women, care and adorning of the body were given special importance.

Then again, common baths have been around since time immemorial. From **Roman spas** to **Japanese water baths** and continuing with **Turkish steam baths**. The bathing ritual at the ancient public baths could last for hours. To begin, the pubic hair would be anointed with oil for an agreeable aroma.

Get the room ready for some afternoon delight!

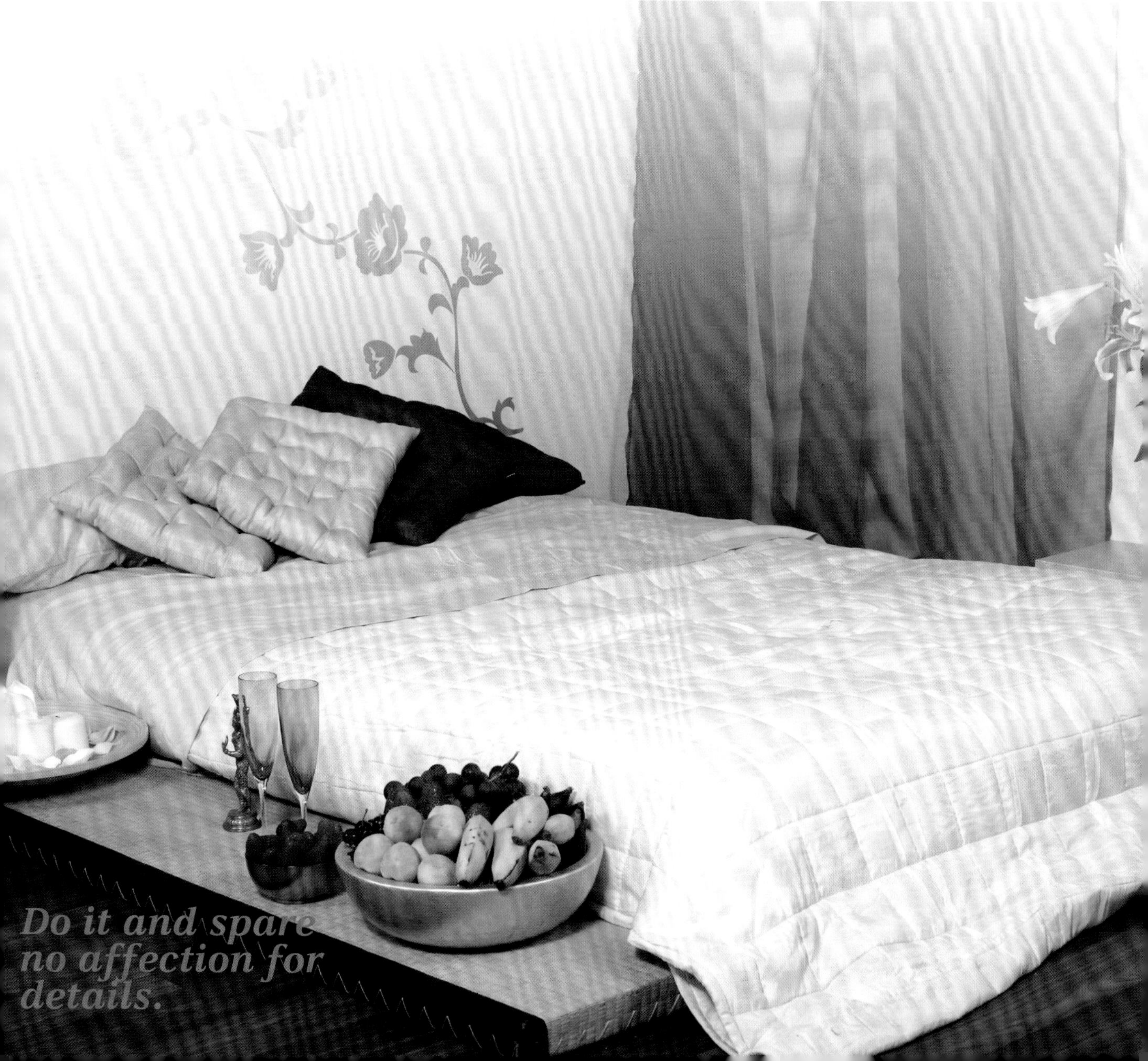

Do it and spare no affection for details.

A Sexy, Hot Bath

Cleopatra undoubtedly received Marc Antony in her bath. It seems she had the habit of bathing in the milk of a female donkey to keep her skin smooth and young. Like Cleopatra, you can invite your lover for a couple's bath. An aromatic bath is the best way to get rid of stress and tensions. Sinking yourself in scented hot water will open the gates to erotic pleasure.

We'll assume you've already chosen who's going to begin the massage. Make a blend for the bath water using bath oil and a couple of drops of essential oil (don't put essential oils directly in the bath water without an emulsifier or the skin might become irritated).

If you need an idea, we suggest two blends that are super-sensual: Aphrodite's Secret and The Secret of Venus.

Essences for Pure Pleasure

Aphrodite's Secret

Mix 2 drops of sandalwood, 1 drop of neroli, 2 drops of Ylang Ylang, and 5 drops of bergamot with two tablespoons of whipped cream and two of honey.

The Secret of Venus

This is a very sensual blend. Mix 1 tablespoon of bath oil with 3 drops of patchouli, 2 drops of jasmine, and 5 drops of orange.

Pour the mix into the almost-full bathtub, then add a bit more water. Light some candles, grab a warmed bathrobe, and go get your partner. Invite them to partake in a tantalizing bath. You can soap them up and enjoy exploring the nooks and crannies of their body and other places that await your touch.

After a while, get into the bathtub with your partner. Sit facing him/her or behind them, depending on the size of the tub. Enjoy the sensation of the water and when you leave the bath to dry, take turns drying each other. Put on your bathrobes and go together to the bedroom or wherever you have chosen. For the massage, you can either clothe yourselves or remain nude.

After a hot bath the skin and muscles are relaxed and ready for a nice massage.

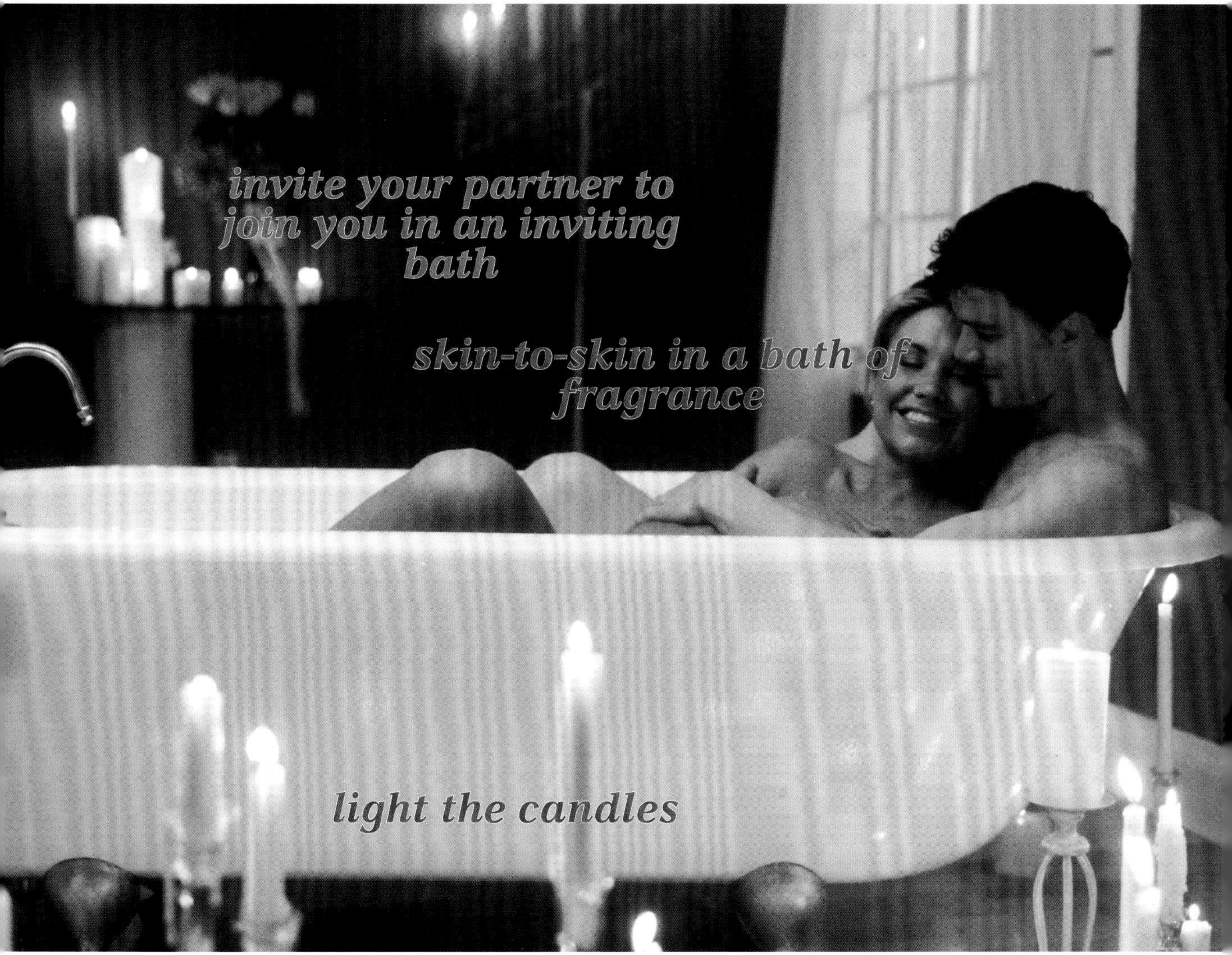

The best way to end a hard day at work and a gift to your senses.

Aphrodite's Back Massage

The massage we are about to show you is gentle and includes the whole body. Your partner remains silent, using only pleasure sounds to communicate. He/she is allowed to growl if they feel either excessive pressure or anything disagreeable.

The massage room must be kept at the right temperature. Don't forget colored scarves, an oil heater, candles, flowers, and prepared oil blends in a tray.

Step by Step

- Ask your partner to lie nude face down on the bed or, even better, on a layer of blankets spread across the floor. Give him/her a cushion that they can put under their head.
- Tell your partner they're about to embark on a sensual odyssey. Use relaxing music and provocative items that will awaken their desire. Tell him/her that they will be more disposed for a seductive massage with fine aromatic oils.
- At first, just let your partner smell the massage oil to excite their sense of smell.

the massage oil will begin to stimulate their sense of smell

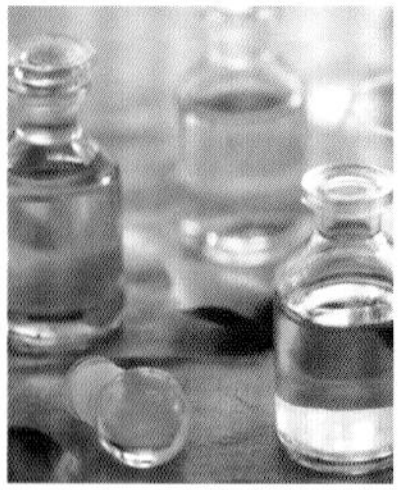

Silk Scarves

- Next, get your partner's sense of touch involved. Go over his/her entire body with a silk scarf from head to toes. Use one that's hot and another that's cold. Use different colors. Orange and red are perceived as hot; yellow, green, and blue are cooler. White is neutral and imparts a sense of relaxed fluidity.
- From time to time ask your partner if he/she feels cold or hot. Remember they are allowed to answer using only inarticulate sounds.
- Softly slide the scarves from top to bottom all over their skin until they shiver with an enjoyable chill. Let your partner enjoy this with eyes closed.
- Remember there are several very sensitive points that lie along the spinal column and buttocks that react positively to tactile stimulation.

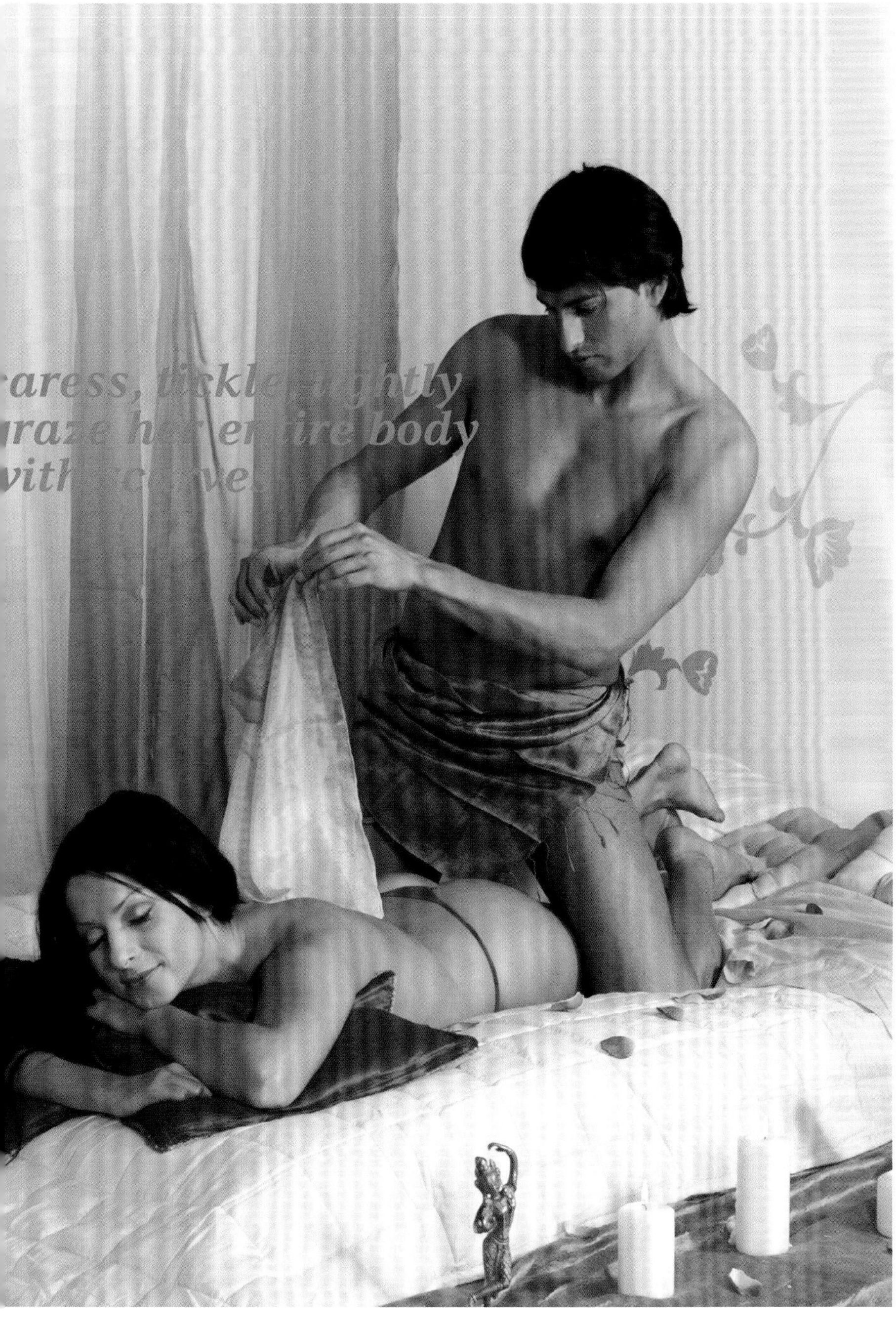
caress, tickle lightly
graze her entire body
with

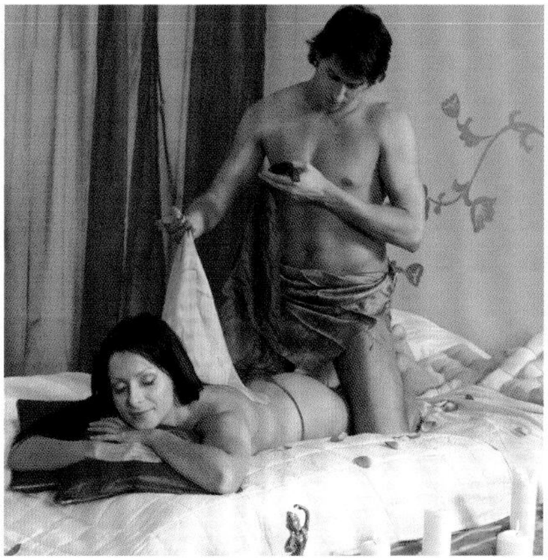

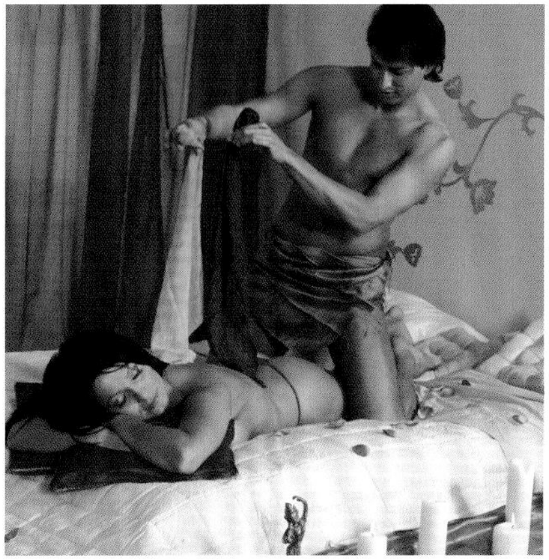

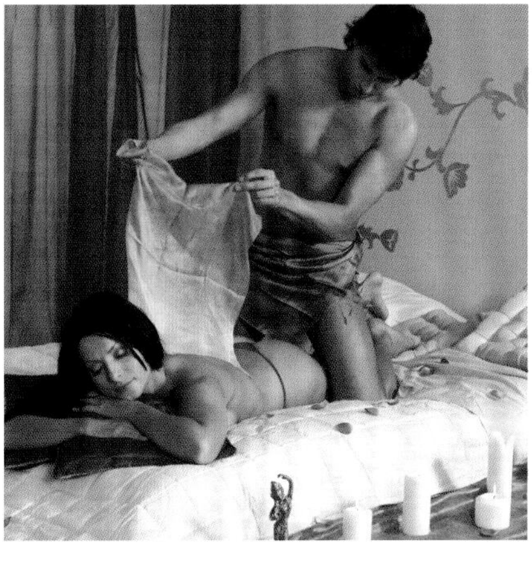

Playing with Brushes and Feathers

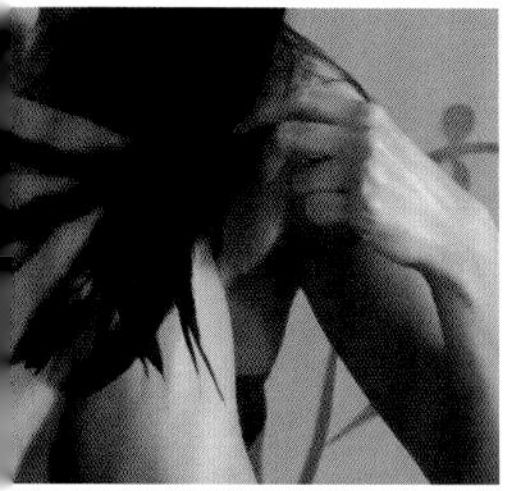

go over your partner's body, caress it all over tenderly

Sit on your partner's left. Take a makeup brush and draw small "figure 8s" in the area of their neck and shoulders.

1. Begin in the center of the back and slide the brush sideways up to the right shoulder. Outline your partner's shoulder blade then return to the center of the back. Then go across the back to the left shoulder. Draw around the shape of the left shoulder blade and return to the center of the back.

2. Use the brush all over the back area, settling on the nook that lies just above the buttocks. When you arrive there draw large "figure 8s" that cross the spinal column. Start in the center and then go out all the way to one side, and then the other.

3. You can go from "figure 8s" to circles, best of all in the region of the buttocks. You can even use two brushes at the same time.

Now use your brush on your partner's hands and arms. Begin on the shoulders. Draw "figure 8s" along the arm and forearm, reaching the fingertips, then returning along the same route to the shoulders. Your brush strokes should be large and wide.

After a while, sit on your partner's other side and change arms.

Make sure your partner is satisfied with the rhythm of your movements. They should be neither too fast nor too slow.

Now take your brush and start at the very top of the spinal column, going down its length making small "figure 8s" all the way to the butt cheeks.

Take two vertebrae and draw a circle around them. Go down the spinal column this way, two vertebrae at a time, starting from the top and going down slowly.

Draw "figure 8s" on the sacrum. You can use two brushes at the same time. Spend a good amount of time here. Remember this is a sensitive spot with a number of points of sexual stimulation.

Trace circles on your partner's butt with a brush and go lower making eights from the exterior of the right thigh downward to the ankle.

Trace "figure 8s" on the inside of your partner's thighs using the brush. Go from the bottom upwards, and then down again on the outside part of the right thigh.

Then stimulate the inside of the thighs with brushes, going from top to bottom. Finish by drawing circles on the inside of the ankles. Move the brush down to the soles of the feet until you reach your partner's toes.

Now exchange the brushes for feathers or silk gloves and repeat the above process step by step.

Gentle tickles with feathers and brushes is a perfect complement to massage.

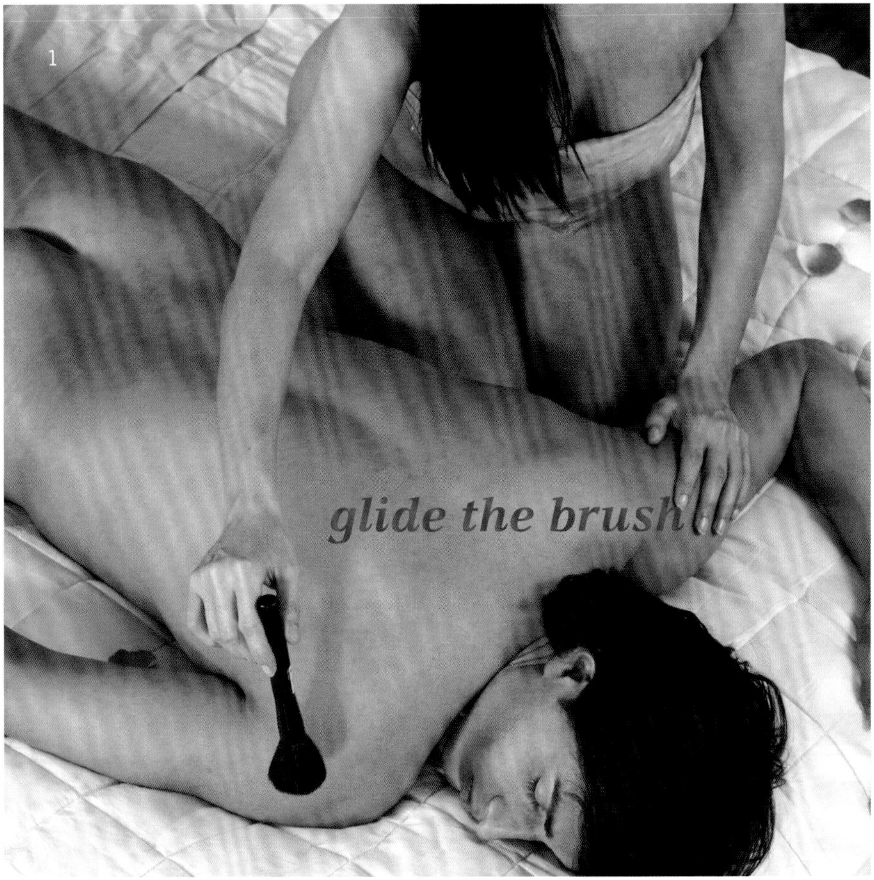
1
glide the brush

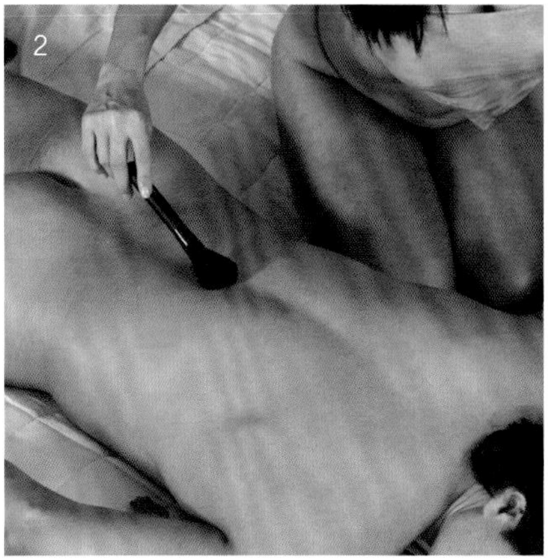
2

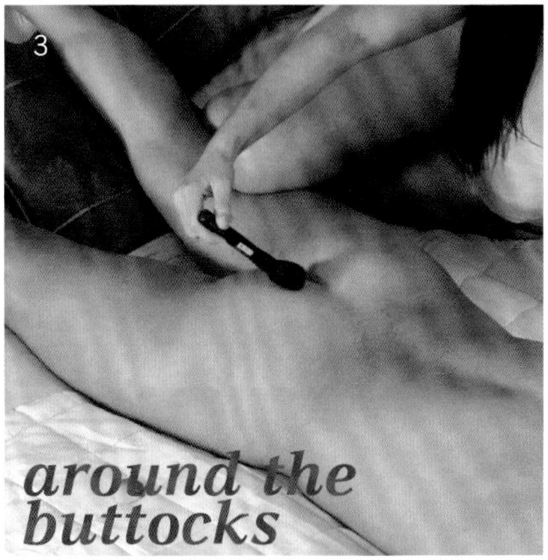
3
around the buttocks

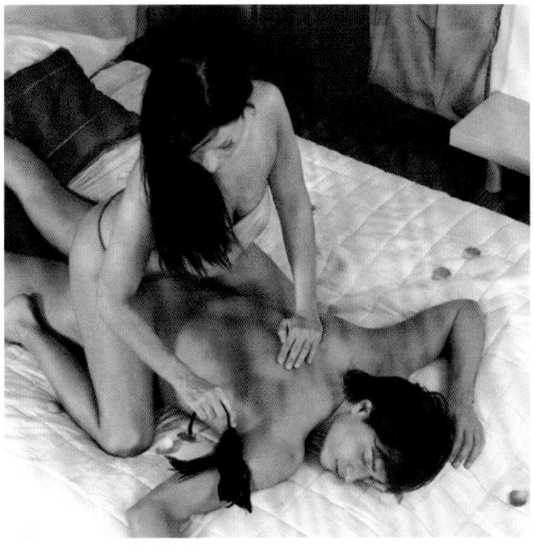

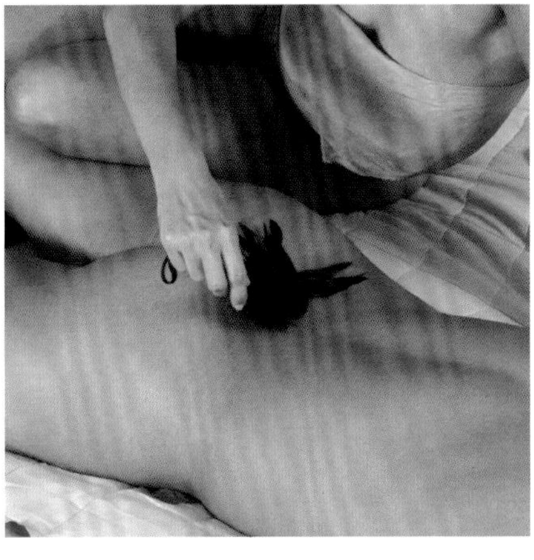

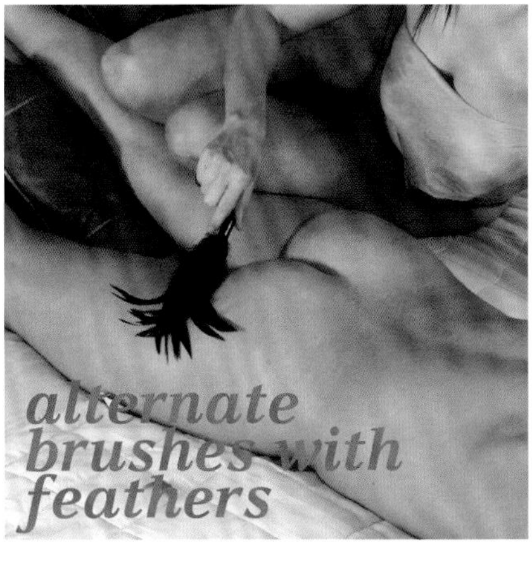
alternate brushes with feathers

Using Your Hands

- Your partner's body is now perfectly ready to receive a hand massage. You can begin working the whole posterior of your lover's body as we've just described, but this time use hands, fingertips, and thumbs instead of feathers and brushes.

- It's important to use enough oil to keep the motion fluid and rhythmical. This way you avoid unpleasant tugging on the skin of your partner.

- Give enough time to the most sensitive areas. Remember the sacral bone. Knead it deeply. Your partner will always thank you for this. . .

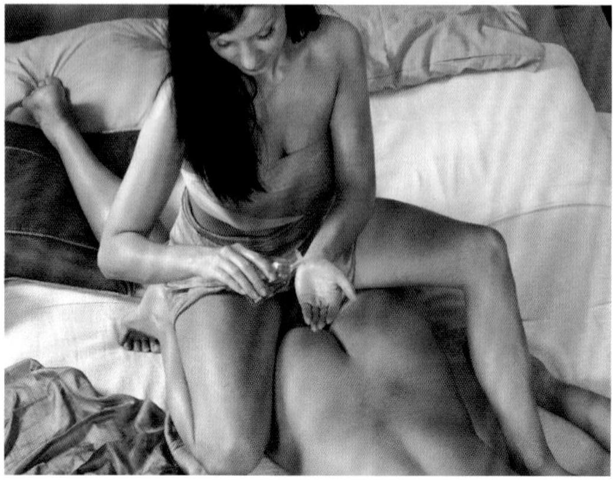

use enough oil

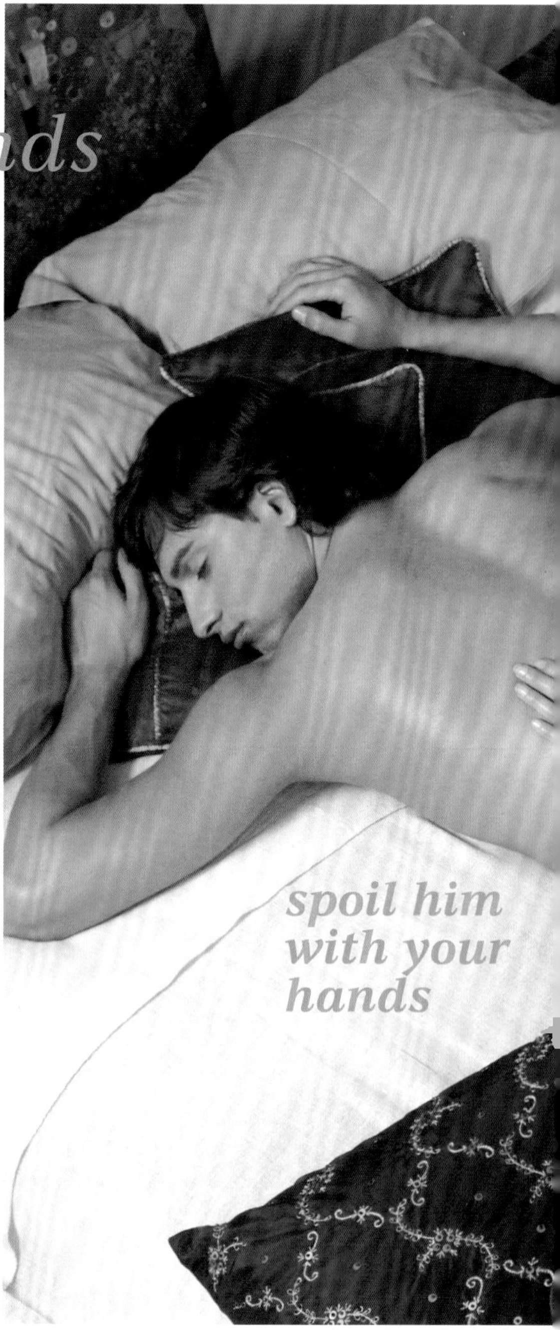

spoil him with your hands

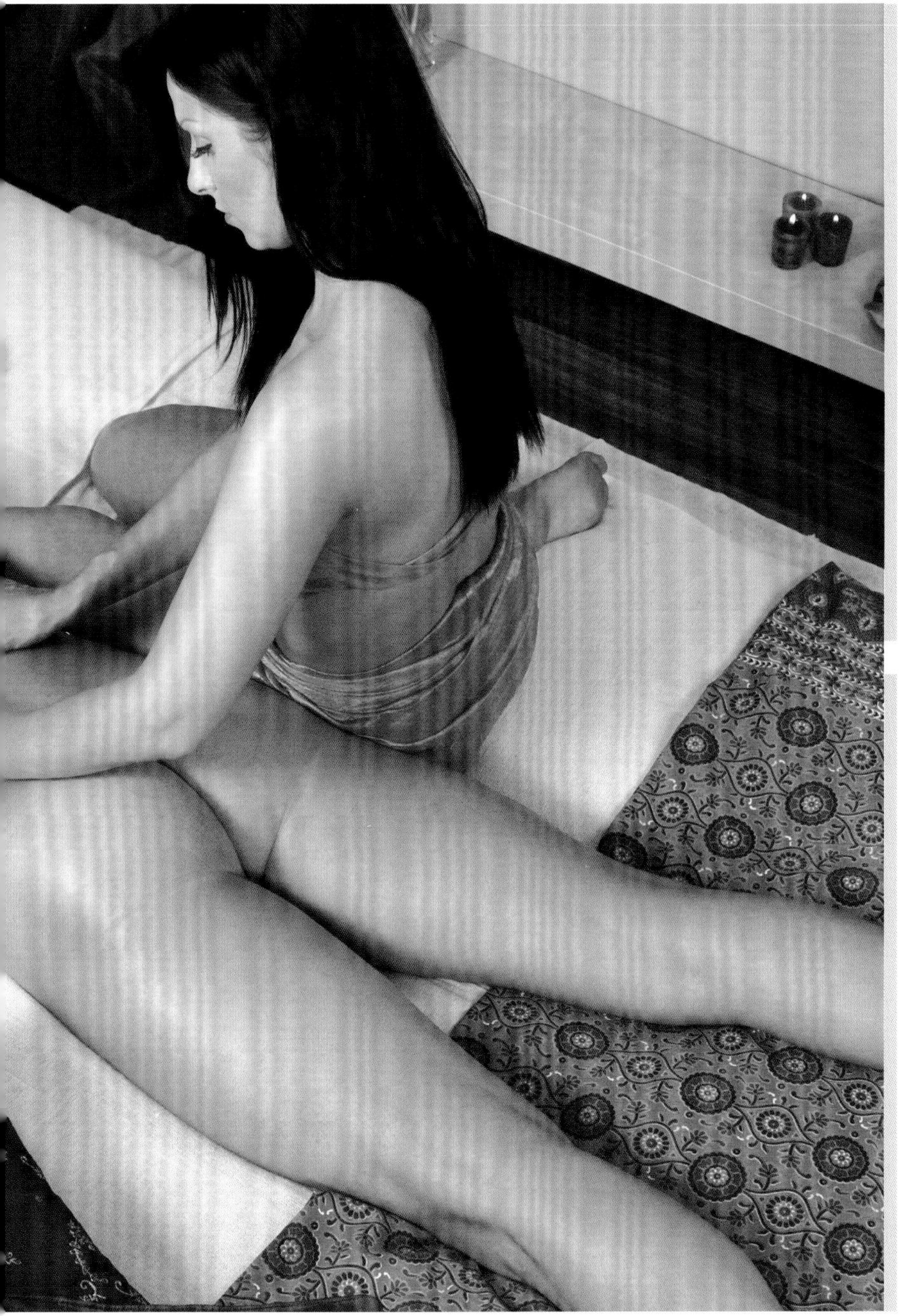

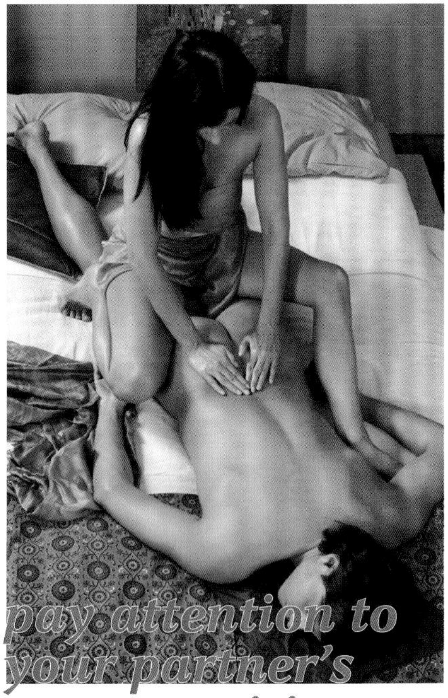

pay attention to your partner's most sensitive areas

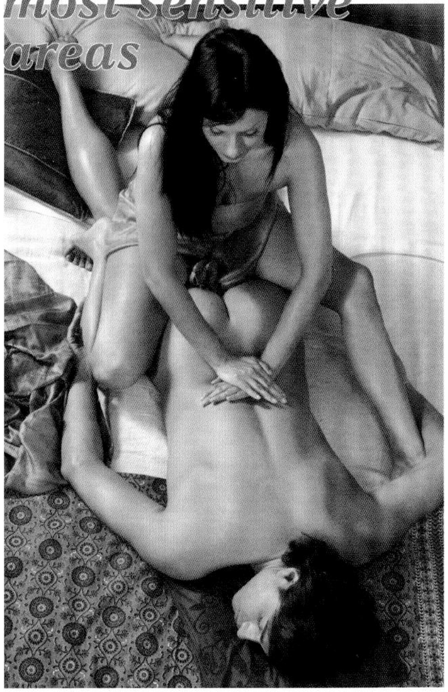

Silk Caresses on Chest and Abdomen

After such an extensive treatment of your partner's body it is only right that you ask him/her to return the favor to you. The front is the most sensitive part, especially for women. It is quite likely she will like the experience of fine silk on her breasts and genitals.

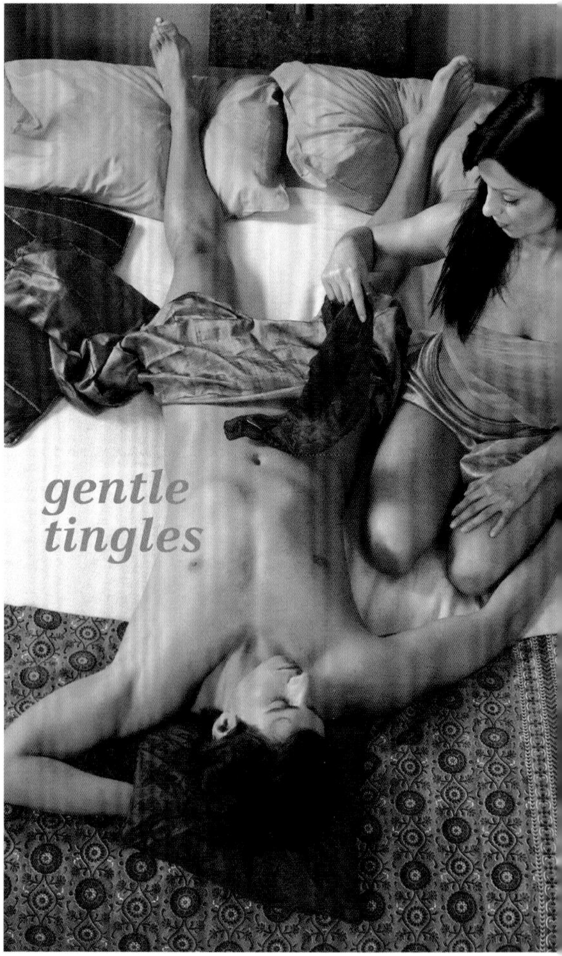

Silk Scarves

- Slide scarves and handkerchiefs all over your lover's body. Include their arms and legs. Go over the other zones that are especially sensitive such as breasts and genitals.
- Be especially delicate when you caress the inside of your partner's thighs.
- Tell your partner to close his/her eyes and alternate using cool and hot handkerchiefs. This way you will extend the excitement phase.

Turn on your lover's desire and rub him/her with silk.

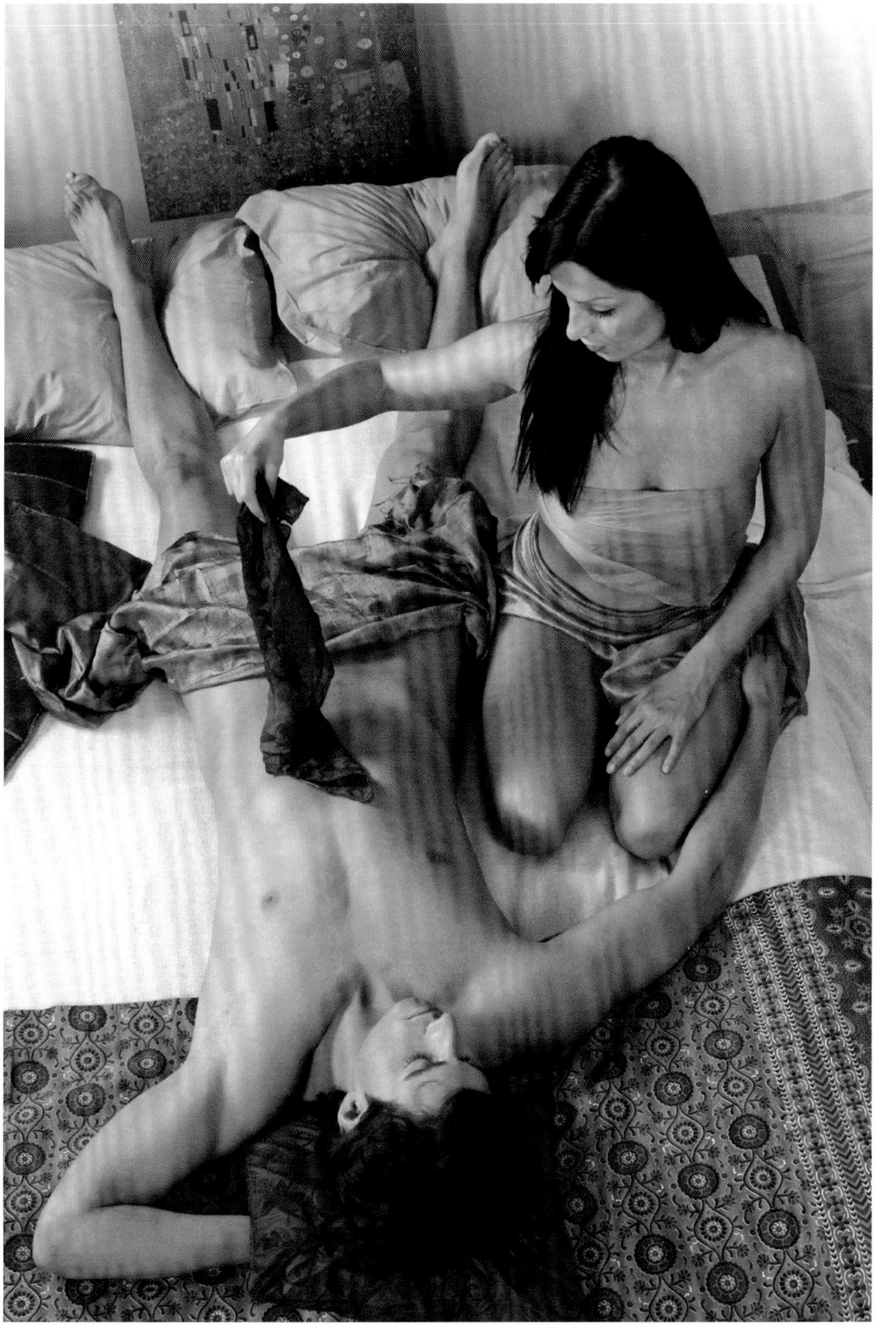
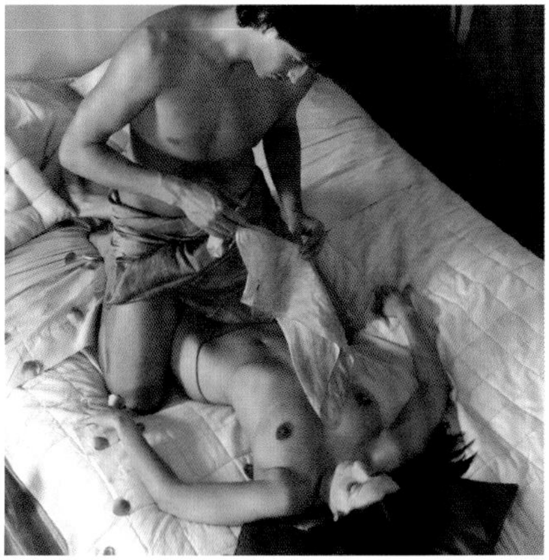
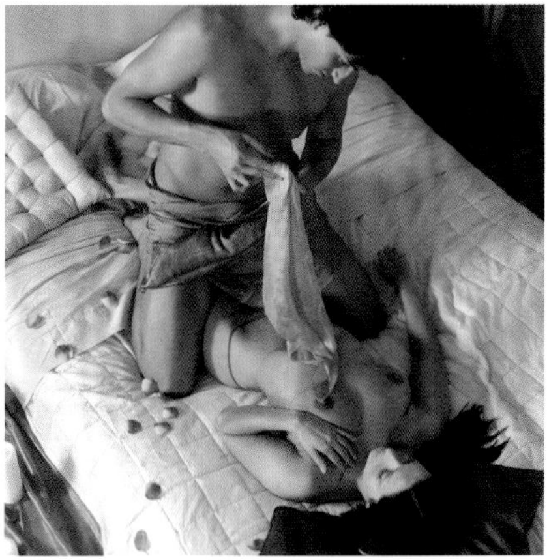
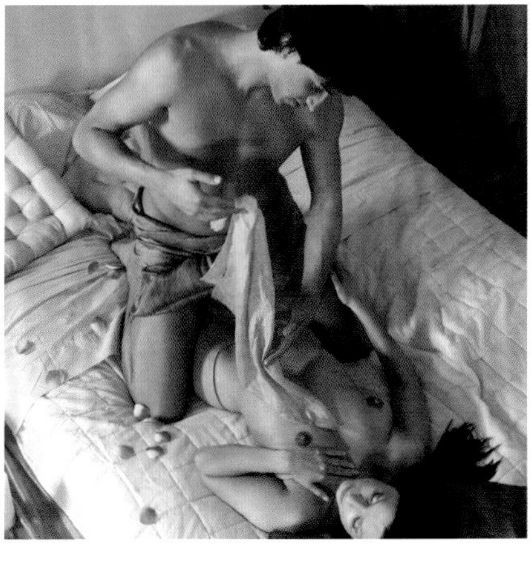

Tracing Your Desire on Your Partner's Skin

1. Sit behind your lover's head and run over his/her forehead with two brushes, starting in the center and going outwards towards the hair.

   Keep one brush still in the center of your partner's forehead while you brush all around. Repeat this movement several times.

   Outline the area around your partner's eyes. Then go above the cheek bones to the area between the eyebrows, ending at the forehead again. Do this several times.

   Now run the brush around the mouth, stopping at the upper lip and then moving to the area between the chin and lower lip and moving next to the jaw.

   Go down the sides of your partner's neck (you can use two brushes) with small, circular movements until you reach the shoulders. Then go over the collarbone and finish between the breasts, moving from inside to outside.

2. If your partner's reactions tell you that these movements are stimulating, you can repeat them with a makeup brush, feathers, or silk gloves. You don't have to use all the items you have chosen. If you prefer, you can go straight ahead to the massage.

3. Continuing, circle your partner's chest area from right to left with "figure 8s" or even draw small circles from the center of their chest outwards using brushes, feathers, or silk gloves.

   Now move to the right arm with wide, stretching circular movements and work your way down to the fingertips. Then go back the way you came.

   After a while, go back and repeat the process with the left arm.

4. Next, concentrate on the solar plexus, torso, and abdomen. Draw circles clockwise around your partner's navel.

5. Very gently stroke your partner's groin area, then her Mount of Venus or his penis. You can use feathers or very soft brushes here. It is very exciting. Nevertheless, keep in mind that before you get carried away, it could be very interesting to hold off from any sexual act and continue with the massage. This will allow desire to grow much more intensely.

   Continue massaging downward on the legs until you reach your partner's toes. Do this several times.

6. Now go on and draw "figure 8s" on the outside of their leg with feathers or brushes. Then do the same on the inside of the leg and then both legs at the same time, outside and inside. Repeat several times.

   To finish, do "figure 8s" all over your partner's feet.

Alternate using your hands with feathers or brushes.

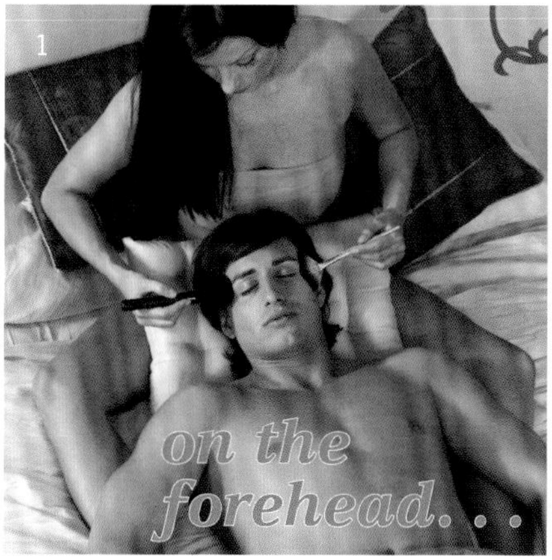
1
on the forehead. . .

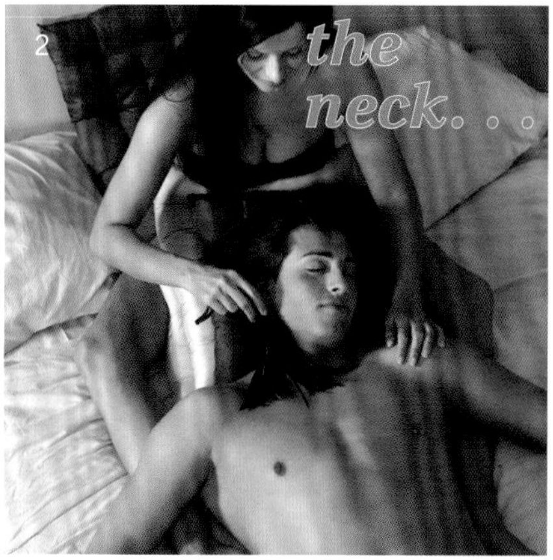
2
the neck. . .

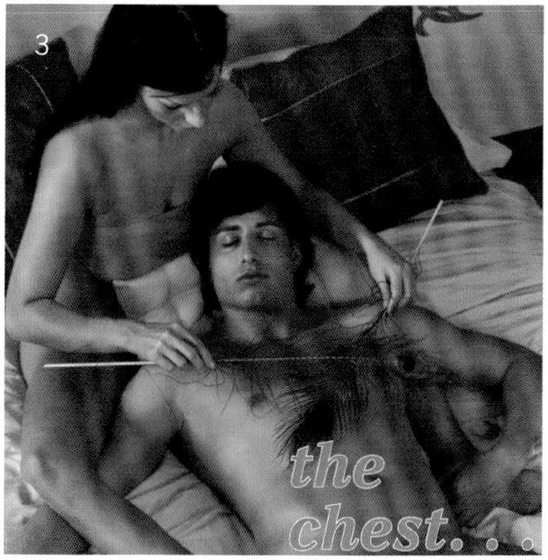
3
the chest. . .

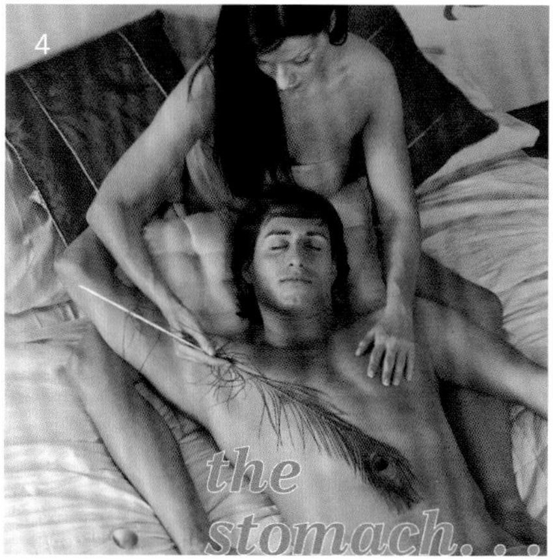
4
the stomach. . .

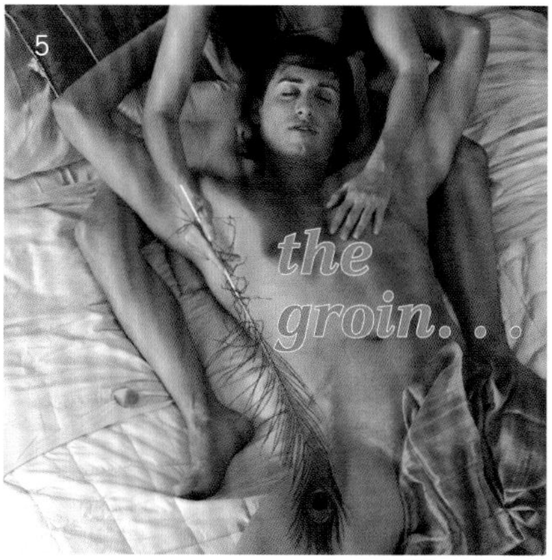
5
the groin. . .

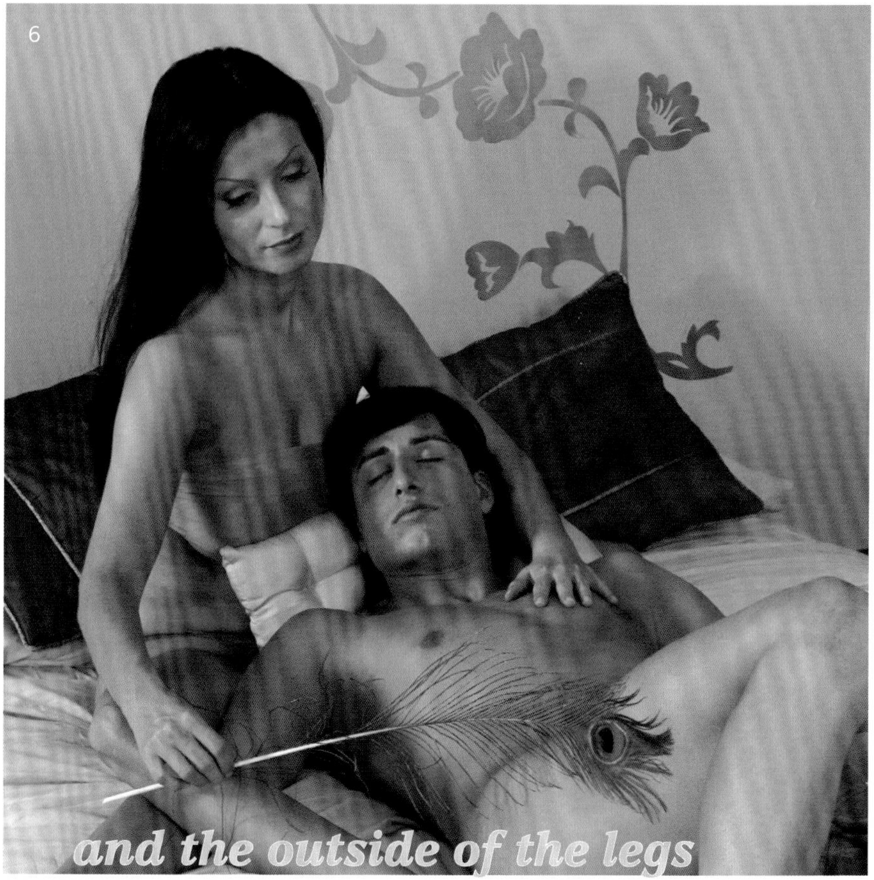
6
and the outside of the legs

An Intense, Finishing Massage

Your partner is now ready for a deeper massage with aromatic oils.

You can now repeat all the steps we've just finished using circular kneading. Of course, you can concentrate on only those areas that interest you the most.

1. At the finish, gently tug on your partner's toes and then warm up both feet in your hands.

2. If you want to give your partner a special treat, ask him/her to turn and place yourself behind their head. Put massage oil on your hands and forearms and rub, making "figure 8s" up their spine and upwards and out so that an intense wave of pleasure travels all over their back.

Do these movements several times, making sure to finish this massage by going over your partner's whole body.

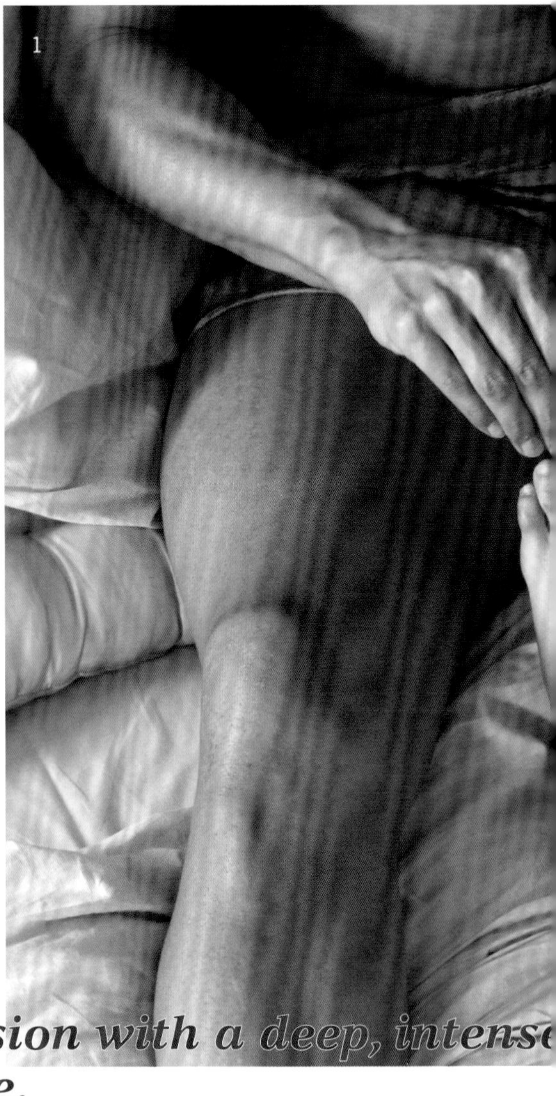

It's important to finish the session with a deep, intense massage.

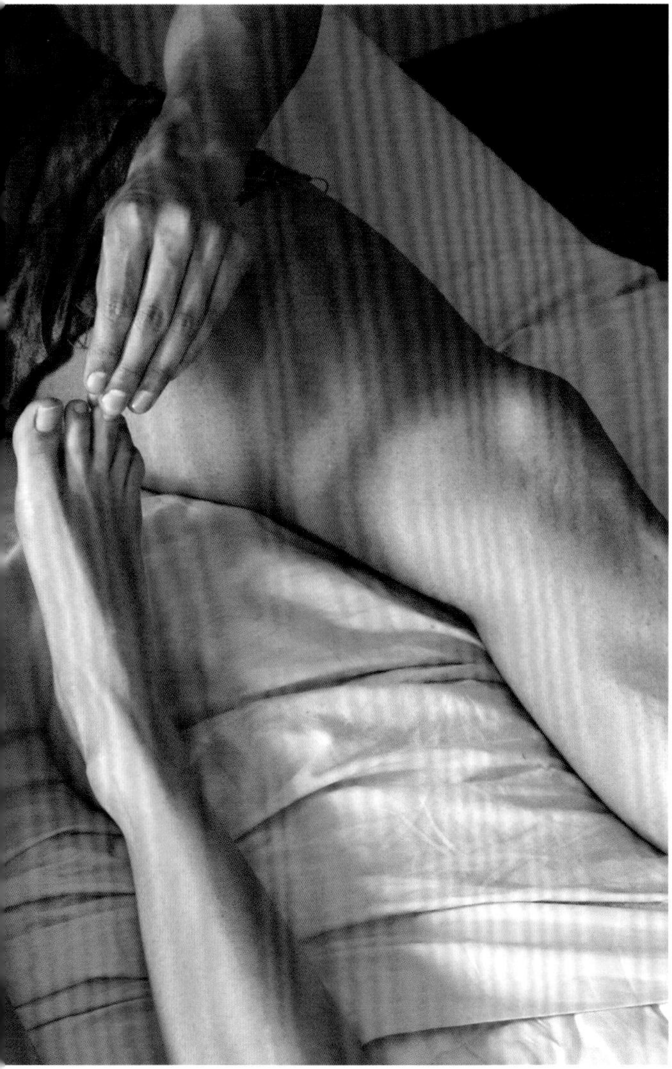

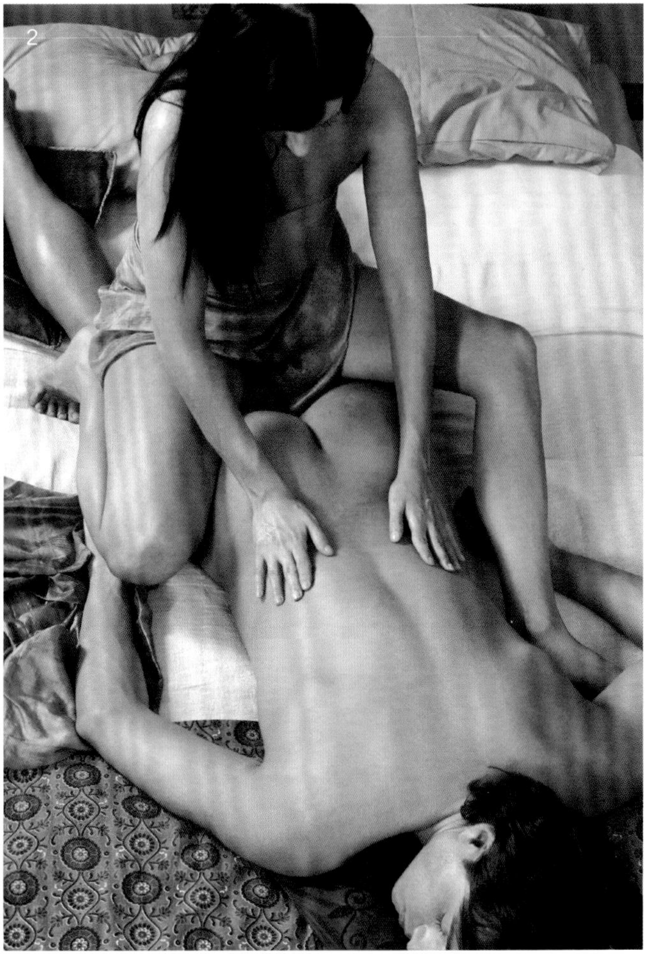

And Then?

After this complete massage, both of you have neared sensory ecstasy and are now totally filled with loving energy. You can take a short break, or go for another high point. Whatever you choose will promote intense bonding between you as lovers. Have a glass of champagne or nibble on something to regain your strength. Perhaps it's time to change roles, or maybe you would like to explore the following erotic variant . . .

Body on Body

Continuing, we offer a delicious variation on the massage we have just completed. This time we will use not only hands, but our entire body. You can massage any part of your partner's body with your breasts, your hair, lips, tongue, or even your breath. You can rub or slide with these on your partner. With your eyes closed, the sense of touch will assume a greater role and your perceptions will be intensely amplified. This variation of erotic massage that uses your entire body as a tool for pleasure implies undertaking a real voyage of exploration of your lover's body.

Close your eyes, use your imagination, let go, and this massage will become something unforgettable. It is highly probable you will end up making love after this.

Step by Step

Oil your entire body so you will be able to slide easily on your lover.

Your partner lies face down with his/her arms on their head.

1. Place your hands at the side of their legs and sink your chest between his/her thighs.

Use your arms for support and slowly glide upwards on your lover's body.

Continue by lying on your partner with your belly on their lumbar area.

2. Support yourself on your forearms and turn on your axis, first 40 degrees and then 90 degrees. Then massage your partner's gluteals and lower back with your belly.

Resume your initial position and remain laying a couple of minutes with your arms on top of your partner. This will produce a pleasant sensation of well-being. If you think your weight will be too much, support yourself on your forearms.

After a while, make snake-like, undulating movements with your body on your partner's back and gluteals.

3. Next, use your lips and tongue to cover your partner's shoulders with kisses and then work downwards.

Make sure to use your forearms and keep sufficient oil on your hands.

Knead you partner's buttocks and lumbar area with care.

4. Continue by sitting astride his/her buttocks and hold your partner between your thighs. Then slide your buttocks on your partner's and also on their lower back, moving upwards.

Repeat a couple of times more. You can also trade places at this point.

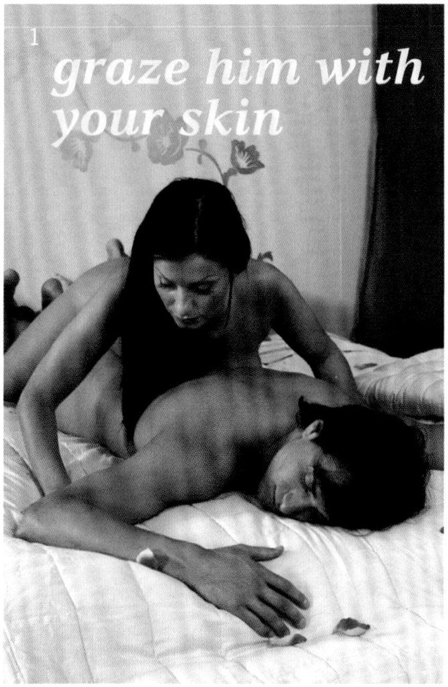
1
graze him with your skin

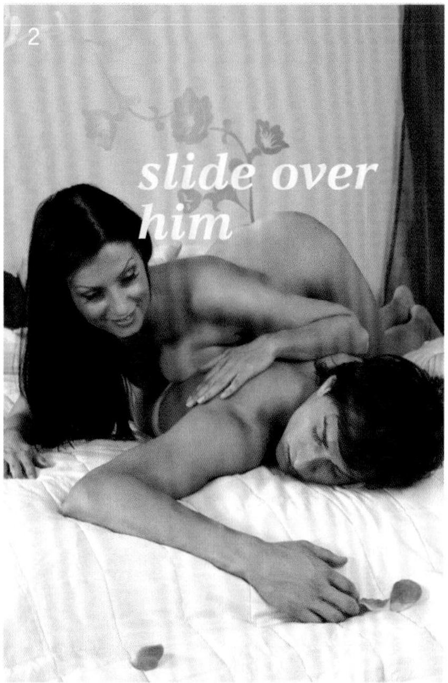
2
slide over him

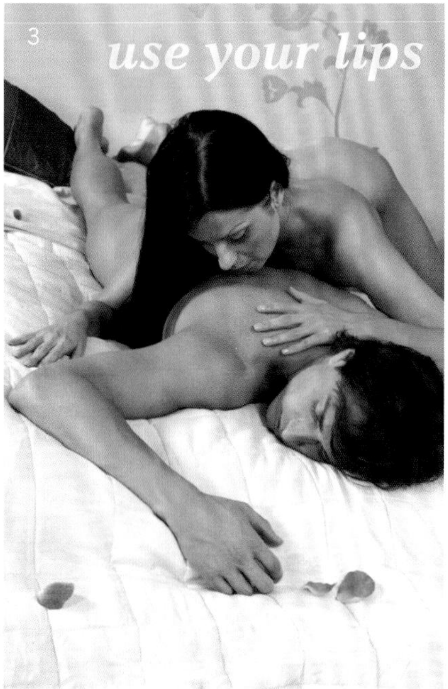
3
use your lips

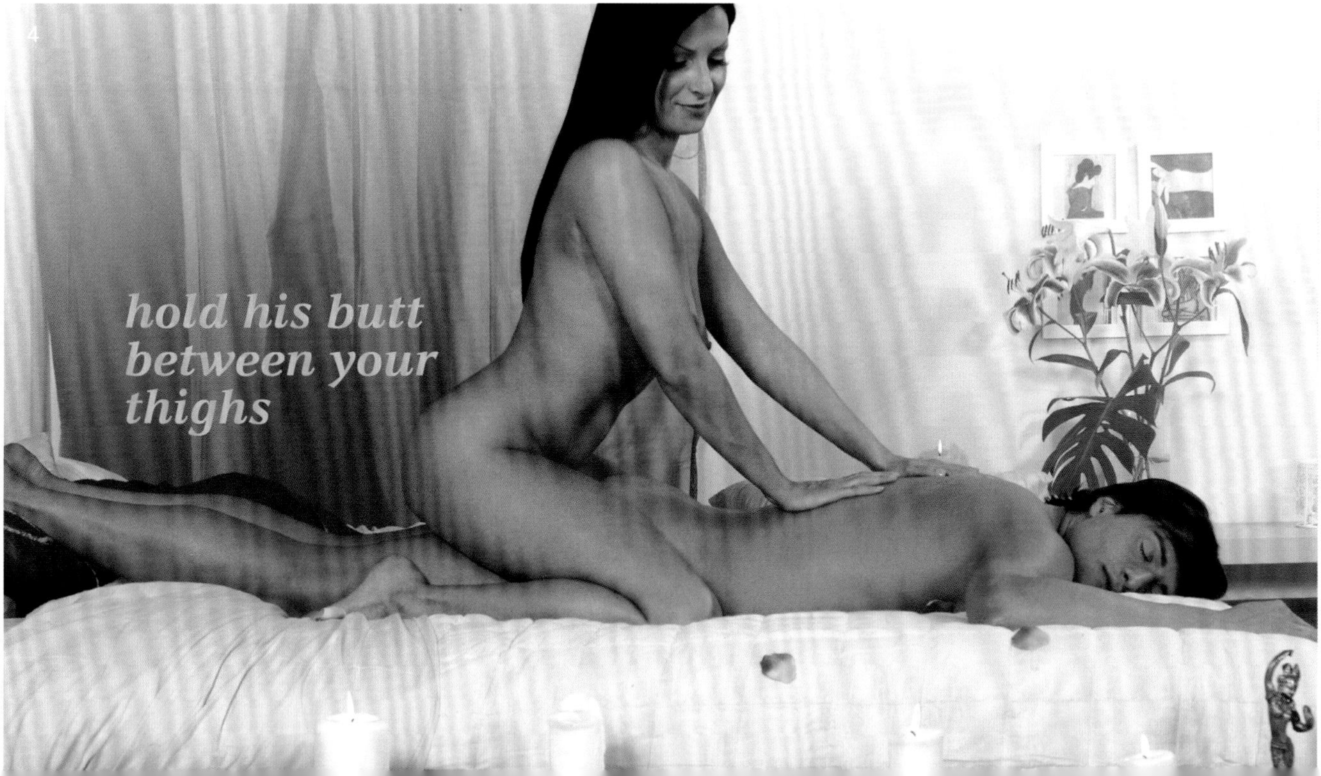
4
hold his butt between your thighs

Intimacy and Bonding

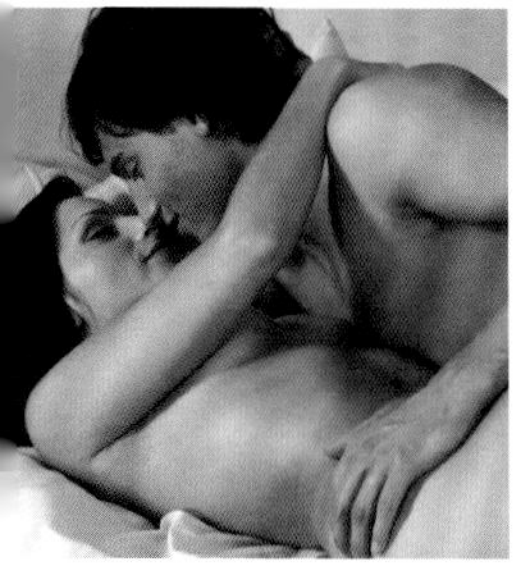

These special days are an occasion to better and more deeply know the body of the one you love and discover his/her desires and preferences. Little by little you will form a bond that will allow you both to share the deepest secrets of your souls. Encourage your partner to share his/her fantasies and dare to reveal your most personal intimacies.

After the massage it is more than likely you will want to make love. It's possible you won't want another massage, and so the one who has received will start off the next time. It will be fine if you remember to switch roles. Remember that in love it is as important to give as to receive.

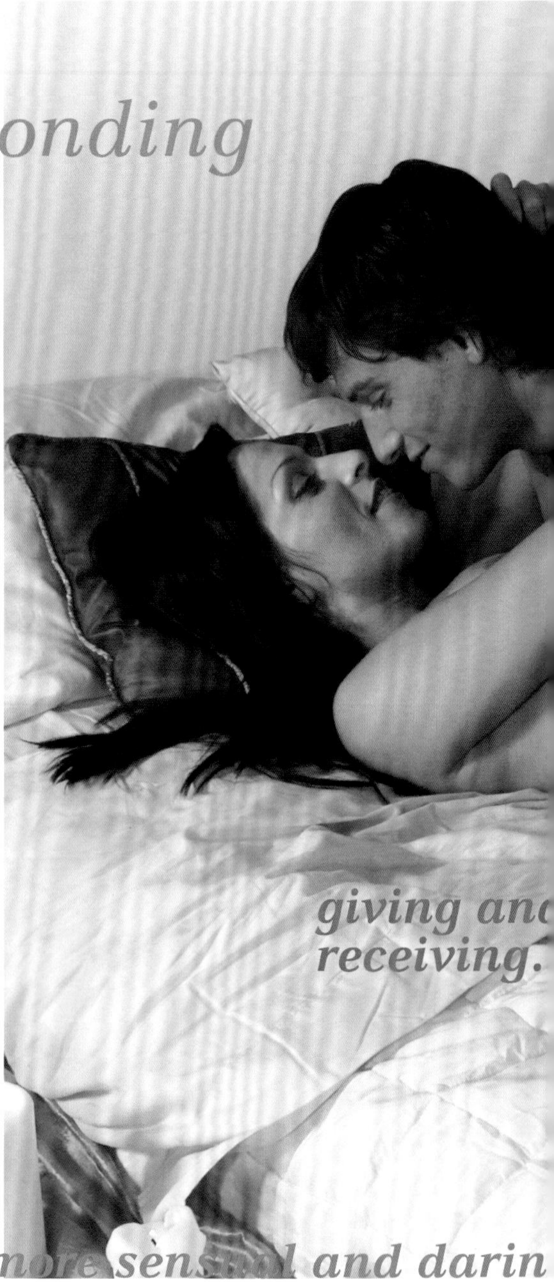

giving and receiving.

After the massage you can try more sensual and daring caresses.

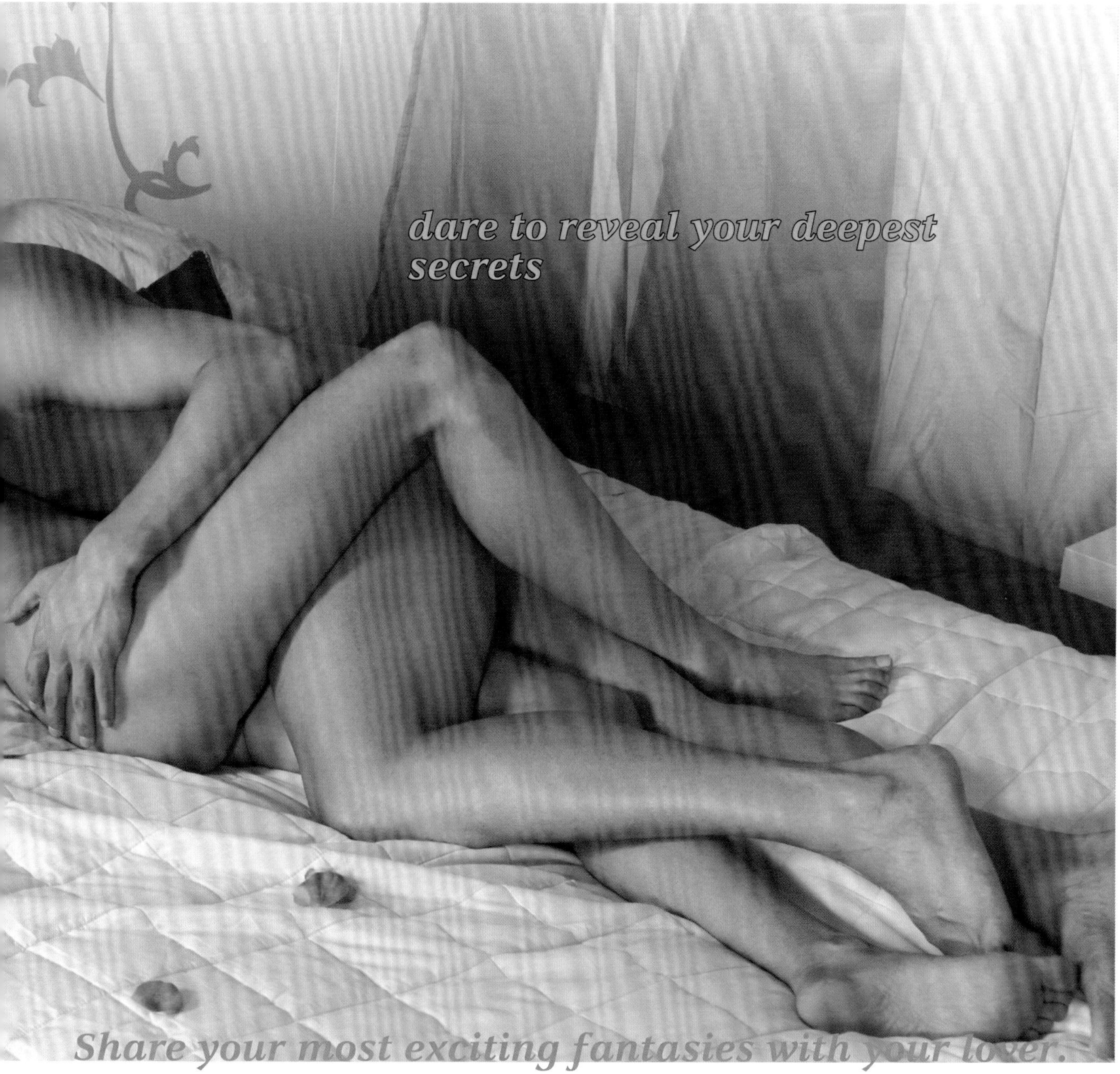

dare to reveal your deepest secrets

Share your most exciting fantasies with your lover.

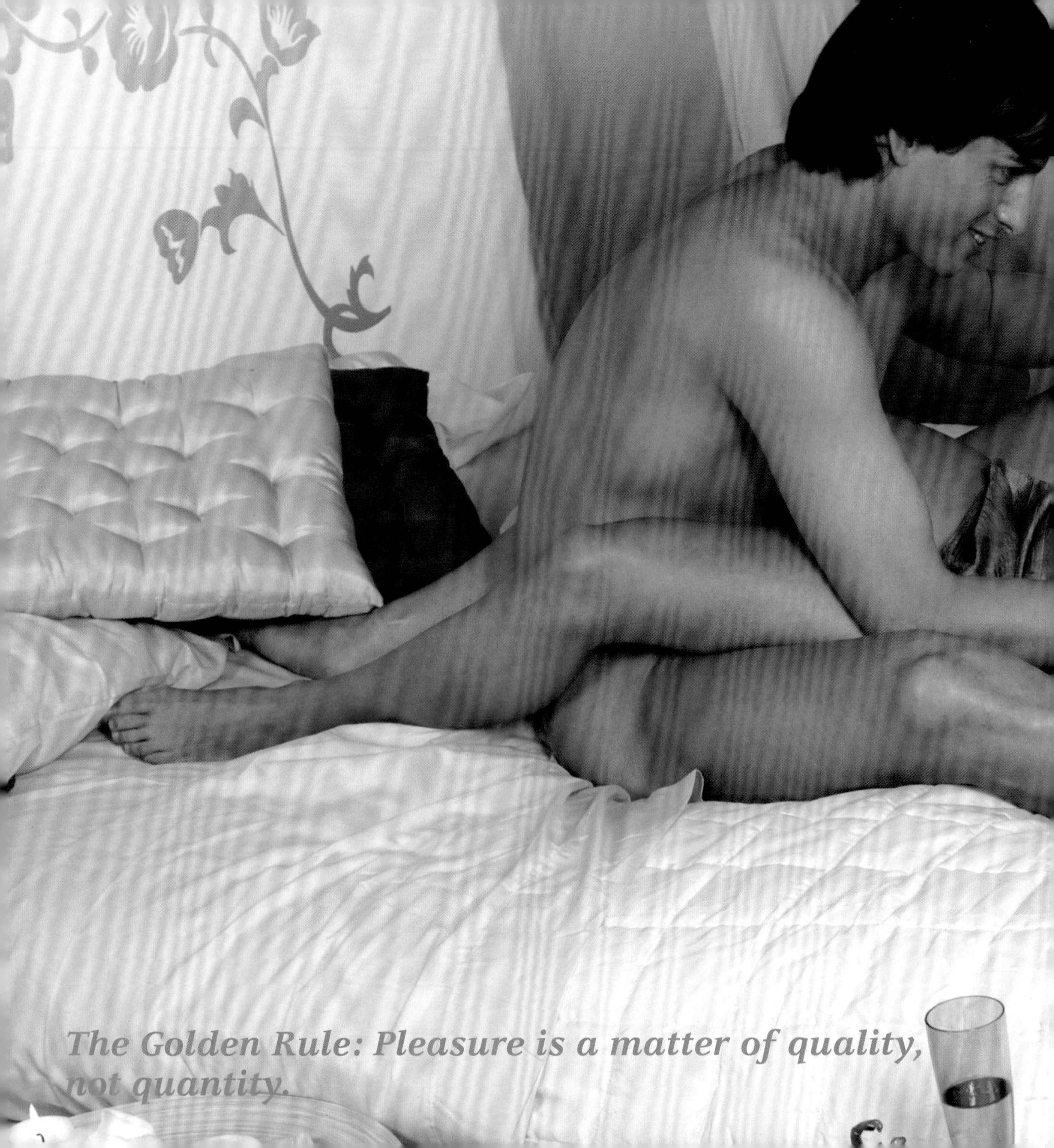

The Golden Rule: Pleasure is a matter of quality, not quantity.

An Hour of Pleasure

SIX QUICK MASSAGES

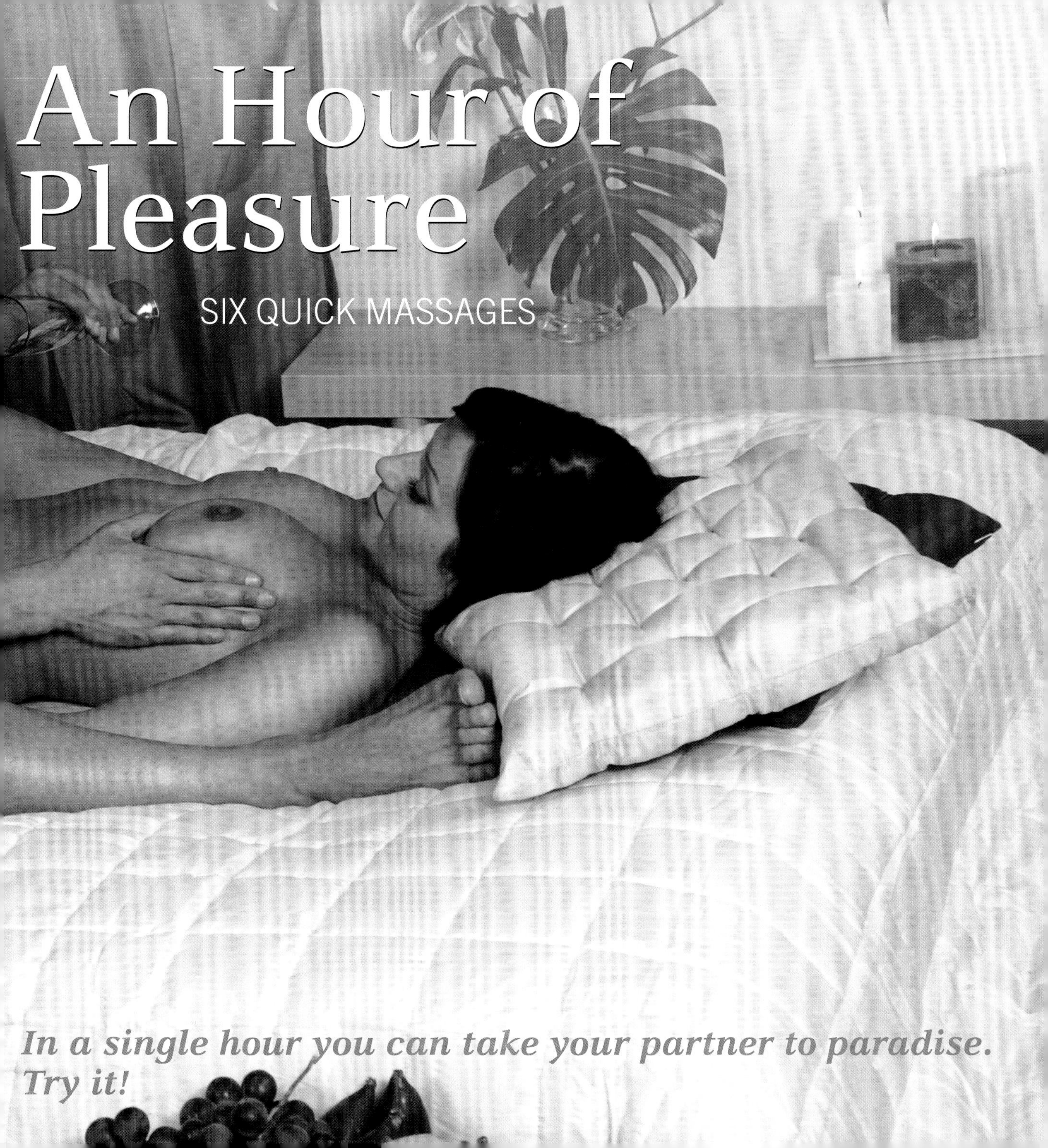

In a single hour you can take your partner to paradise. Try it!

Gluteals and Lumbar Area

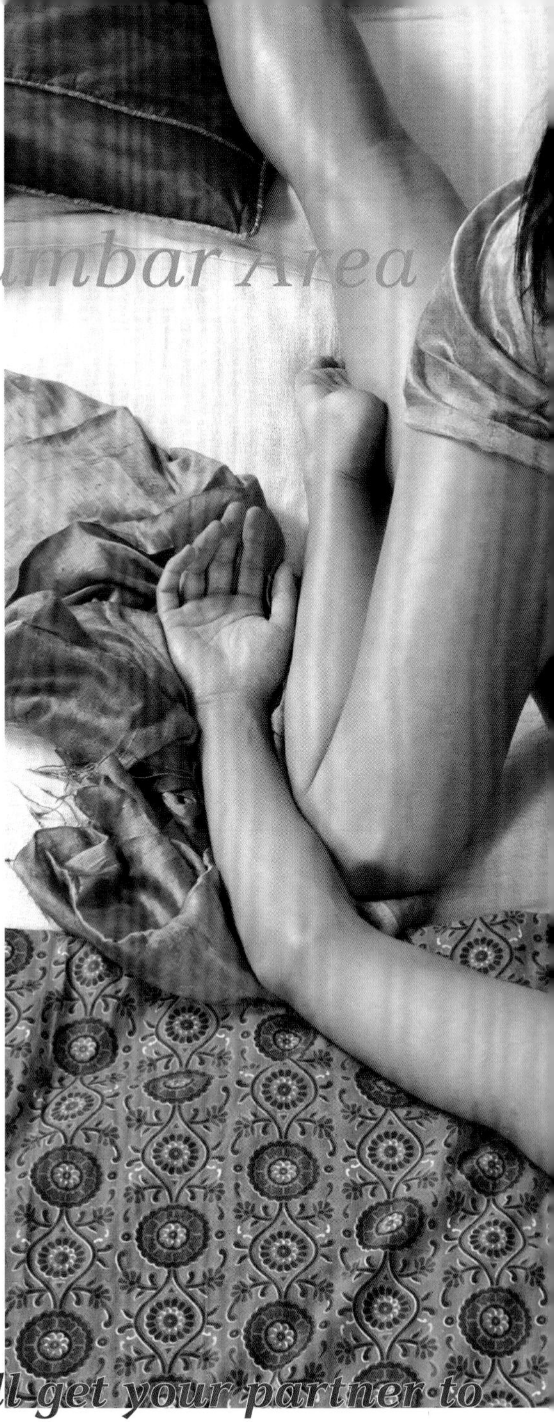

You already know that massaging the lumbar area and the gluteals is something especially erotic. This time we will include an important new element.

- In addition to using **fingertips, thumbs, and palms of the hands,** we will now use the **"Mount of Venus."**
- Massaging the gluteals with the genital zone is incredibly exciting for both partners.
- This time we suggest you choose a **blend of oils that contains sandalwood or jasmine**. This will maximize the erotic charge of the situation. Remember to keep the room temperature comfortable.
- Have available **two feathers, a brush, and several scarves.**

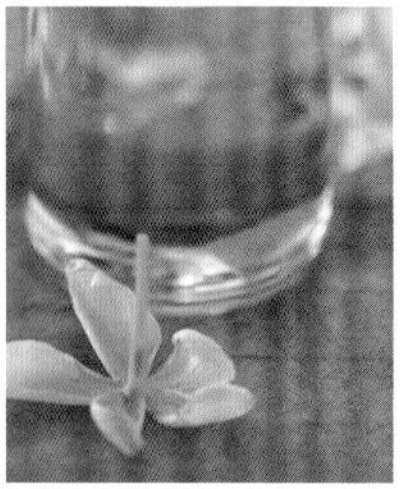

With this erotic massage you will get your partner to maximum excitation in record time.

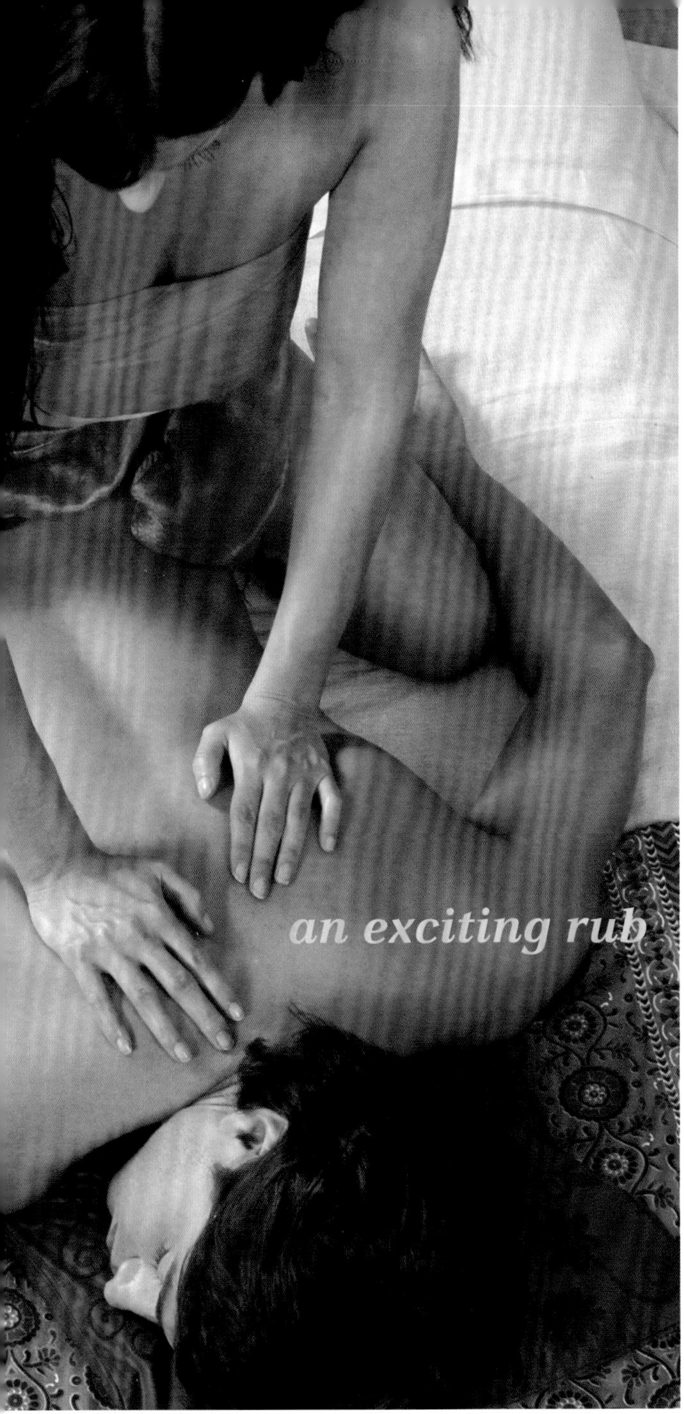
an exciting rub

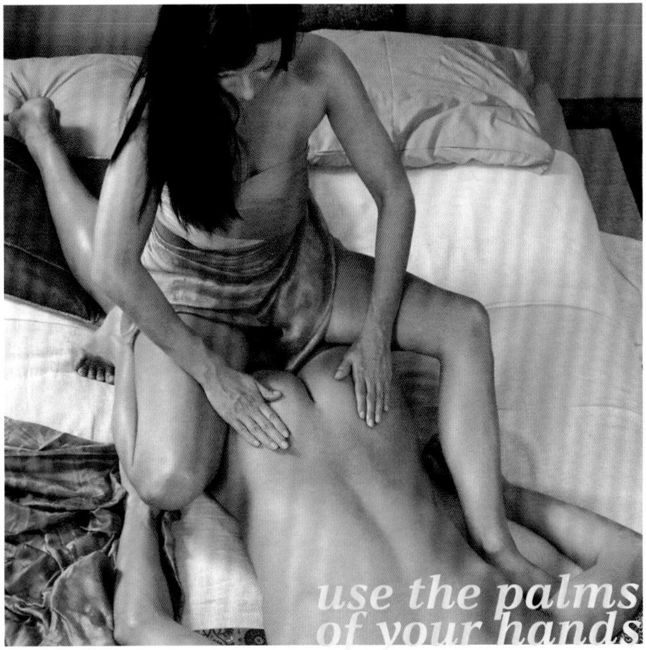
use the palms
of your hands

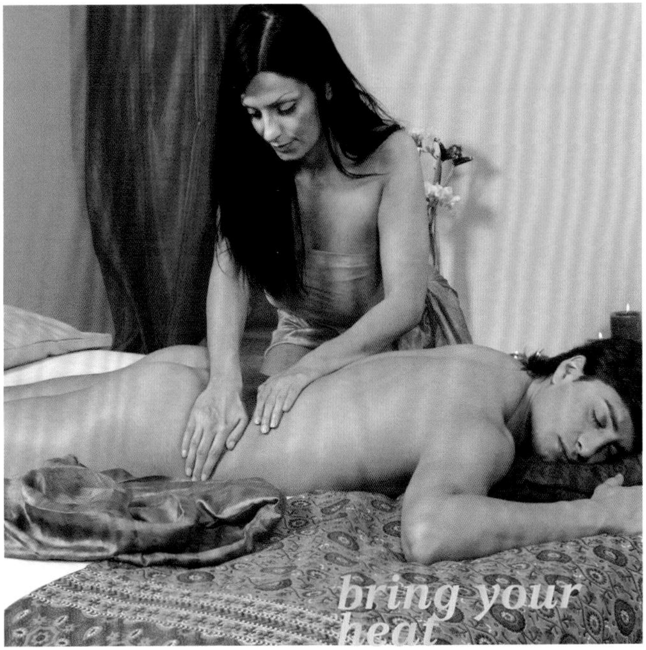
bring your
heat

Step by Step Gluteals and Lumbar Zone

Your partner is stretched out on their stomach with their arms relaxed along their sides.

1. Sit on your partner's right and put your hands on his/her back. Tune in to their body and get ready to give a massage.

2. Put sufficient oil on his/her back. Ask if they like the aroma as well as the pressure of your hands and the temperature.

3. Softly massage the lumbar zone with your fingertips, going upwards until you reach the neck. Then continue down your partner's arms until you reach their fingertips.

4. Continue by drawing soft waves with your fingertips, starting to the right of the spinal column and going outwards and then in toward the spine again. Do this ascending your partner's back. Repeat the same sequence on the left side.

5. Then slide your fingers from bottom to top on your partner's back. You will see how this arouses exciting sensations for your partner.

Now concentrate on the lumbar area. Place both your hands there with the thumbs side-by-side. Remember that at the level of the navel there is an area that, according to Oriental wisdom, contains highly stimulating points.

Make circles with your thumbs over all this area and change the pressure to what your partner likes.

Pay attention to your partner's reactions or just ask them how they are doing. Repeat the circular movements several times. You can use mouth or tongue or feathers and brushes. These will enhance the effect of your circular strokes.

6. Then use both hands to vibrate the point opposite the level of the navel.

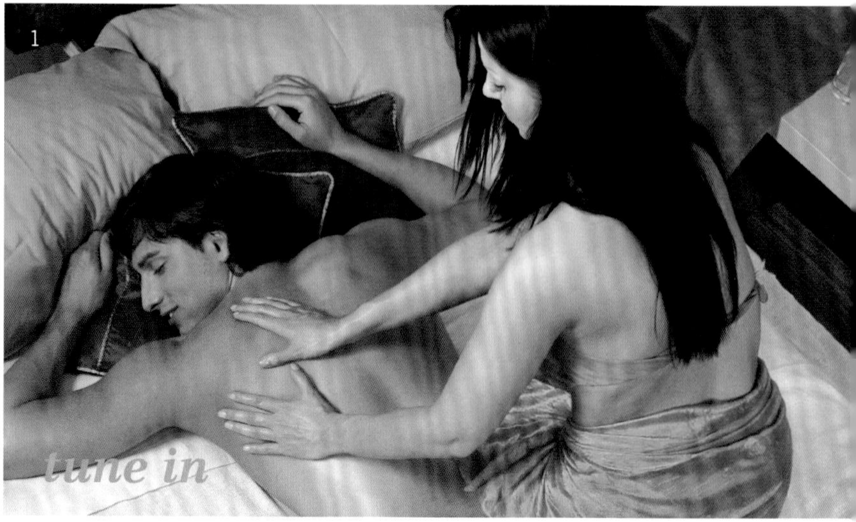

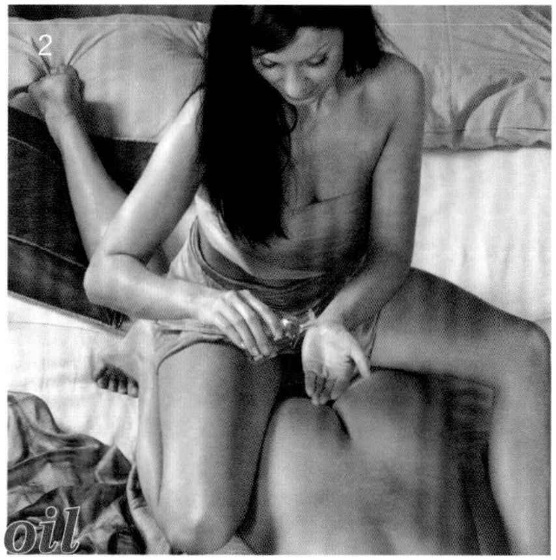
2
oil

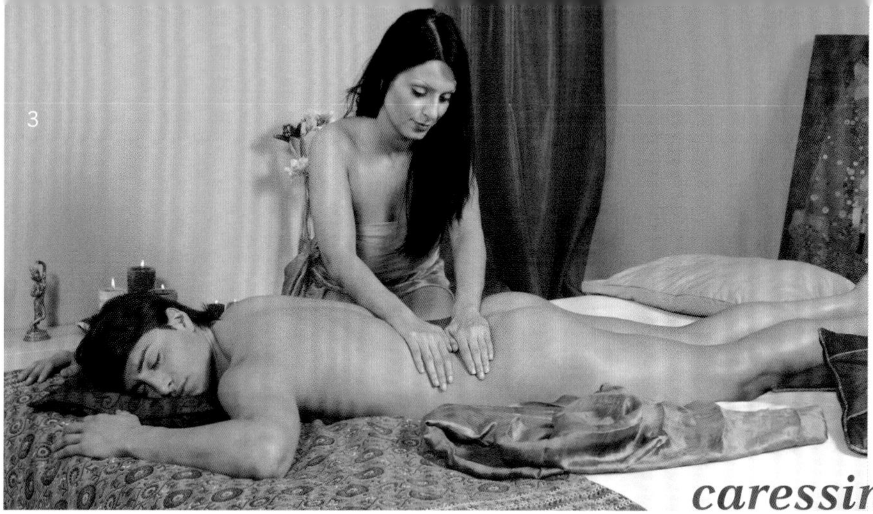
3
caressing

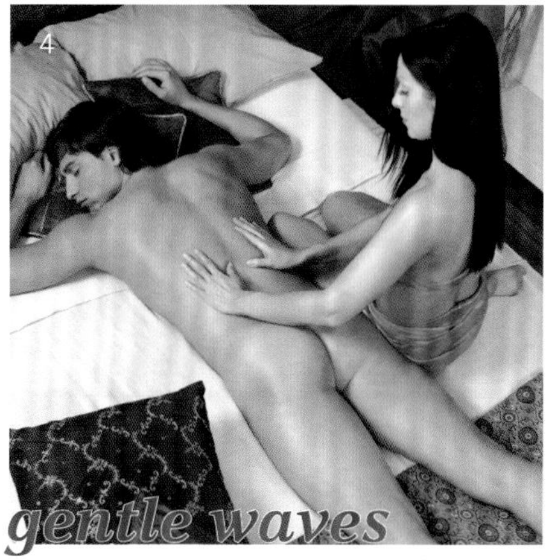
4
gentle waves

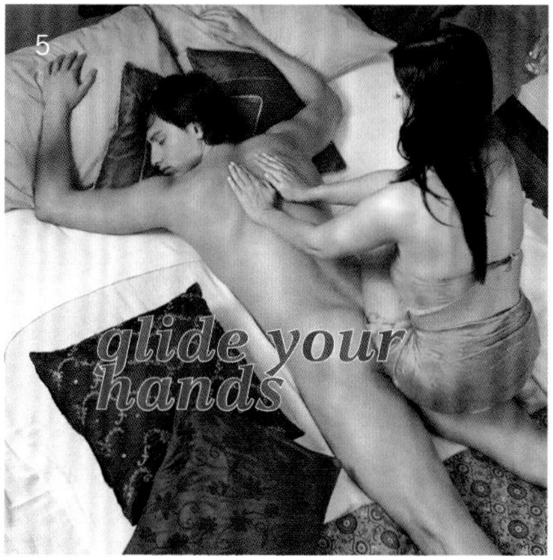
5
glide your hands

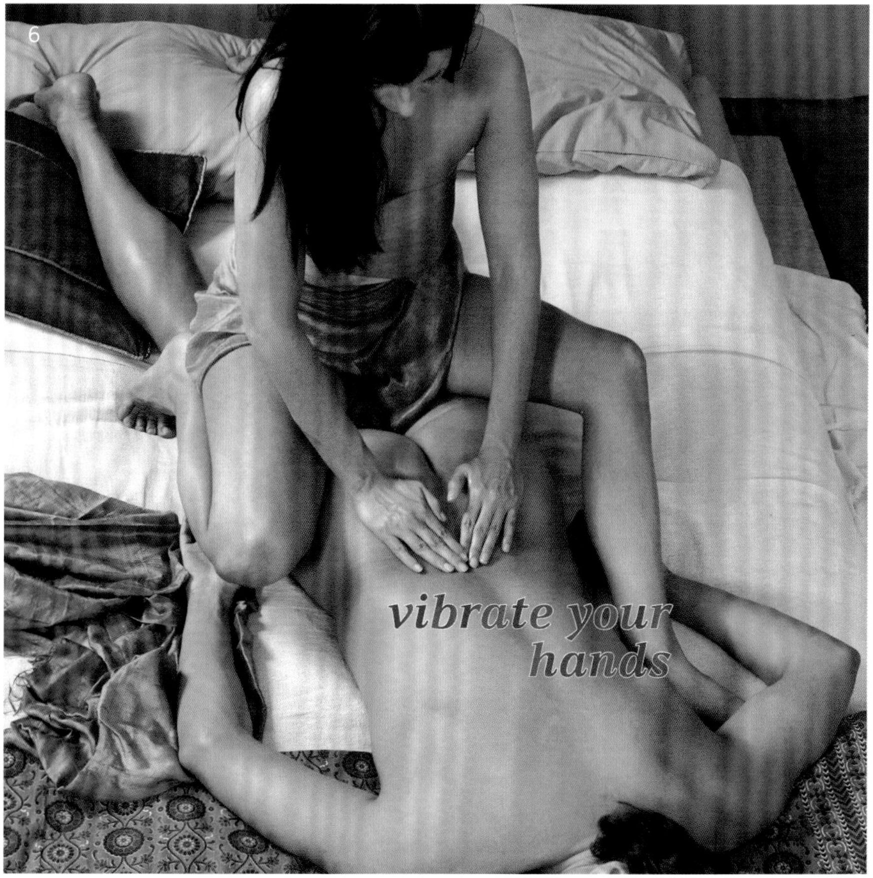
6
vibrate your hands

7. Put your hands on your partner's gluteals and make gentle circular movements inside to outside over the whole area.

Ask your partner if they like the intensity. Circular pressure on the butt is always a pleasure. Spend some time on this area.

To continue, use the base of the palm of your hands to apply gentle pressure. Knead like a cat does when it's preparing to nest. Go from below upwards until you arrive at the sacrum.

8. Now apply pressure with your left hand on your partner's left gluteal and your right hand on the right butt. Alternate the pressure one side at a time.

Then knead and massage both buttocks with soft, wide movements. This will alleviate the tensions that have accumulated in this area. Take your time with this and verify what pressure is adequate.

9. Take the right butt and make wave-like movements along the meridian points. With your left thumb, ply the skin against your right hand and continue with this wave of pressure.

10. Now push your right thumb against the edge of your left hand. Alternating your hands will form an undulating movement that will go from the pelvic area to the sacrum.

Work both gluteals the same way. You can sit astride your partner's thighs or change sides.

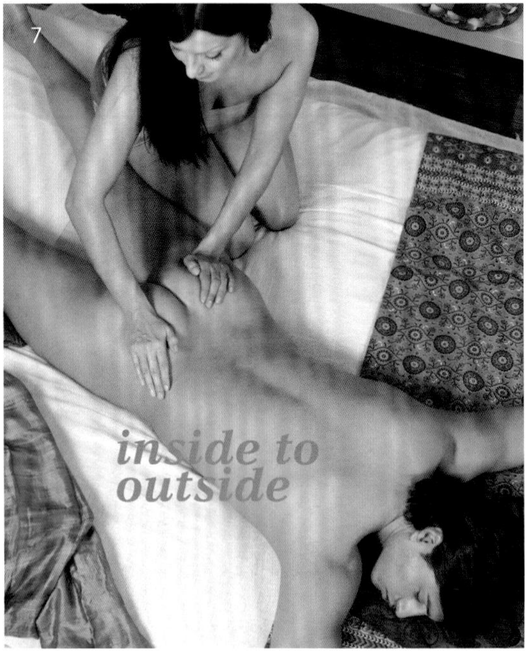

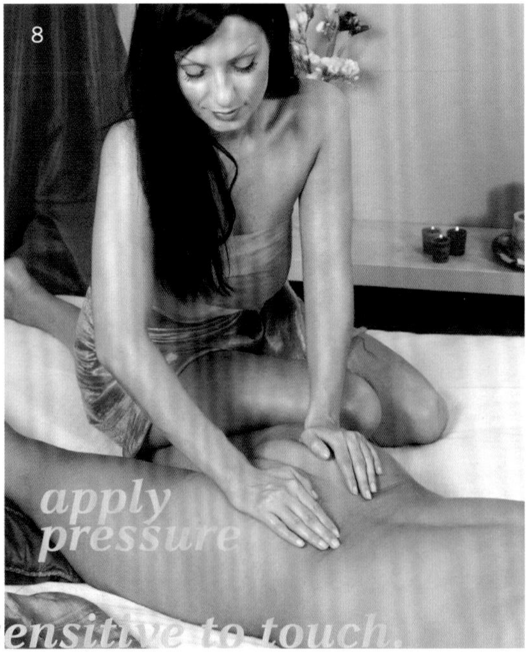

A man's gluteals are extremely sensitive to touch.

9

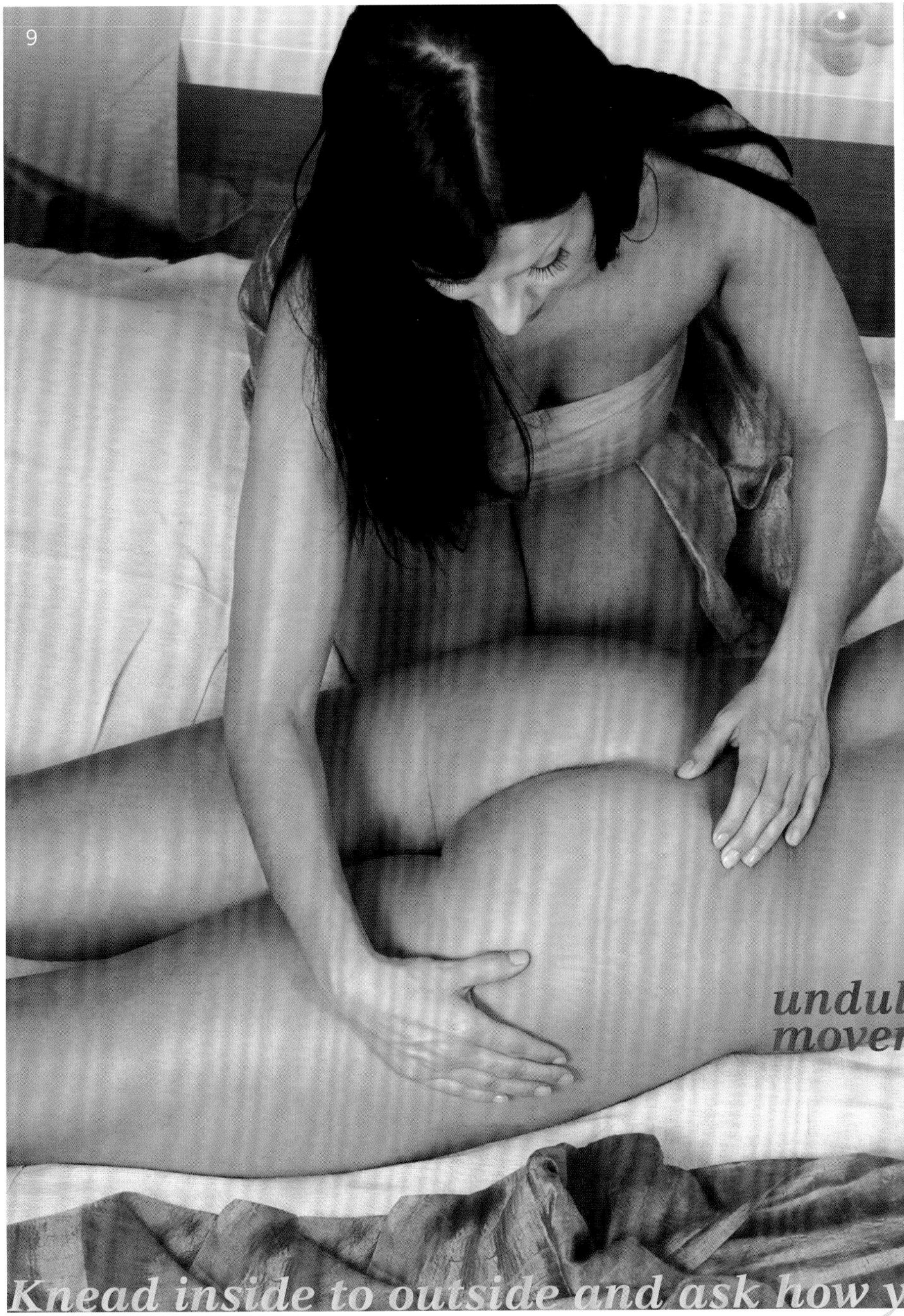

10

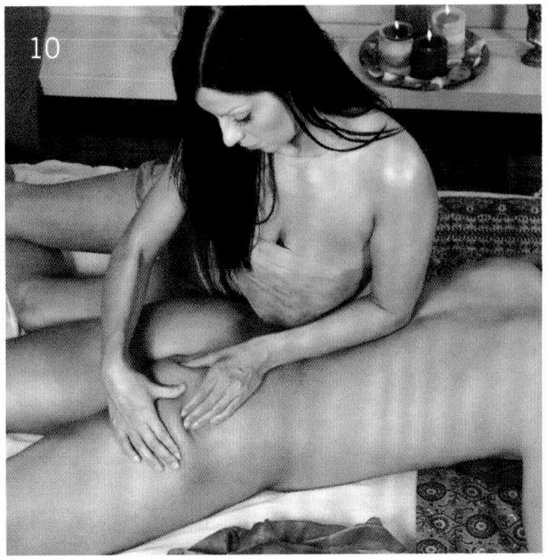

undulating movements

Knead inside to outside and ask how your partner likes it best.

A Delicate Tingle

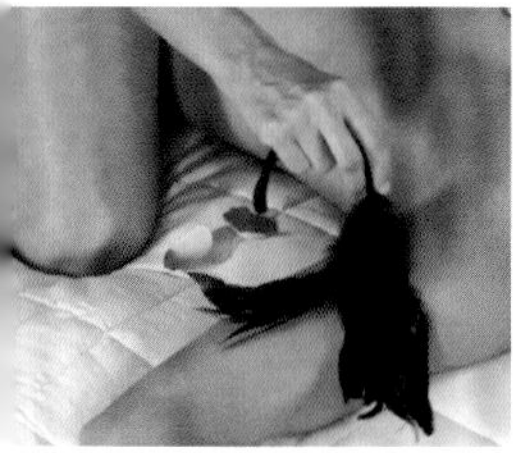

Use a feather and then a brush to trace wavy lines like you did before. Your lover will tremble with pleasure.

1. On the upper part of the buttock, in the sacral area, draw "figure 8s" with a feather and then with a brush. Make sure the motions are done slowly. This will produce a sensation that is both relaxing and exciting.

2. If you want to give more intense stimulation, use a makeup brush to deal with the wider area.

Take your time and ask your lover where they like it best. By this time your partner's sensitivity will have increased considerably.

3. Take two feathers and run them over the exterior of his/her butt up to the pelvis and then over the sacrum to the loins.

Move the feathers together toward the spinal column, cross them, and then go back to the pelvis. Do this several times.

You can end either with a massage or draw out the last tracings with the feathers on your partner's belly.

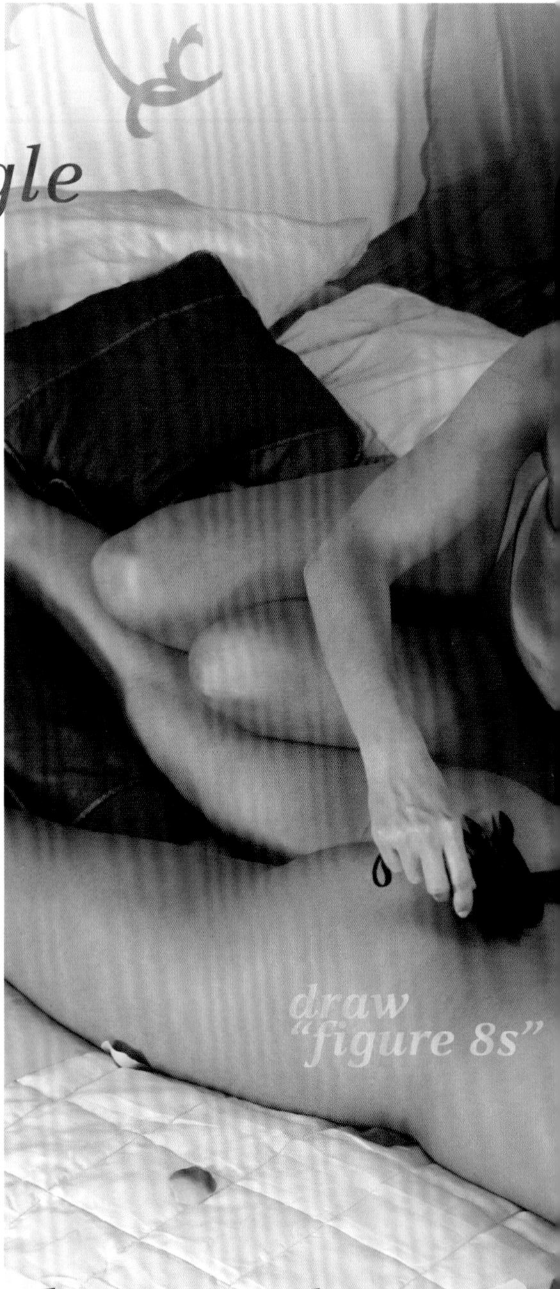

Make your partner tremble with pleasure and go over

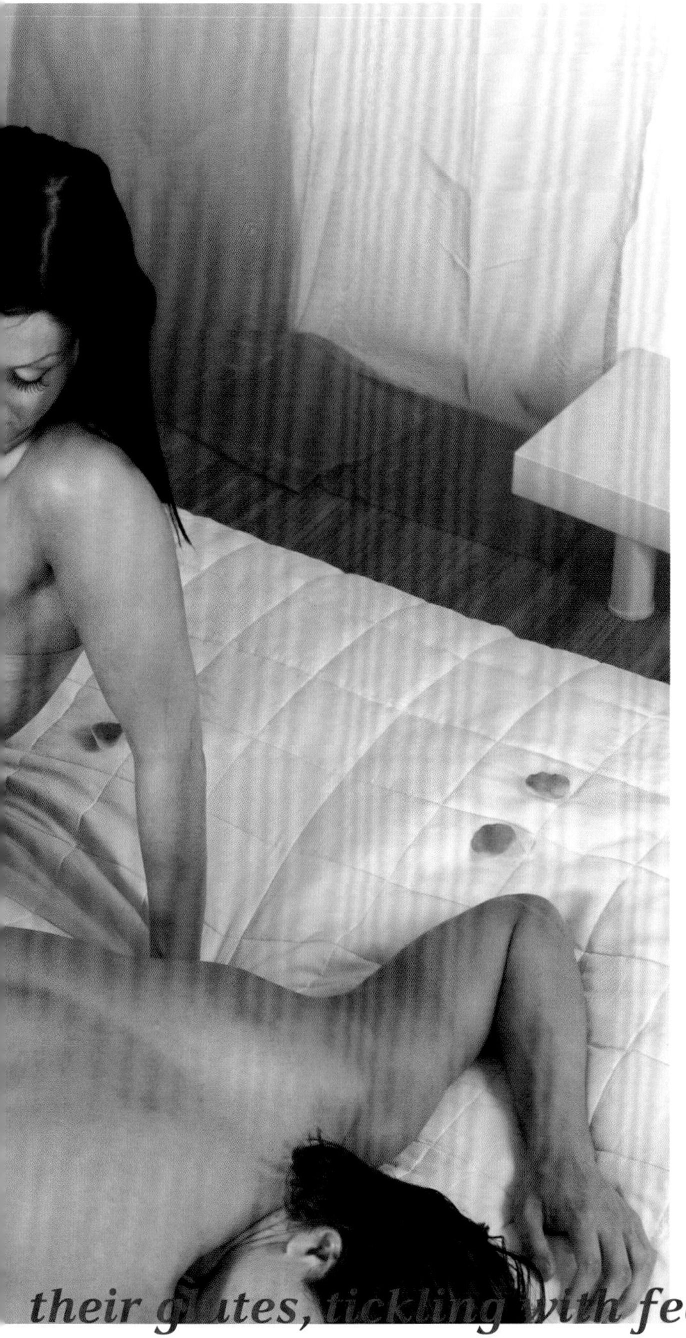

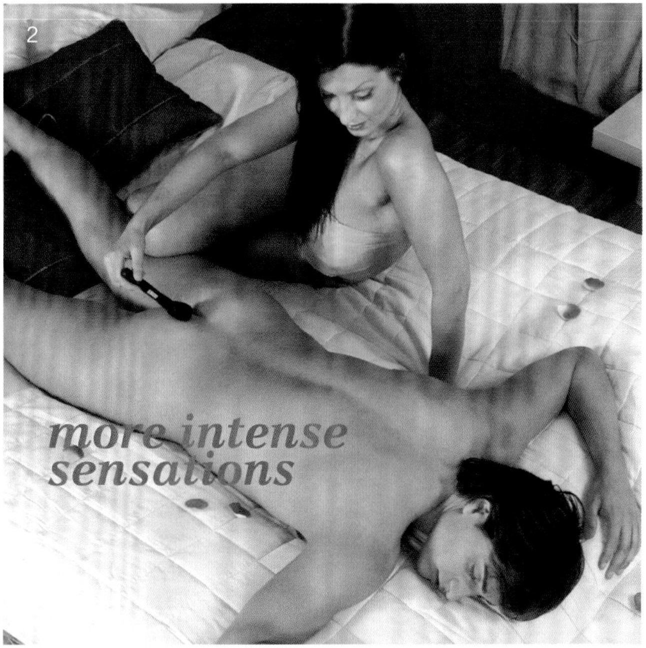

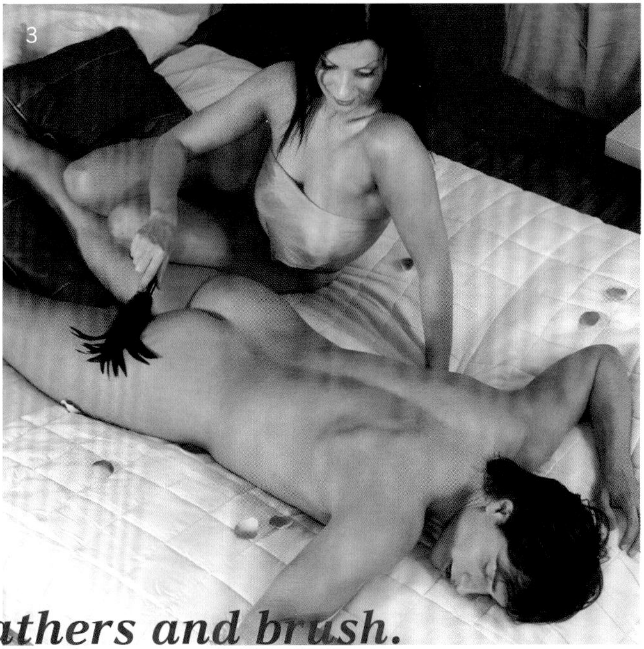

their glutes, tickling with feathers and brush.

A True Delight

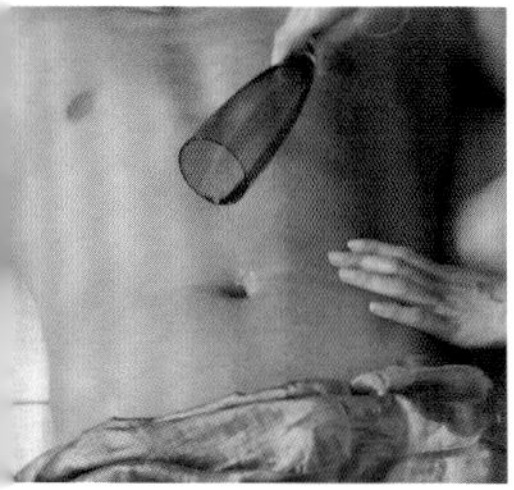

A massage of the abdomen is something stimulating and sensual by itself, but you can turn it into something even more enticing and appetizing. Simply add **champagne, yogurt, honey, or a fruit smoothie**.

The skin surrounding the navel and groin area down to the genitals is extremely sensitive. Experiencing the lips and tongue of your lover on this area can bring you to a really unusual level of excitement.

The pleasure goes both ways. To lick goodies from your partner's skin is very stimulating.

Preparation

- To prepare the **strawberry purée**, blend 10 ounces (300 g) of ripe strawberries with one-half glass of **champagne**. Put the resulting purée in a decorated jar or other container.
- You can add 2 drops of orange essence and 1 drop of vanilla extract. This will give the mix a more refined taste and aroma.
- If you want to try **honey**, just pour the amount you want into a little bowl.
- For this enjoyable and playful massage, **have your partner lie on a towel**. Keep in mind that strawberry stains are especially hard to remove.
- Have ready **two silk handkerchiefs**, feathers, and brushes. It is best to first stimulate your partner with these and later attempt the honey and strawberry mix.
- This time don't use oil for the massage. Place an **oil heater** in the area to provide an aromatic backdrop to the room.

Enjoy a refreshing banquet on your lover's belly!

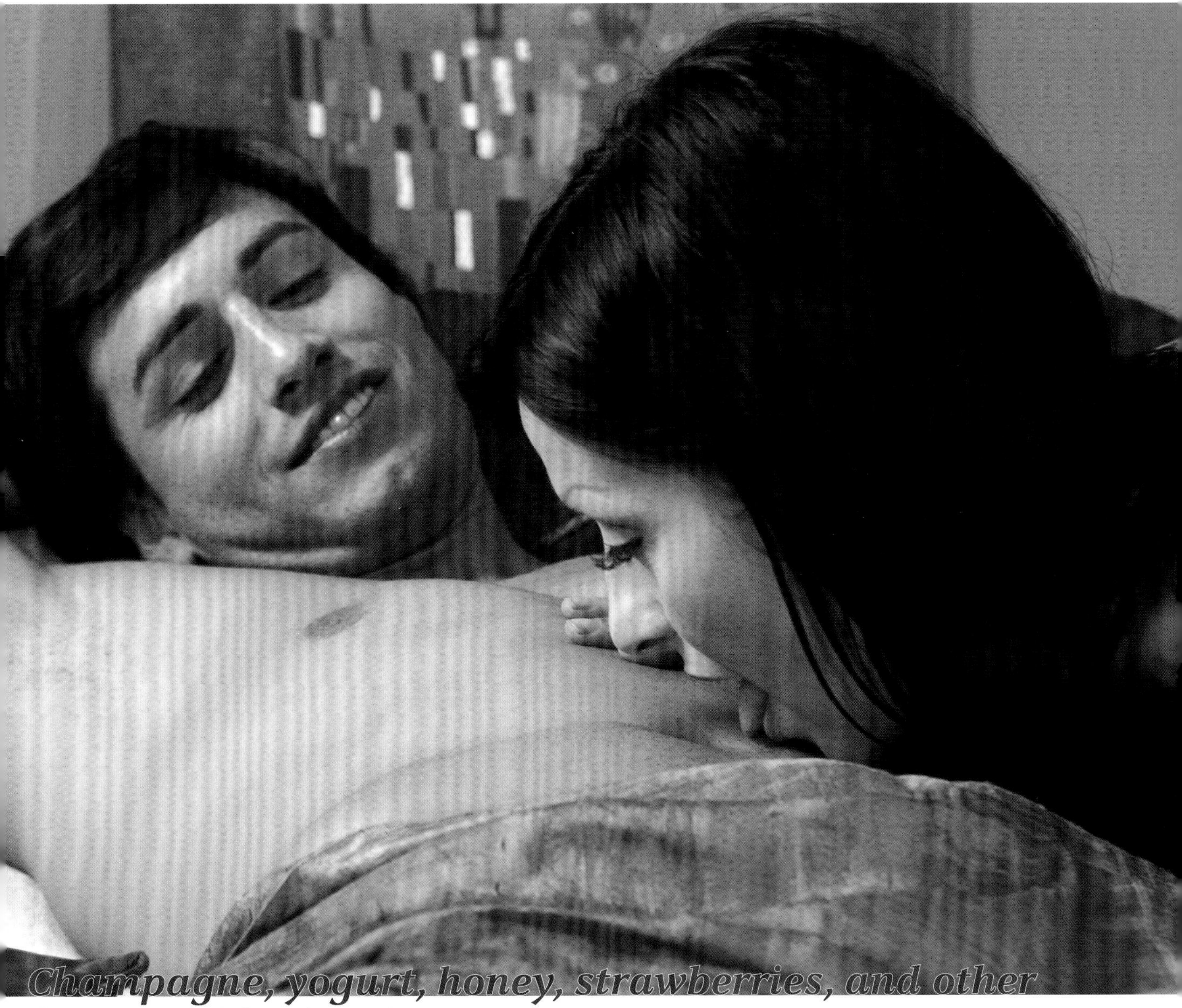

Champagne, yogurt, honey, strawberries, and other fruits will ignite the passion.

Step by Step: A True Delight

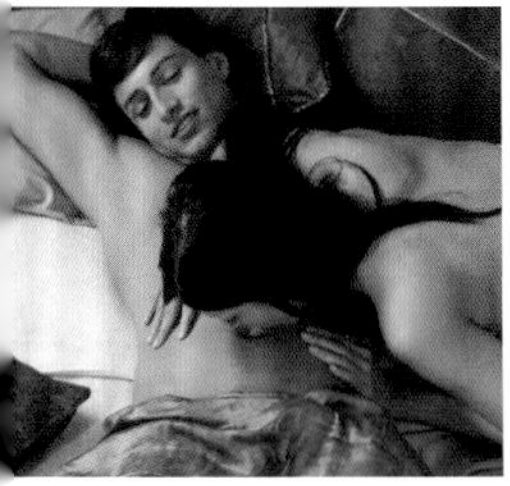

Your partner should be lying on his/her back, relaxed. If you notice any goose bumps, cover their chest with some scarves.

1. Begin by tracing large and small circles around your partner's navel with a silk scarf. Go clockwise.

Then move on to the solar plexus area and later on to the genitals.

Using a second scarf, make small circles at the level of the navel and upwards and outwards along the groin, passing over the Mount of Venus, and then back to the start.

Repeat this pattern several times. Change rhythms and make the cloths move in opposite directions.

Your partner will totally enjoy these slow and sensual movements of silk.

Later exchange the scarves for a brush and run over your partner's abdomen with circles, outward or inward.

If you've chosen a makeup brush, begin drawing small circles and gradually increase their size. If you see your partner shivering, press a little harder.

After this, you partner will be ready for new thrills. Get the strawberry purée and ladle it onto his/her belly.

2. If you prefer to use just honey alone simply pour it using a spoon and draw circles or even a heart around their navel as a sweet declaration of love.

Then give yourselves a special treat by licking the goodies directly from their belly. Use your tongue and go over the abdomen down to the genitals. This way you will announce the pleasures to come and cause much excitement and the desire to continue.

Lick and enjoy running your tongue and lips over this sensitive area that leads to the genitals. You can even go a little bit lower, if you feel like it.

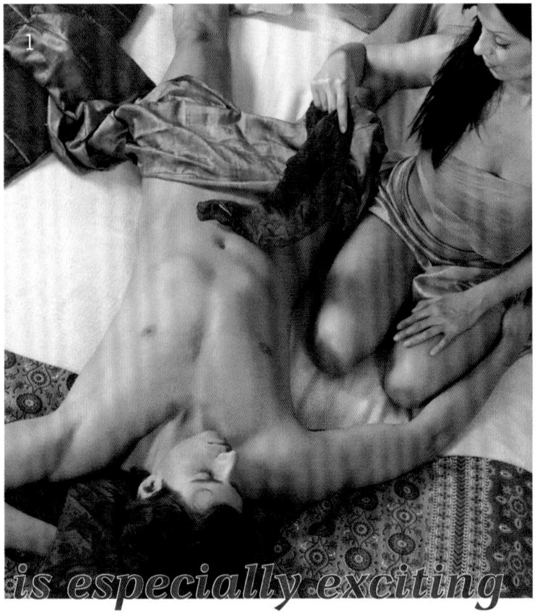

Stimulating your partner's belly is especially exciting and pleasant.

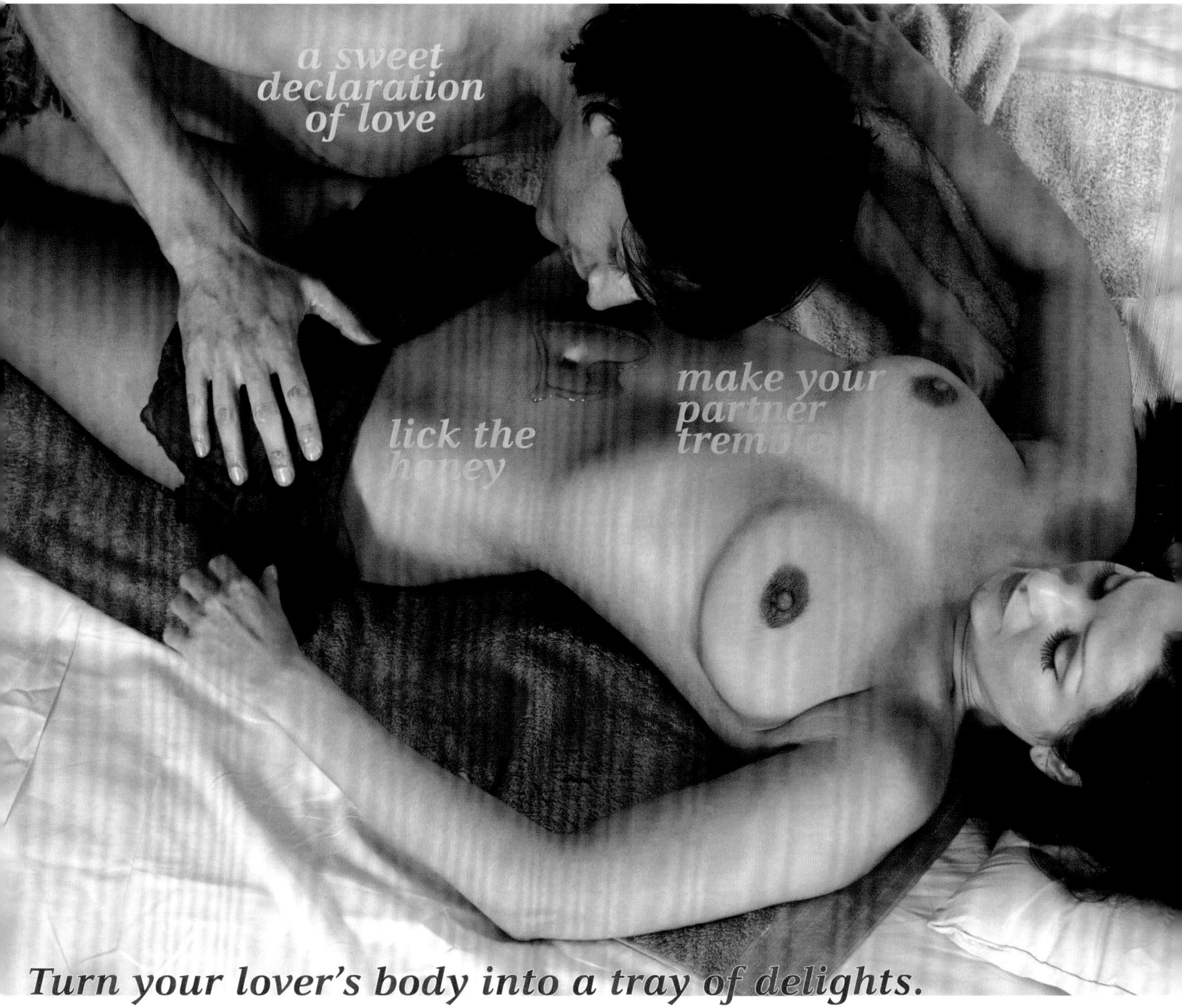

Turn your lover's body into a tray of delights.

Persephone's Green Clay

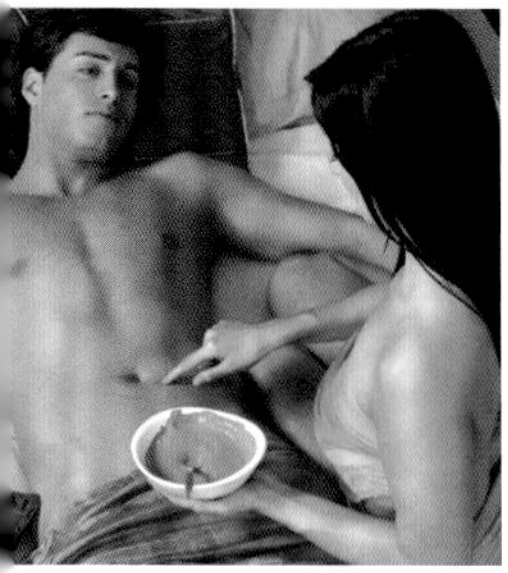

draw circles on their skin as a sweet declaration of love

Moving on, we offer you another playful variety for a pleasant belly massage.

Green clay, in addition to its inviting aroma, has a very luxurious consistency.

It is a total revelation. If you try it, you will want to repeat it.

Preparation

- You can buy **green clay** at virtually any natural health food store. To prepare it follow the instructions and simply mix the indicated amount of lukewarm water with the green powder.
- It's a good idea for the one receiving the treatment to lie **on a towel** to catch any drops.
- You will also need **two silk scarves and a broad brush** so you can begin with the same stimulation we showed you involving the strawberry purée or honey.

Step by Step

1. Start with the silk scarves and later with the brush in the same way we indicated in the "Step by Step" section of the previous massage.
2. Continue by applying green clay using the three fingers of your right hand. Spread it over the abdomen with either one or two hands.

Make circles around the navel with one hand. Make the circles progressively bigger and ask your partner how he/she is feeling.

3. You can let your imagination go when you paint with green clay. You can draw shapes, letters, or even a declaration of love. Take your time and enjoy, using various movements, and sliding your hands over the clay any way you like, with pleasure.

Use your thumbs to draw a line from the navel to the genitals and back by way of the groin to the navel again. Go over this route several times.

When you finish, remove the clay with a bath mitten and scented warm water. You can use essence of myrtle or rose (Aphrodite's favorites). You lover's skin will feel as smooth as silk.

If this massage has enticed you to try even more things, you will find a schedule of special treats for both him and her in the following material.

The pleasing aroma and exquisite touch of green clay

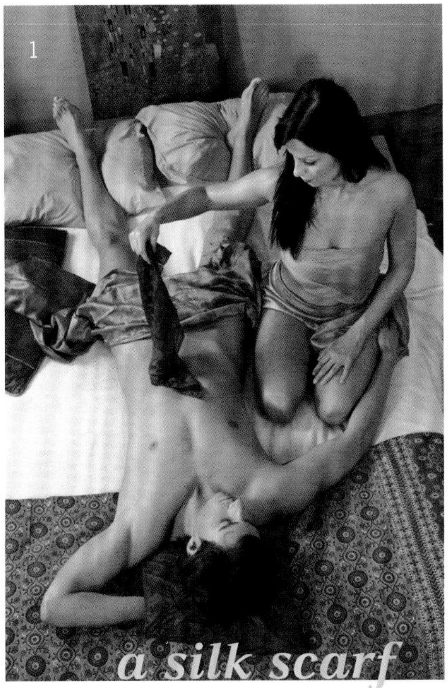

1

a silk scarf

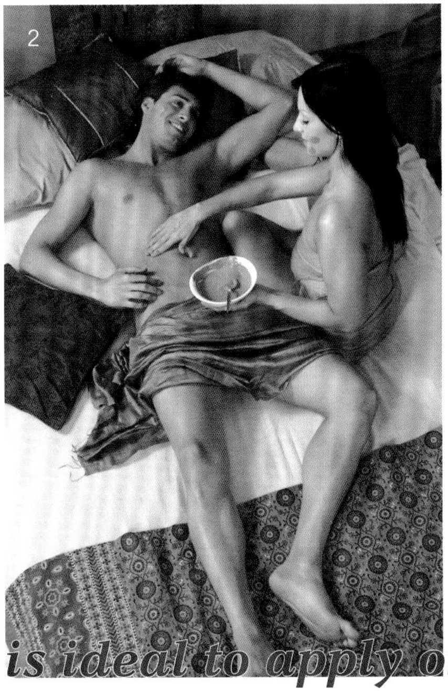

2

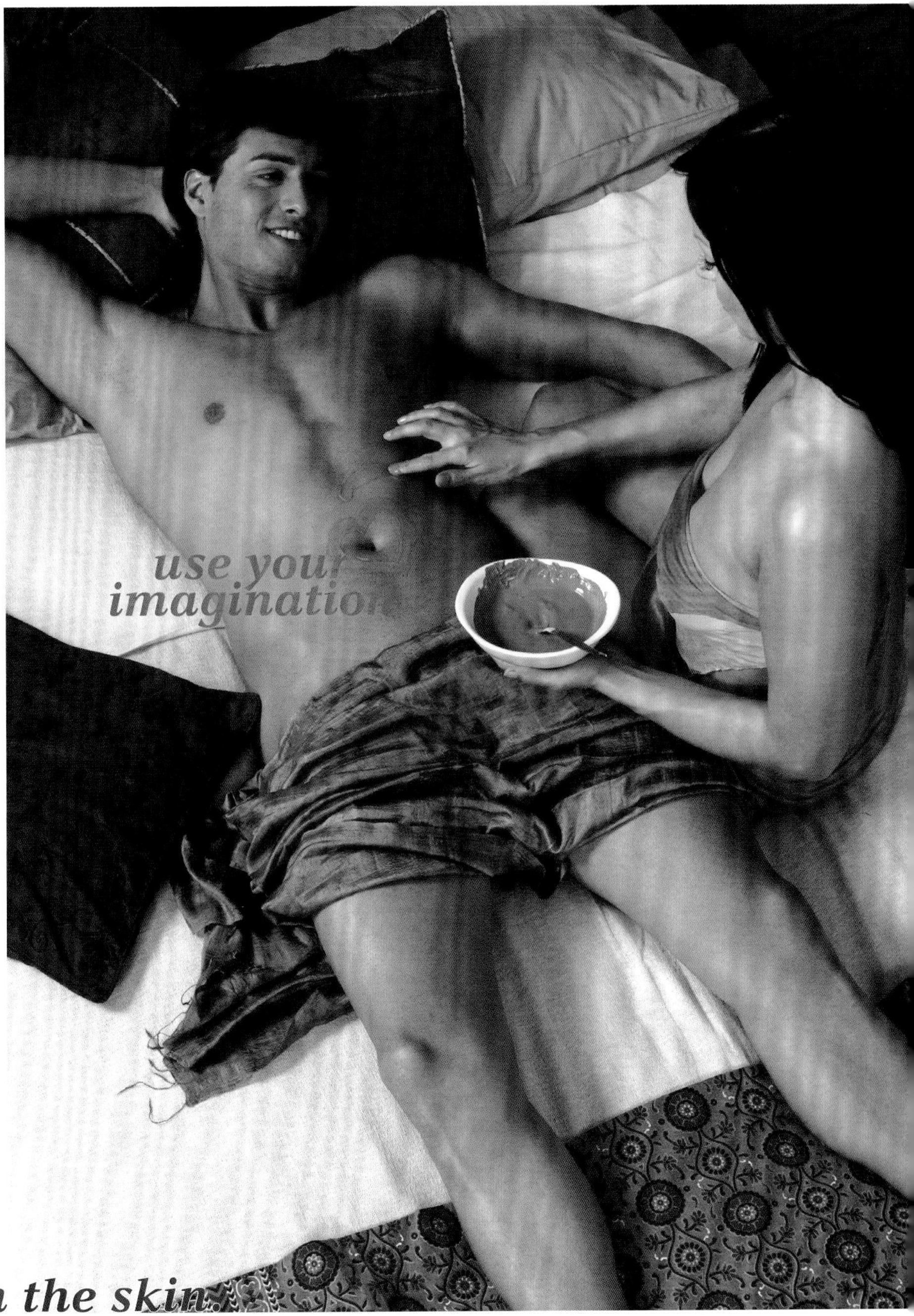

use your imagination

is ideal to apply on the skin.

Semiprecious Stones for Him

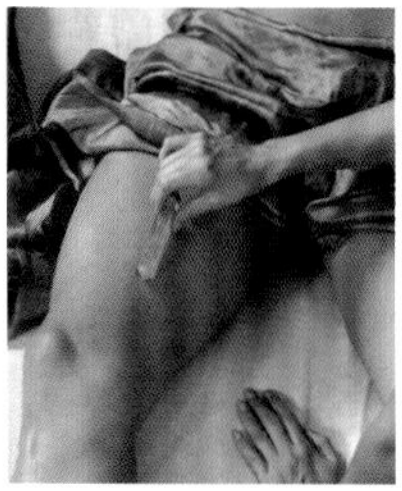

gently draw "figure 8s" with the crystal . . .

Now we will describe a massage for the thighs, ideal after our journey over the abdomen. It is a very exciting massage, suitable for both him and her, but this time we are going to concentrate on him.

Preparation

- You will need **silk scarves** and some semi-precious stones. Most common are **quartz crystal, amethyst, or rose quartz**, but you can choose whatever suits your taste and pocketbook. You will find these stones at the jewelers, stores that sell spiritual/esoteric items, or gem shops.

- Keep in mind that each stone has specific beneficial properties relating to health. It is said rose quartz promotes tenderness, quartz crystal furthers energy flow, and amethyst is for harmony. We are not interested, right now, in these properties, but in the stimulating effect that results from putting these smooth, cool stones on your partner's skin.

Step by Step

Begin by running the scarves on the inside of his thigh going from the knee to the genitals. Then go from the groin to the outer part of the thigh and back again to the knee. Repeat this pattern several times.

Continue by making small circles with the stone on the inside of the right thigh from the beginning of the leg to the kneecap.

Repeat the same circular movements on his left thigh and make sure to go over the points of sexual stimulation that lie there.

Now draw "figure 8s" with the point of the crystal. Do this on the inner part of the right thigh from the knee to the groin.

Pass on next to the exterior of the right thigh and down to the knee making "eights" and then returning up the inner part of the thigh.

Repeat this circuit several times, always beginning with the knee and ending with "eights" on the groin.

Repeat the entire process on both legs alternately until you notice you have obtained effective sensual stimulation.

Scarves and gemstones

For a final touch gently massage your partner's perineum with your fingertips. The perineum is the area between his penis and anus. It is also known as the masculine "G" spot.

The perineum is extremely delicate and sensitive. Don't forget to ask your companion if he likes you massaging there and how much pressure to apply.

If you feel your partner is too excited and you still want to continue the massage, use a cold cloth or spray scented water on his abdomen or genitals. This has a refreshing effect and will help calm him down and let you continue with these wonderful preliminaries.

To restart his fire you can kiss or caress his points of sexual stimulation.

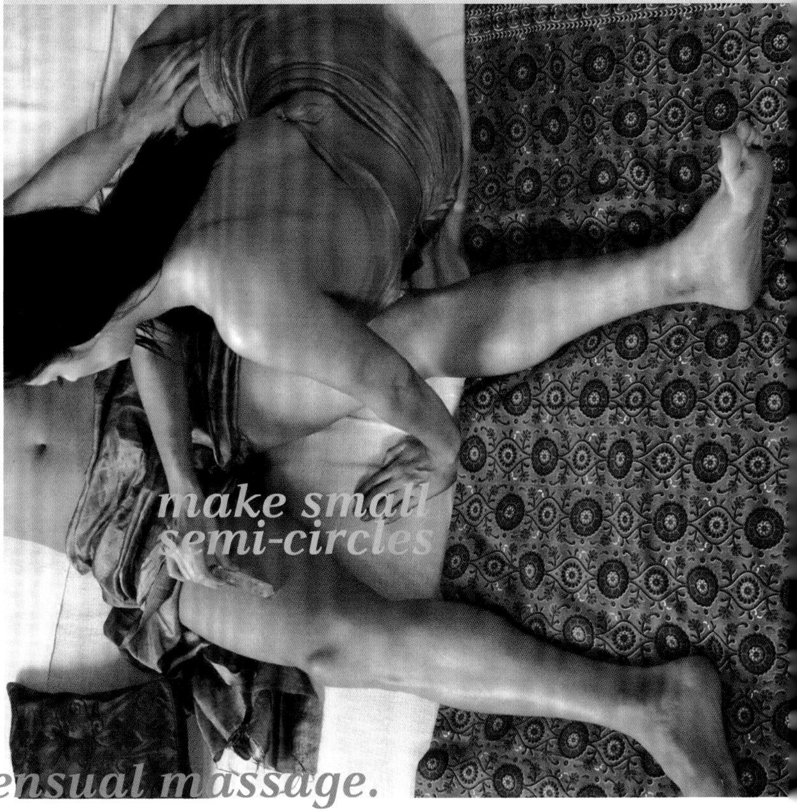

will be perfect for this sensual massage.

Mint Powder for Her

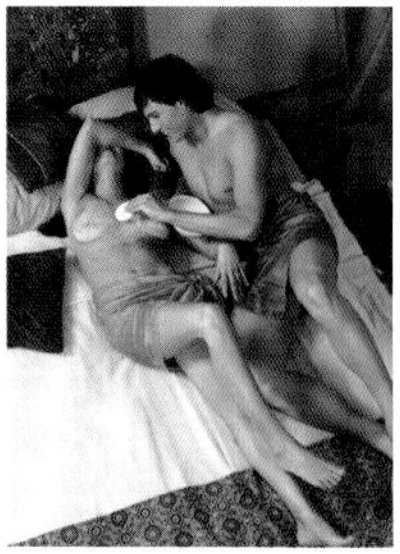

delicate, soft strokes of mint

Here is a chest massage for her using acacia honey. It is the ultimate sensual pleasure for women. Men without a lot of chest hair can also try this.

Preparation

- Take a **pretty crystal jar** and pour in the amount of honey you will need.
- You will also need on hand a pair of **silk handkerchiefs.**
- We suggest you practice massaging with powder. For this you will need **talcum powder and a wide brush or powder puff**. You will use about 2 ounces (50 g) of talc and 1 drop of mint oil that you can mix in a porcelain mortar.

Step by Step

1. Sit on your partner's right. Since we are going to perform a special massage we will start with the handkerchiefs. Use them to massage her breasts, her belly, and her genital area.

Using a tablespoon, drip honey on her breasts, making circles over their contours.

Next, spread the honey with your fingers following the trail of its dribbling. Drip some honey on her nipples and make small circles around their contours.

It's probable by now she is quite excited and her nipples are hard. But the most exciting part for both will be when you suck the honey following its flow pattern.

2. Mint powder is a good alternative to honey. Dip a brush in the powder or use the powder puff and go over her breasts softly and all over their contours.

The aroma and texture of mint powder will awaken her desire.

1

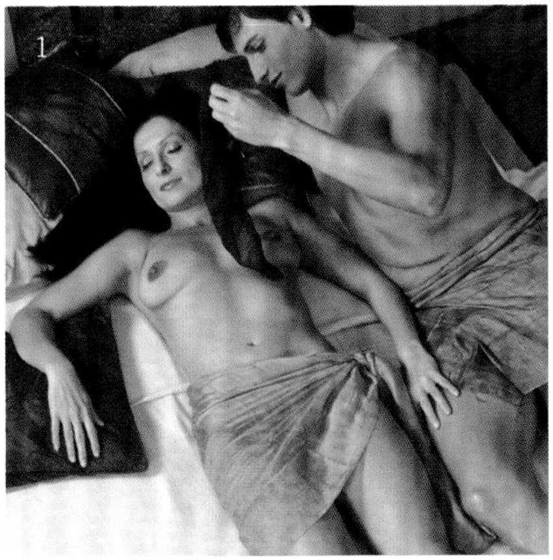

2

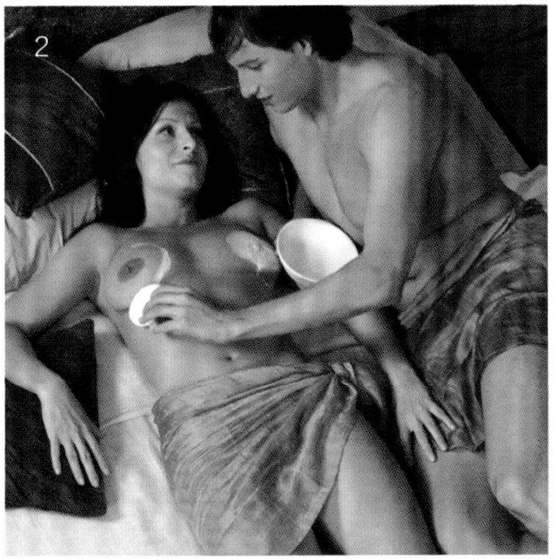

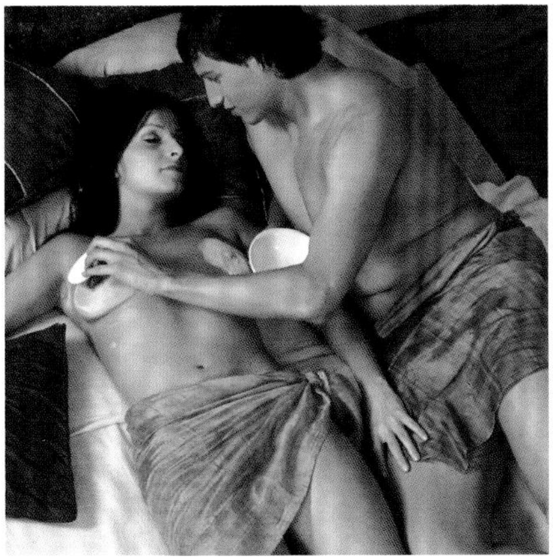

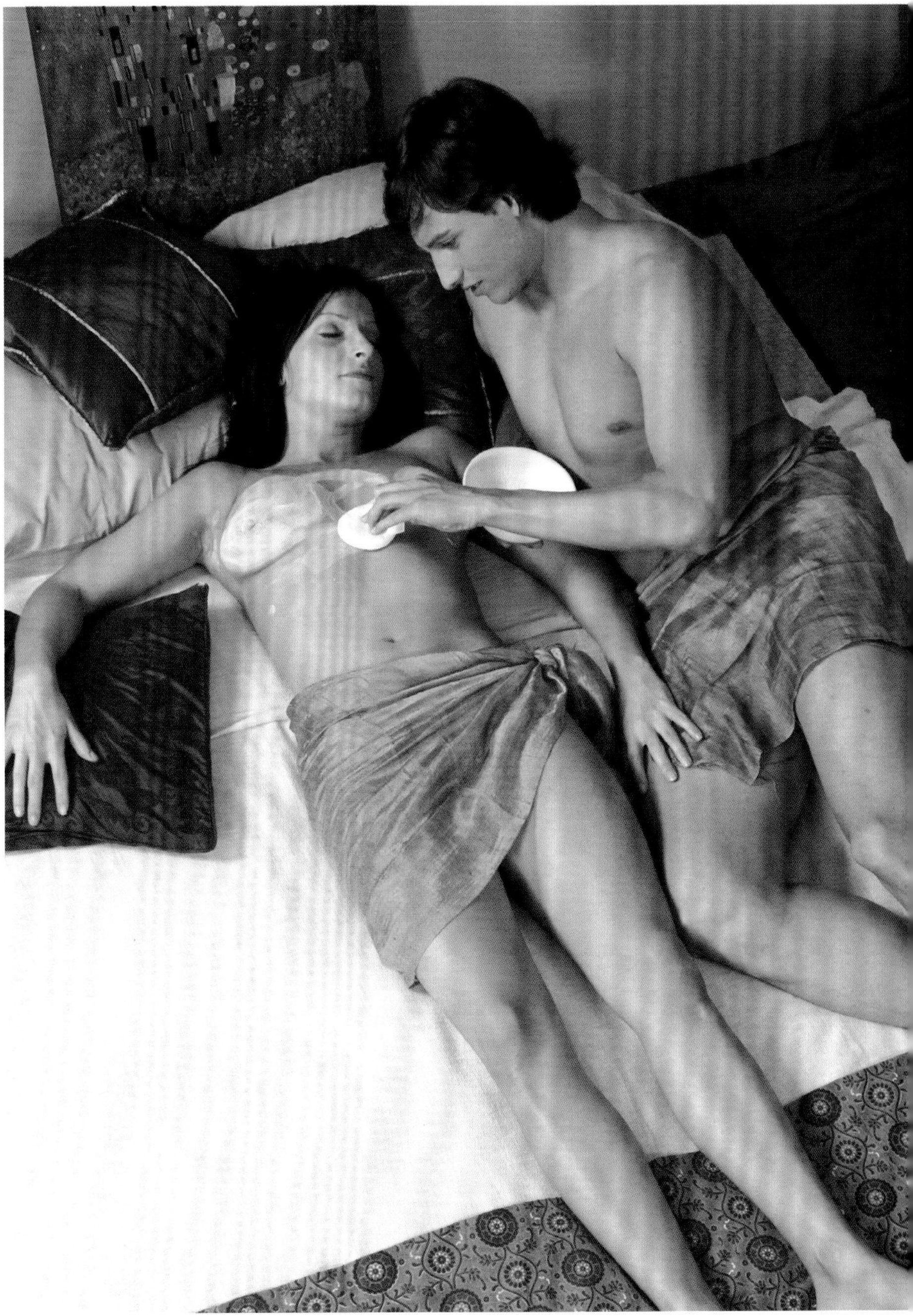

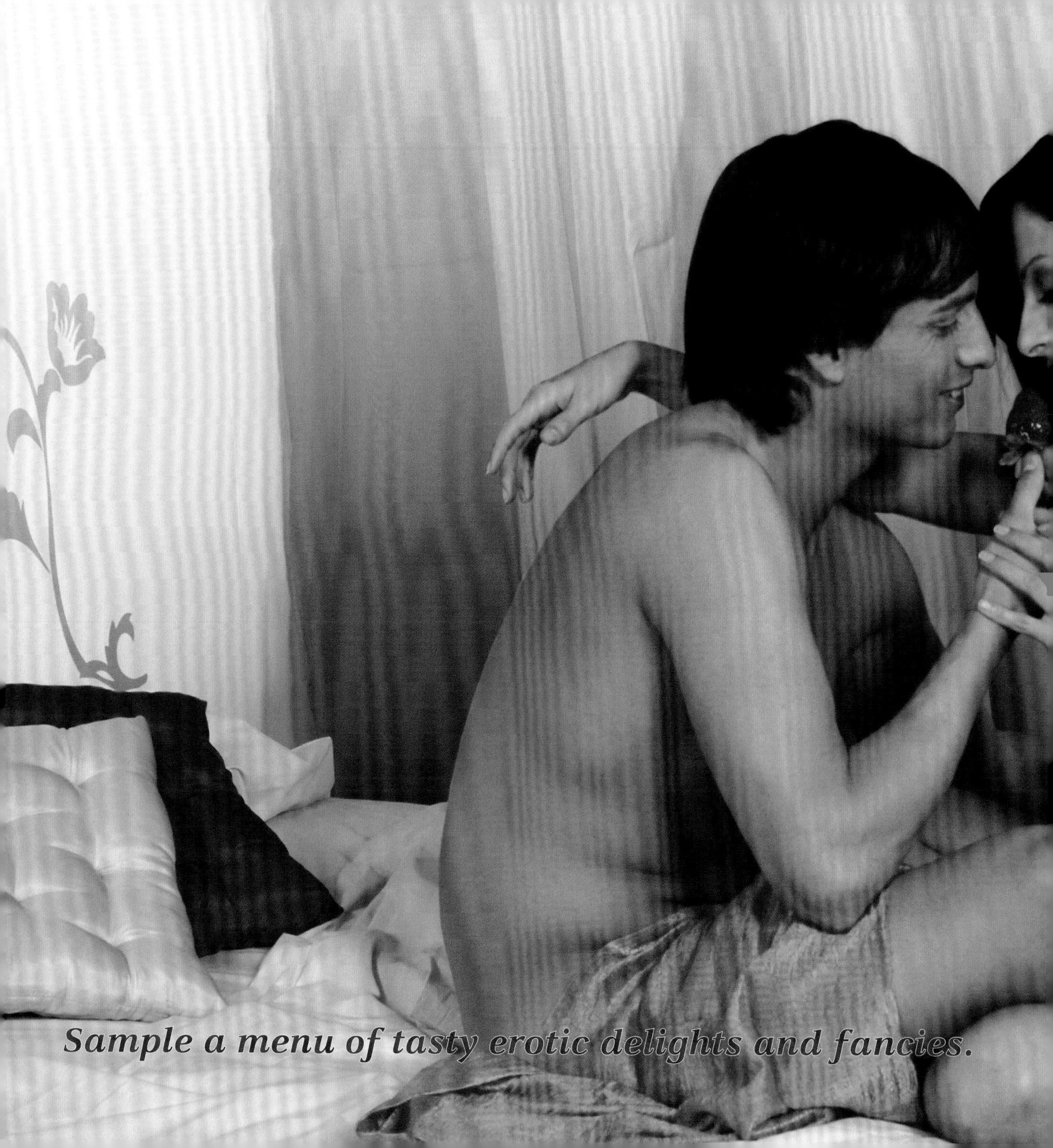

Sample a menu of tasty erotic delights and fancies.

Aphrodisiac Recipes

TO SAVOR TOGETHER

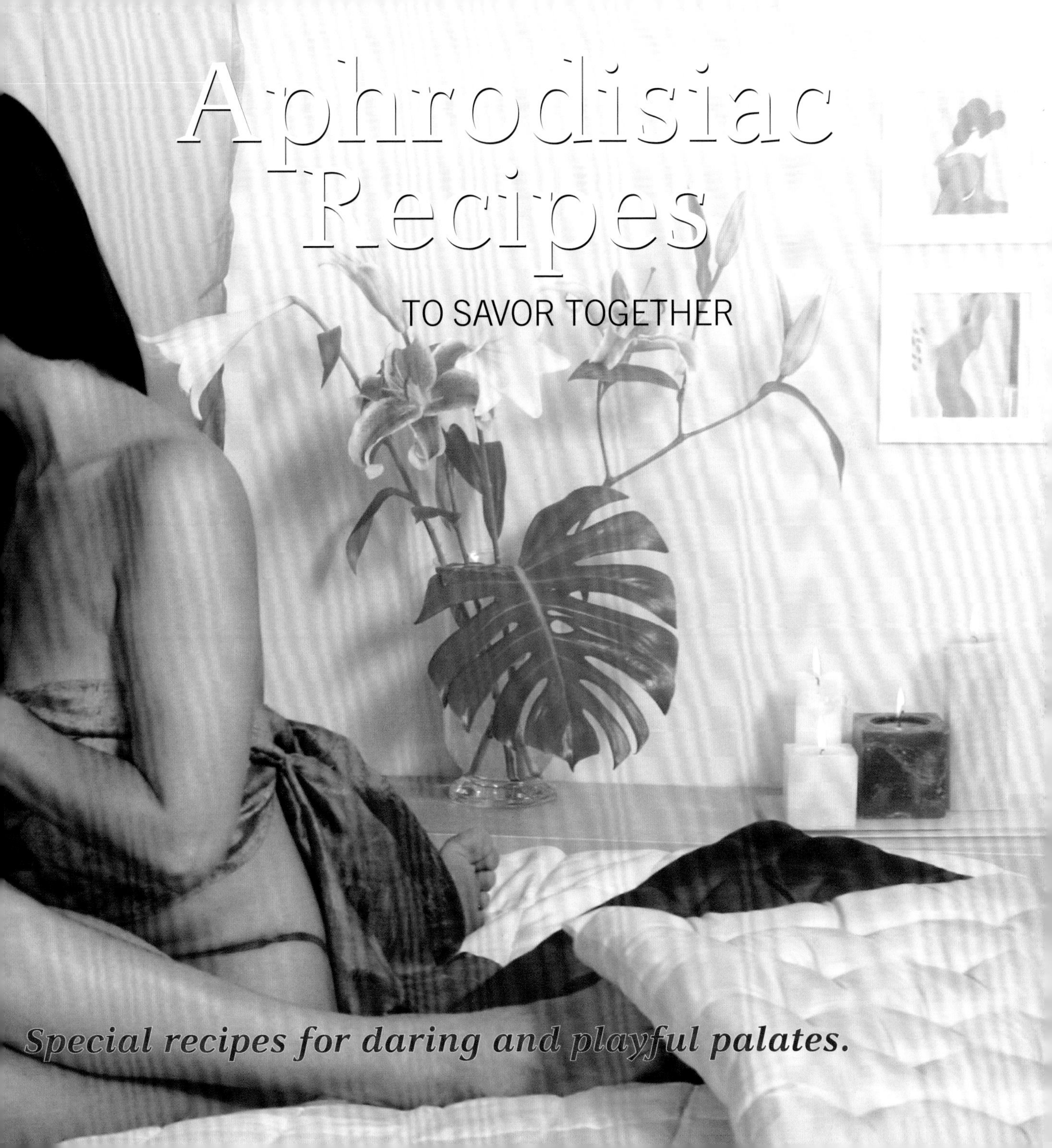

Special recipes for daring and playful palates.

Between-Meal Snacks

Raw Vegetable Dip

Cut up various lengths of **carrot, celery, cucumber . . .** Then make the dip by mixing yogurt with salt, mint, cumin, parsley, cilantro, and a trickle of lemon (all the ingredients are optional except the yogurt and parsley. Feel free to invent your own dip).

Fruit in Melted Chocolate

You already know chocolate is one of the most aphrodisiac of all foods. You can choose **strawberries, bananas, grapes . . .** the fruits you like the most. Wash them and cut them into small pieces and dip them in melted chocolate. Serve them on a little plate accompanied with tooth picks. It will be very tasty if you add 1 drop of pepper oil and 3 drops of orange essence to 2 ounces (50 g) of chocolate.

Tomatoes with Ricotta

Slice three ripe tomatoes in half. Remove the seeds and fill with the following ricotta cream filling:

To Prepare the Cream:

- 4 ounces (125 g) of ricotta or cottage cheese
- 1 tablespoon of sour cream
- one-half tablespoon of lemon juice
- salt, pepper, chopped parsley
- a drizzle of olive oil

Suggestions

You can make this recipe a touch more aromatic by adding 2 drops of orange essence and 1 drop of vanilla extract. Orange pepper seasoning is also something you might try to enrich the flavor of this recipe. To prepare it put 10 drops of orange essence in a non-wooden grinder and add peppercorns and grind.

Make some simple mouthfuls to go along with the massage.

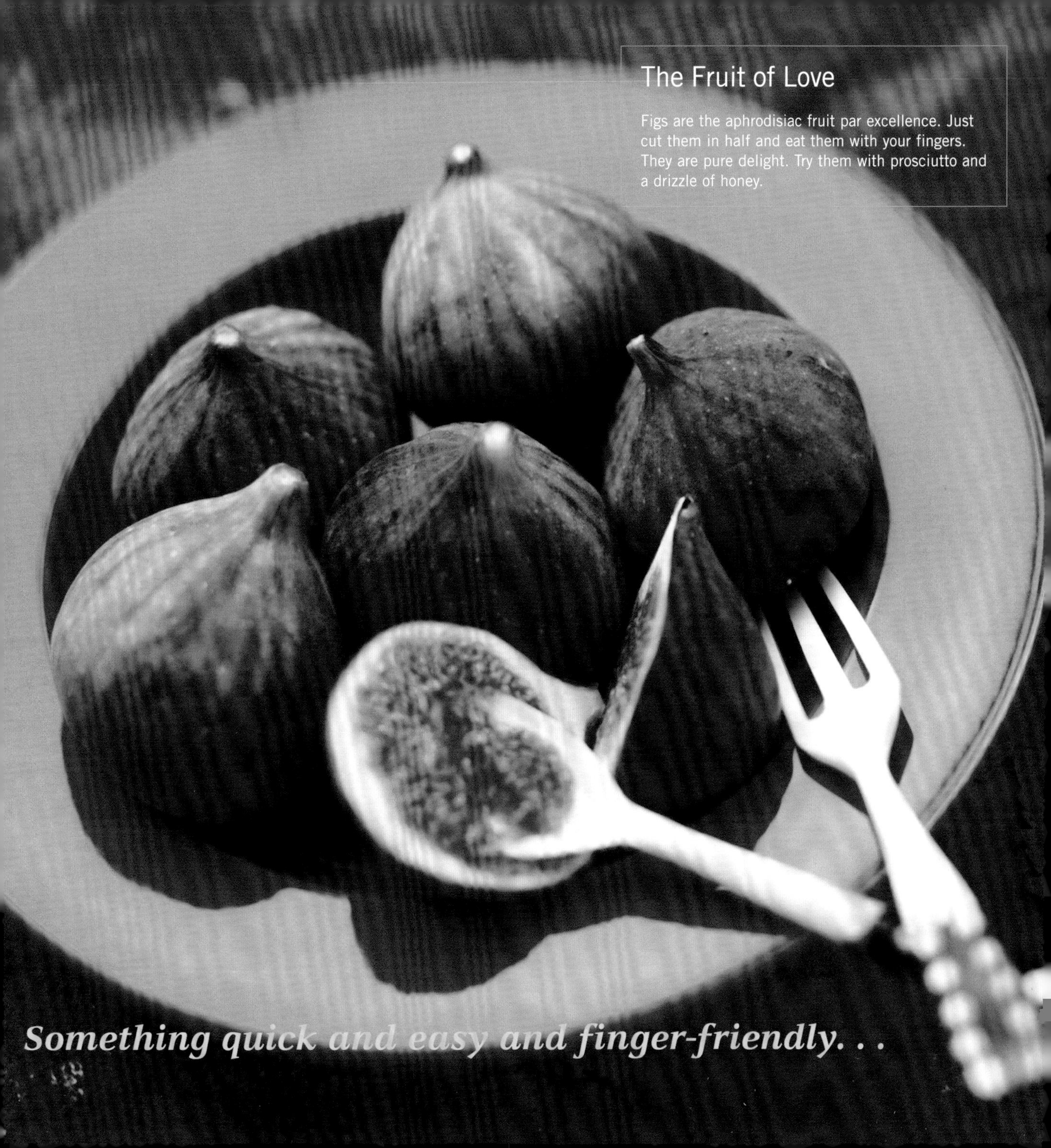

The Fruit of Love

Figs are the aphrodisiac fruit par excellence. Just cut them in half and eat them with your fingers. They are pure delight. Try them with prosciutto and a drizzle of honey.

Something quick and easy and finger-friendly. . .

Olive "Caviar" and Rosemary Potato Rösti

For the "Caviar":

- 6-8 olives of the best quality (organic if possible)
- a pinch of salt
- a pinch of pepper with orange essence

For the Potato Rösti:

- 2 medium potatoes
- 1 teaspoon olive oil
- 1 teaspoon finely chopped rosemary
- a pinch of salt
- a pinch of pepper or pepper with orange essence

1 To prepare the "caviar," pit the olives and chop them very finely. Mash them into a paste. If you wish, you can season them with salt and orange pepper. Hold aside.

2 Skin the potatoes and cut them in slices, not too thin. Mix the rosemary with the olive oil. Add a pinch of salt and pepper.

3 Heat the oil in a pan. When it is heated, add four patties of the potato and fry for a couple of minutes on one side, then turn and continue frying until golden.

4 Divide each patty in four pieces and serve on two plates. Put a tablespoon of the olive "caviar" with the potatoes and decorate with tomato slices and sprigs of aromatic herbs.

An Alternative

A quicker and simpler variation consists in serving the olive "caviar" spread on a piece of toasted bread.

A savory recipe to enjoy without leaving the bedroom . . .

Prawns with Ginger Sauce

This is another voluptuous, savory dish. The prawns are as enticing due to their delicious flavor as to their size and shape. Eat them with your fingers, sensuously licking and sucking them. The prawns provide proteins and phosphorous, which stimulate the pleasure area of the brain.

- 2 spring onions (scallions)
- 1 small piece of ginger root
- 1 tablespoon of sherry
- 1 tablespoon of ginseng syrup or 2 tablespoons of soy
- 4 large shelled and veined prawns
- 1 teaspoon of lemon juice
- 1 drop lemongrass essence
- 4 drops of "orange in love" natural aroma (orange oil, vanilla extract, and rose oil)

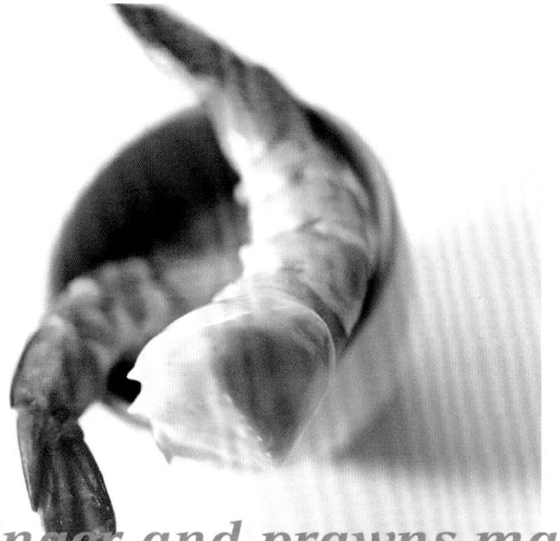

1 Pour 2 drops of "orange in love" on a moistened cutting board and spread it. Peel the onions and chop them very fine. Peel the ginger root and chop it finely or grate it.

2 In a small pan, mix the onion, ginger, sherry, and ginseng syrup. Add the shrimps and cook for a couple of minutes, covered.

3 Let it rest a minute and then add the lemon juice, the lemongrass essence, and another two drops of "orange in love." Let this cook another half-minute.

4 Serve the prawns with jasmine or basmati rice.

Ginger and prawns make an aphrodisiac pairing.

"Asser Roman" Egyptian Cocktail

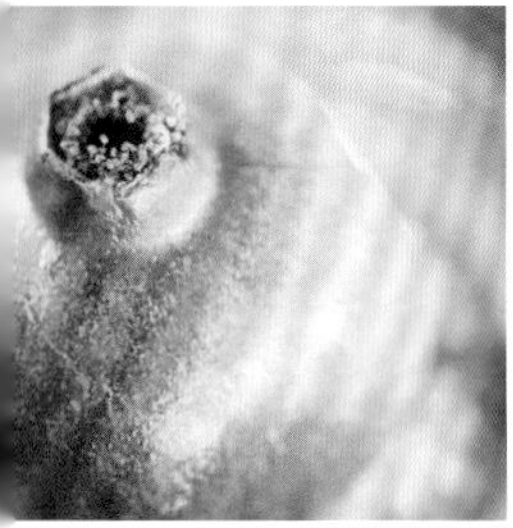

This cocktail, an ideal aperitif, is a famous love potion of Egyptian origin. It was very popular in the time of Cleopatra and is still greatly appreciated for its fruity, aromatic taste and aphrodisiac virtues.

- 2 large pomegranates
- 2 teaspoons of rose water
- 2 glasses of chilled water
- a bit of honey
- 1 or 2 tablespoons of lemon or lime juice
- 3 or 4 drops of "orange in love" (sold in natural health food stores and some pharmacies)

1 Skin the pomegranates and remove the seeds, then put the fruit in a blender with the chilled water and rosewater.

2 Complete by adding the lemon/lime juice, honey, and "orange in love." Blend.

3 Serve this delicious refreshment in a crystal goblet.

An Invigorating, Aromatic Drink

This drink owes its potent effect to celery and parsley that have always been acclaimed for their aphrodisiac properties.

For One Glass:
- 1 tablespoon of celery juice
- 1 glass of apple or grape juice
- one-half teaspoon of honey of acacia
- 1 drop of essential orange oil
- lemon juice
- chopped parsley

1. Mix the honey with the essential orange oil. Add the celery juice along with the apple or grape juice and mix well in a blender.

2. Moisten the edge of the glass with lemon juice and add chopped parsley. Pour the juice carefully into the glass and it is ready to serve.

This savory cocktail will refresh you both during an erotic massage.

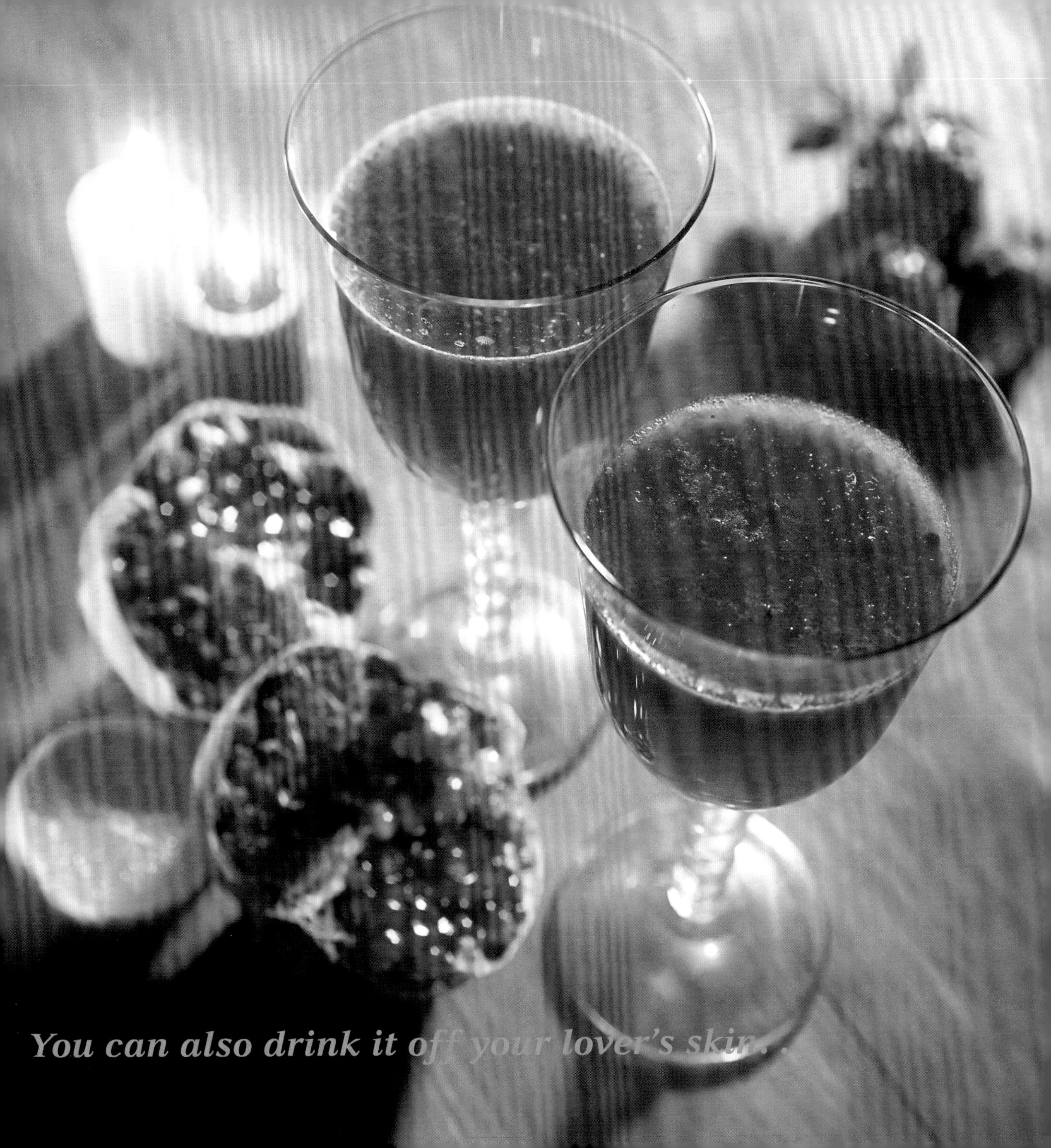

You can also drink it off your lover's skin. . .

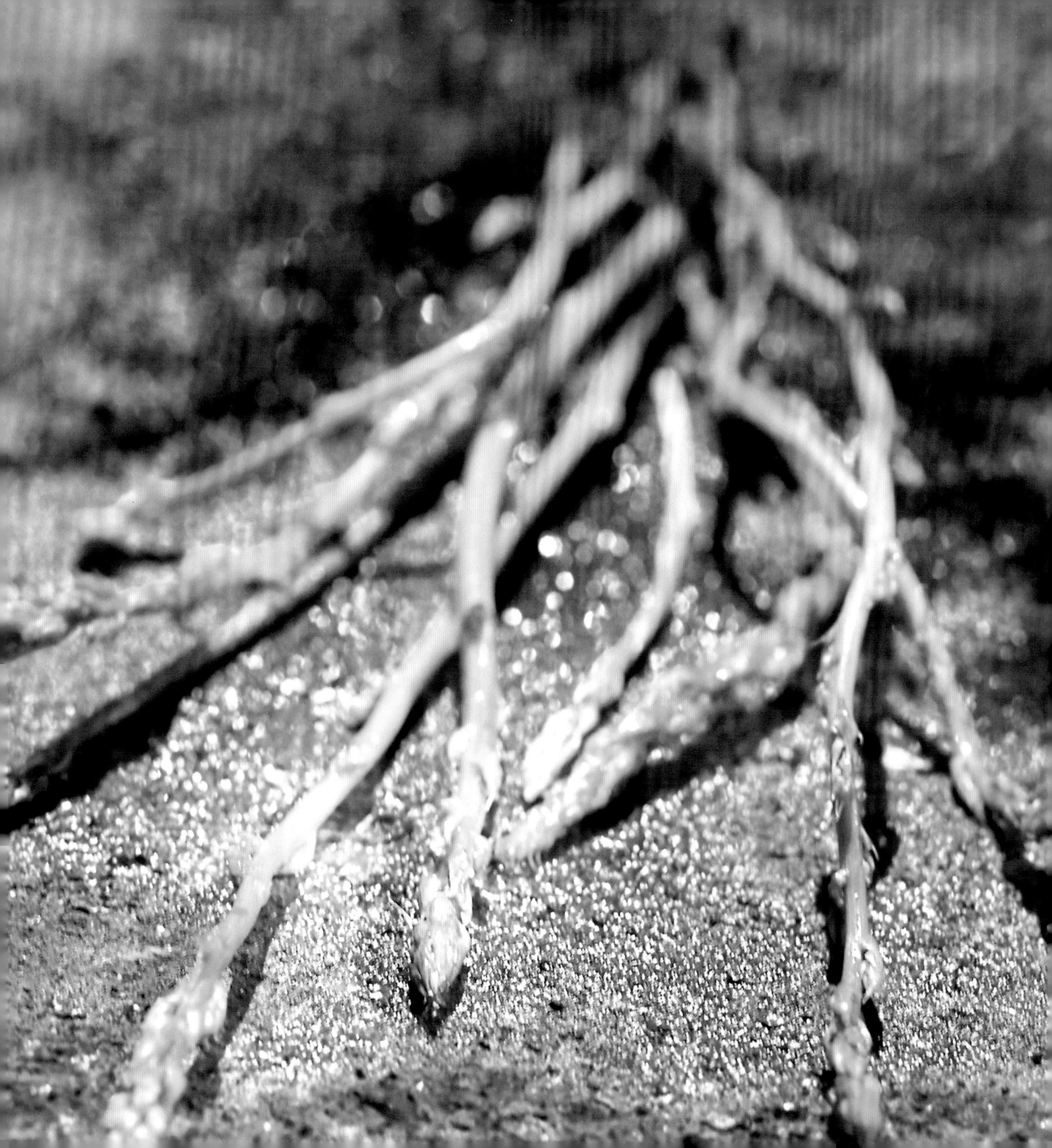

Parmesan Crusted Green Asparagus

Here is a plate that could serve as an alternative to the prawns with ginger dish. The asparagus are exciting not only because of their shape, but for over 2,000 years have been considered to be excellent aphrodisiacs an pleasure stimulants.

- 10 ounces (300 g) of green asparagus
- salt
- 1 teaspoon of lemon juice
- 1-3 drops of "orange in love"
- 1 ounce (30 g) of bread crumbs
- 4 tablespoons of olive oil
- 1 ounce (20 g) of grated parmesan cheese

1. Wash the asparagus and remove the tough part of the stalk on the bottom. Bring them to a boil and then lower the flame to a minimum. Mix the lemon juice with the "orange in love" and add to the asparagus. Let it simmer for 10 minutes. Then turn off the heat and let it sit a few minutes.

2. Put the asparagus in an ovenproof dish and season with orange pepper.

3. Bake "au gratin" for 1 to 3 minutes. It is important to keep alert at this point since the parmesan will quickly turn golden and you don't want it to burn.

4. Serve the asparagus with toasted bread, ciabatta, or baby potatoes. You can boil the potatoes for 15 minutes in salted water with a sprig of laurel while you are cooking the asparagus.

Take an asparagus in your mouth and let your partner nibble on it.

Fruit Skewers Flambé with Sals

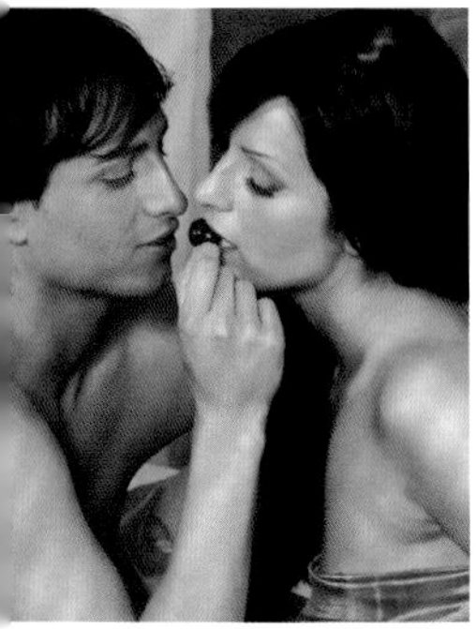

For the Fruit Skewers:

- 1 small apple
- juice of 1 lemon
- 3 drops of "orange in love"
- 4 ounces (100 g) of small strawberries
- 4 ounces (100 g) of grapes

For the Salsa:

- juice of 1 orange
- 1 teaspoon of butter
- 2-3 tablespoons of brown sugar
- 2-3 drops of "orange in love"
- 2 tablespoons of orange liquor or Grand Marnier
- 1 tablespoon of white rum

Suggestion

If you wish to flambé the dessert at the table (a very romantic touch), light the salsa using a long wood taper.

1 Peel and core the apple and cut it into large cubes. Mix the lemon juice and the "orange in love" with the apple so it doesn't oxidize.

2 Wash the strawberries and leave them whole. Do the same with the grapes.

3 Put the pieces of fruit on wood skewers and arrange them on a plate.

4 Put the orange juice, butter, and brown sugar in a small pan and heat the mix until the butter and sugar liquefy.

5 Mix the "orange in love" with the orange liquor and rum and add to the pan and let it heat briefly.

6 Pour the mix from the pan over the skewered fruit and serve as a dessert.

A refreshing fruit dessert for erotic sharing with your partner.

A Love Charm

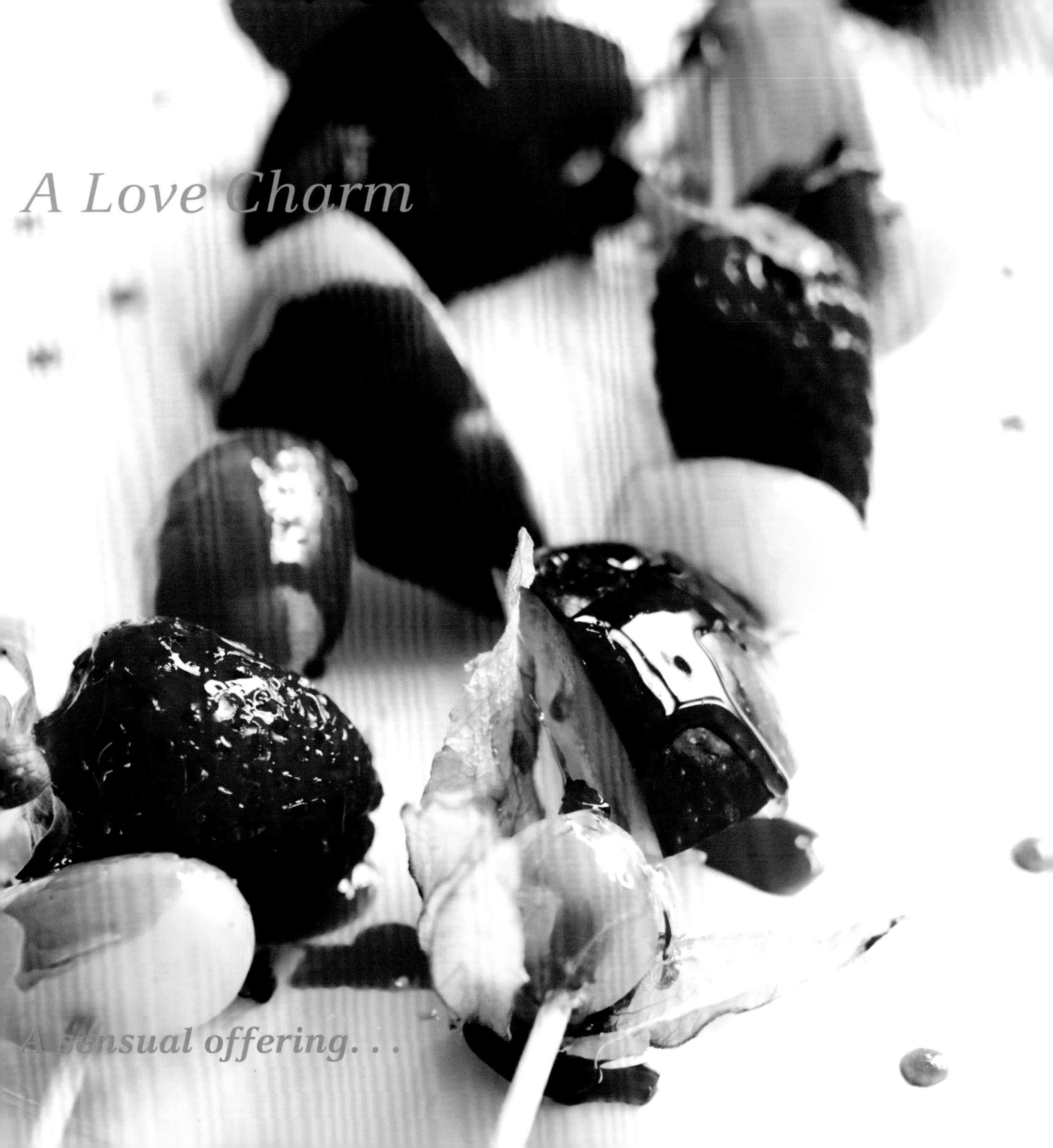

A sensual offering. . .

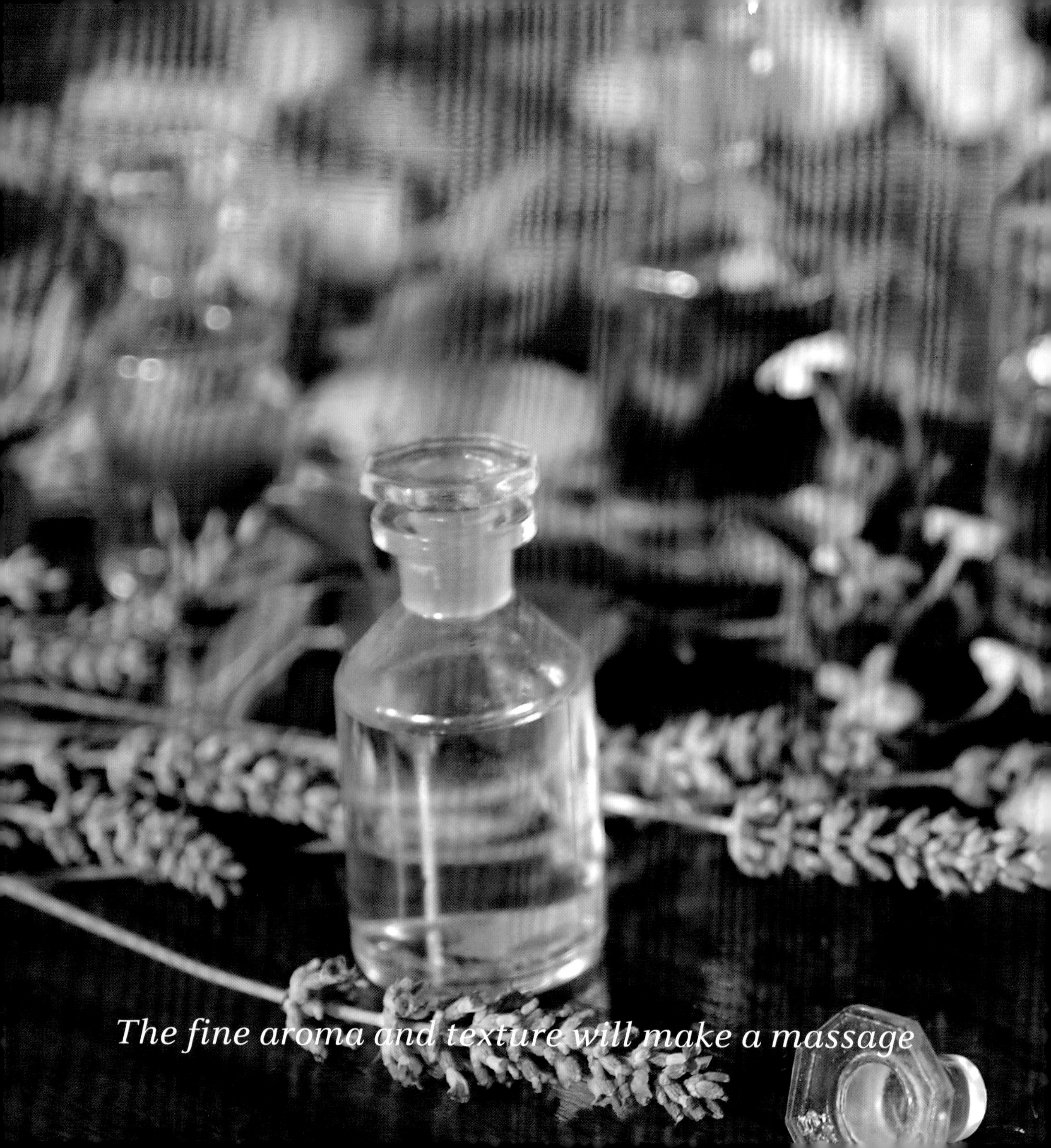

The fine aroma and texture will make a massage

Vegetable Oils

SENSUAL BLENDS

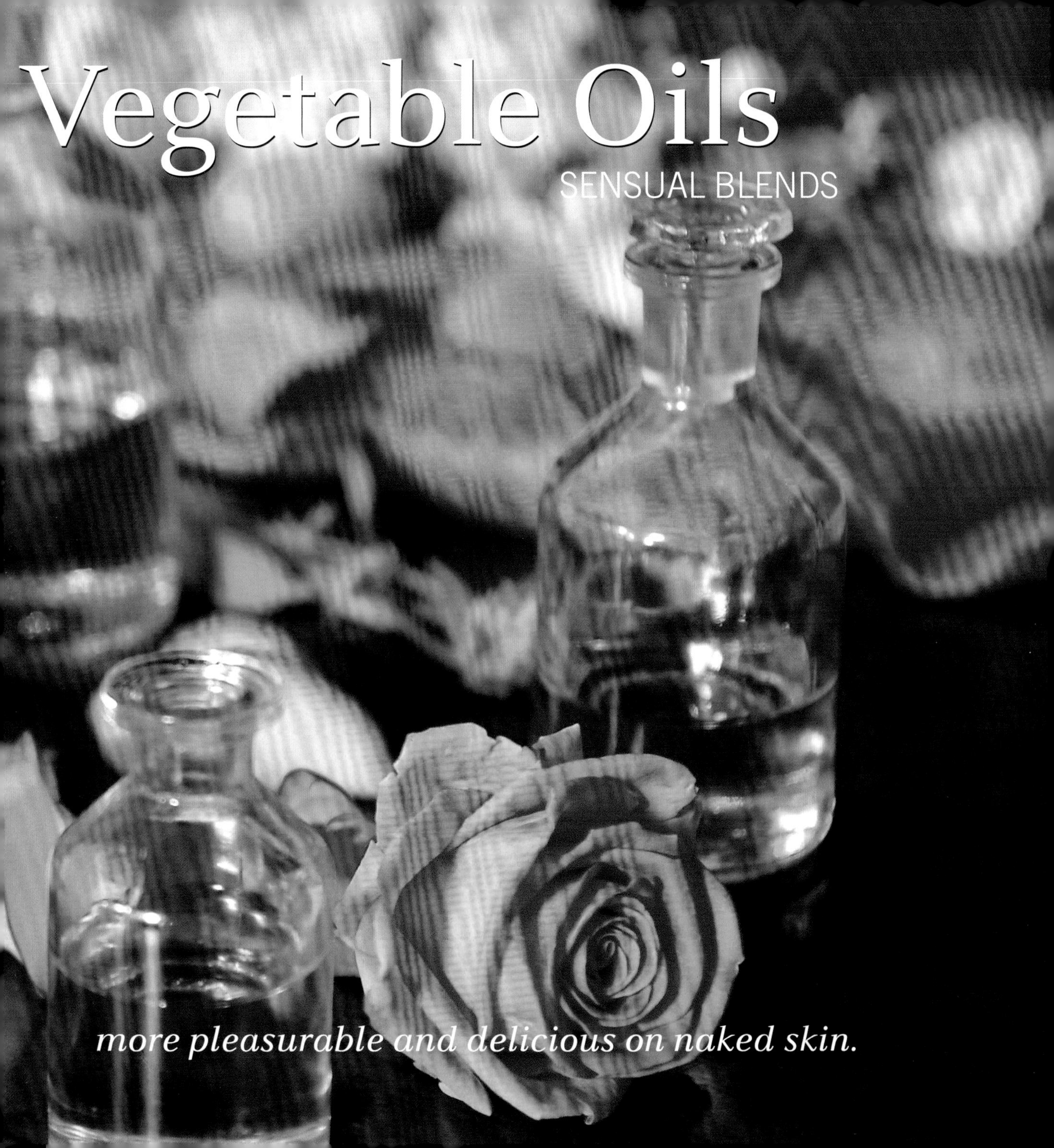

more pleasurable and delicious on naked skin.

About Vegetable Oils

We reiterate that the most important thing to consider when you buy vegetable oils is the **quality**. They should be **cold-pressed**, since this is the only way all components of the oil, fatty acids, lecithin, vitamins, essential aromas, etc, are guaranteed to remain intact.

Fatty acids should be consumed no more than four months after they have been opened and for this reason it is recommended to buy them in small quantities. Most oils are available in bottles of 3 fluid ounces (100 ml) while those of primrose and musk rose are sold in one ounce (30 ml) bottles or even capsules, since they are so difficult to preserve.

Jojoba is an exception regarding its preservation. It does not go rancid since it is a wax. Once opened, you could leave it uncovered for even twenty years and it would still be in good condition.

Attention

You should know that it is not possible to obtain essential oils from flowers such as **lilac, lily, lotus, lily of the valley, or from fruits such as peach or green apple**. These oils are made from synthetic elements and do not have therapeutic or preventative properties. You should not use these synthetics for massage oil.

Essential Oils

These oils are also called "ethereal" oils, an adjective from the Greek which means **"celestial."** These essences are extremely volatile and disperse very quickly in the air.

When we buy essential oils we must pay strict attention to quality and buy only 100% pure and natural products which provide the positive effects we seek for body and soul.

100% vegetable oils are our skin's best friend.

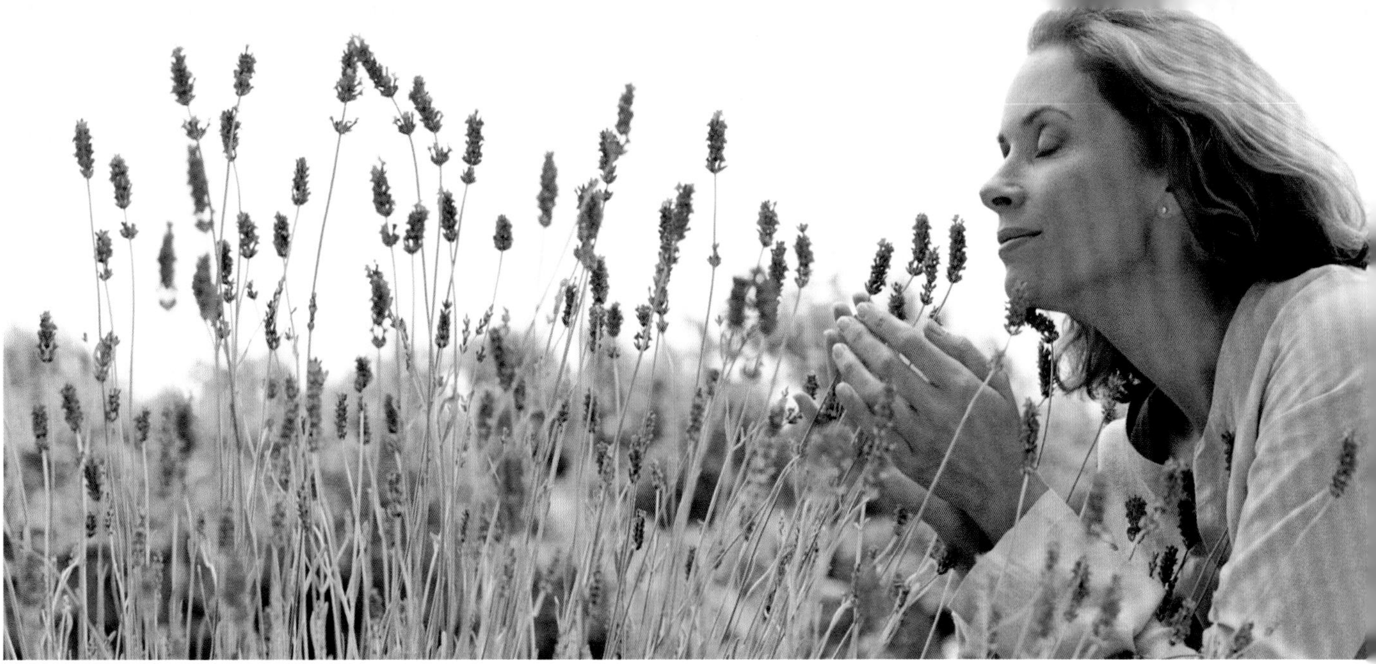

Origin

Essential oils are derived from the **botanical families of mint, myrtle, conifers, *apiaceae* (carrot/parsley family), laurels, and citrus**. These oils are found specifically between the cells of the plant and are conspicuous for possessing special substances (monoterpine alcohol, esters, aldehydes, etc.) which provide therapeutic benefit.

The specific properties of these oils and their function depend on where they are produced in the plant. **They may be produced in the flowers, leaves, fruit, resins, peel, seeds, or roots**.

Another important factor regarding the characteristics of these essences lies in how they are cultivated and varies according to whether they are picked wild, grown in a garden, or are produced using organic farming methods.

Oils from plants growing wild in fields or forests are particularly rich in the desired properties and produce the most intense scents. Organically grown plants also produce essential oils very suitable for massage oil since they are grown without using toxic substances such as synthetic herbicides or pesticides which can alter the plant.

They will not block your pores and are rich in vitamins and nutritive elements.

Their Production

The extraction of the essential oils varies according to their location in the parent plant. The most common method involves **steam distillation,** although there are other methods as well.

Lemon oil, for example, is produced **cold-pressed (expression extraction),** while delicate, costly flowers such as jasmine or tuberose are obtained using **solvent extraction** (a special procedure). Essence of beeswax, cacao, or vanilla are obtained by alcohol extraction.

The Product Label Should Indicate . . .

- if the oil is 100% pure
- the common and scientific names of the plant
- country of origin
- part of the plant utilized (peel, leaves, etc.)
- quantity (metric and English)
- method of production
- harvesting details: if picked wild, grown organically, or grown without using toxic substances
- production control number
- if the oil has been diluted into other substances (it should indicate specifically what has been added and what percentage of the mix it occupies)
- any warnings concerning safe use according to law and any possible effects from inappropriate use.

Quality Criteria

Low cost is not one of the virtues associated with essential oils. To obtain one drop of pure rose essence requires thirty roses, so keep in mind that three-hundredths of a fluid ounce (1 ml) will cost between $25 and $50.

You can be relieved, however, since to make a massage oil blend one drop of essential oil is usually enough, so intense are the properties of these marvelous essences.

One should be wary of buying these products at too cheap a price. Quality is always reflected in the price and the most important thing is that the essences are produced without any toxic substances. These will nullify any good qualities of the oils.

Here are some guidelines for recognizing quality in essential oils: the aroma must be very close to that of the plant that produces it; the vial that contains the oil should be dark to protect it from light; the price of the essence should correspond to the type of oil and its availability.

Simply inhaling the aroma of essential oils relaxes the senses.

Preservation and Shelf Life

As we mentioned previously, essential oils should always be kept in **darkened glass vials**, generally brown in color, since the essences are very susceptible to light, air, and temperature.

Keep them in a **dark and cool place**, outside the reach of children, since there is a risk of intoxication.

Most of these oils have a shelf life of **three to five years**. Some, such as rose or cedar essence, get better with the passage of time and can last for ten years, or even longer.

Citrus essences, on the other hand, are delicate and should be used within six months maximum (you can also use these for household cleaning tasks).

Tolerance

It is important to remember that essential oils **should not be directly applied to the skin or mucosa without diluting them since they will otherwise cause irritation.**

There are exceptions, however: lavender essence, rose essence, rosewood, and sandalwood are among them.

With citrus essences it is a good idea to try a bit on your elbow to see how your skin tolerates it.

To do this, mix 1 drop of citrus essence with almond oil and apply to your elbow. If there is no reaction after fifteen minutes, you can use it in your massage mix without concern.

Evaporation

Essential oils can be classified into three categories according to the time it takes for their scent to evaporate.

Rapid evaporation indicates the scent of the oil is gone after two to three hours; **medium evaporation** applies to the scent lasting up to eight hours; **slow evaporation** means the scent will last up to seventy-two hours.

The ideal would be for a massage oil to contain essences of all three evaporation types. For sensual blends, it is better to use essences of a medium evaporation profile.

Smell can cause a calming effect throughout the entire body.

Oil Base for Massages

Remember that for all massages it is important to use only 100% natural vegetable oil bases of the best quality.

Do not buy any that contain petroleum by-products such as petroleum jelly or mineral oil, since these form a film that is relatively impermeable and don't allow the skin to breathe and, in addition, have no health benefit.

Vegetable oils, on the other hand, are a wonderful gift of nature. **They are obtained from living germinal material such as berries, fruit, nuts, and seeds using the cold-pressed method.** Skin tolerates these very well and benefits from their use since they contain ingredients that build up the skin's natural oils.

The following oils are especially recommended for erotic massage and combine very well with the essential oils.

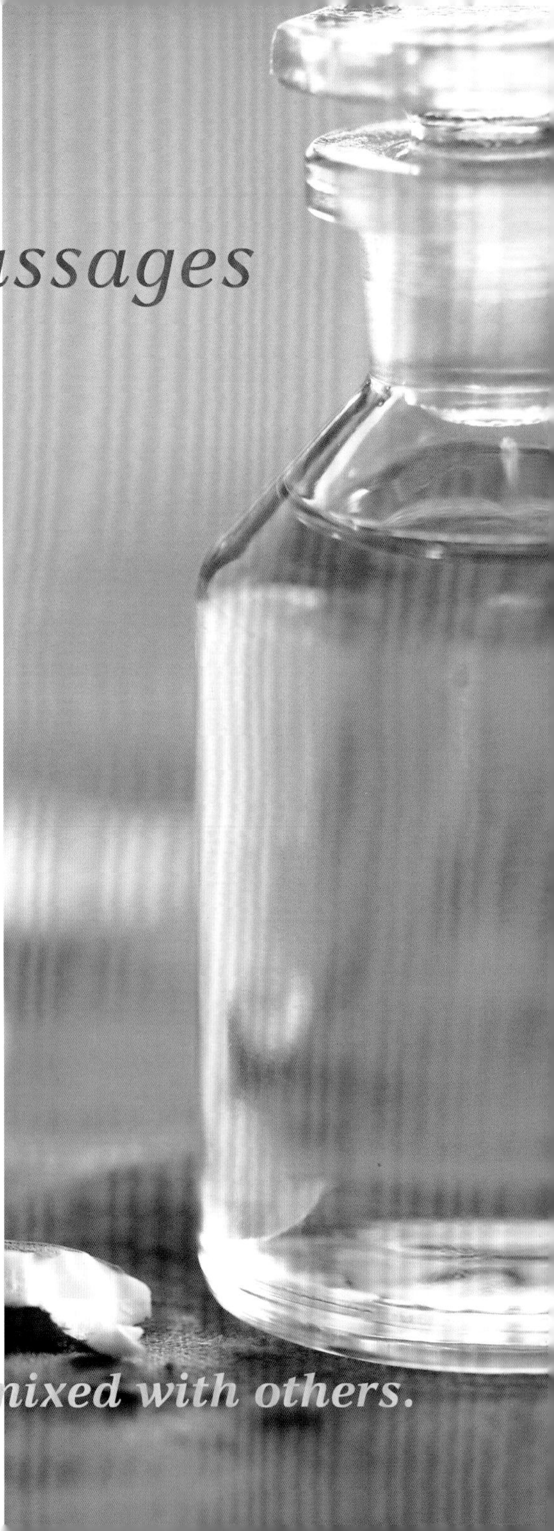

These oils can be used alone or mixed with others.

Almond Oil

This is the classic base for massage oil. It is obtained from the shells of the almond. It has a high content (80%) of oleic acid that allows easy coating of the skin and leaves a protective and nutritive layer. In addition, almond oil contains 15% linoleic acid, an unsaturated fat that helps maintain skin elasticity. Almond oil is highly beneficial to the skin, including the most sensitive type. It is especially recommended for dry skin. The wonderful smell of almonds is an added gift.

Apricot Oil

This is obtained from pressing apricot pits of mature fruit. It is equivalent to almond oil regarding its hydrating and nutritive qualities. In fact, it is a good idea to mix both oils for application to the chest and face. The ratio should be one part apricot oil to three parts almond oil.

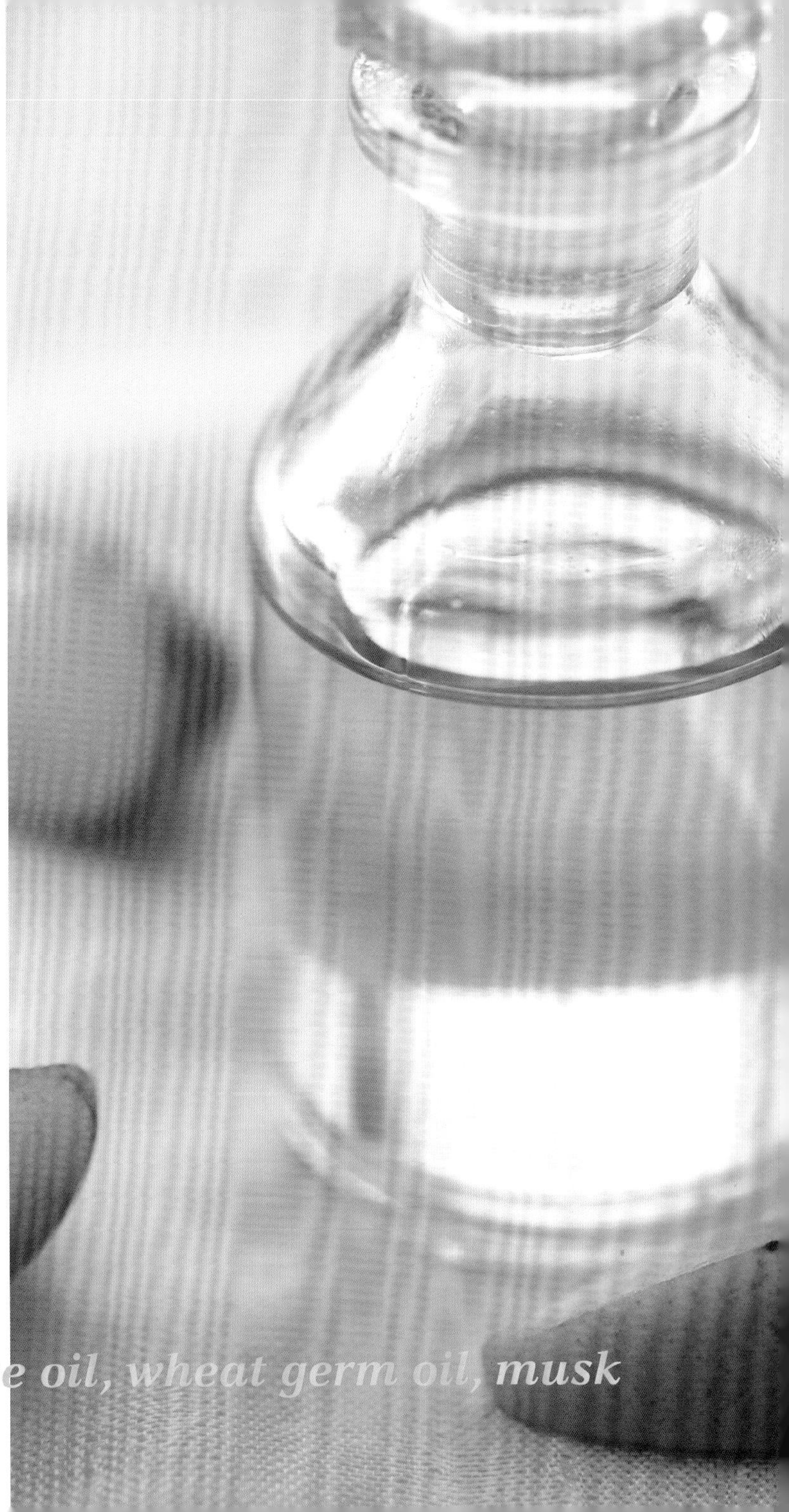

For example, with borage oil, wheat germ oil, musk rose . . .

Jojoba Oil

Jojoba oil is obtained from the vegetable wax of the jojoba fruit. It should actually be called jojoba "wax," but at room temperature it is liquid and to all appearances is not distinguishable from oil. It contains over 50% wax, is low in both oleic and linoleic acids, but has a great amount of minerals and vitamins that help protect the skin.

Jojoba oil stabilizes the skin's pH and regulates the ratio of oil to moisture in the skin. Jojoba is effective for all types of skin, from the driest to the oiliest. It contains vitamin E, which strengthens connective tissue and helps prevent the formation of wrinkles. Jojoba oil maintains moisture levels and it is recommended to moisturize the skin before using it, if possible using an infusion (a liquid that contains plant elements obtained by steeping the plant or flowers). The ratio for jojoba with other massage oils is one part jojoba to four parts of the other oil.

Musk Rose Oil

Musk rose (or rosehips) has been an oil relatively unknown until recently, but which is now gaining attention for the interesting properties it offers the skin. It is obtained by pressing the small seeds of the plant and has an intensely acerbic aroma.

It contains 40% linoleic acids and 40% polyunsaturated alpha-linoleic acids. These are involved in cell membrane function and stimulate skin regeneration. They reduce water loss in the skin and support sweat gland function.

Musk rose is also known for its anti-inflammatory properties.

Musk rose should also be used in small amounts, one part musk rose to five parts of other oil bases.

This oil is a luxury, not referring only to its price, but also due to its regenerative effect on the skin. It is ideal for the face, neck, and chest area. It is best to buy it in capsule form or in 1 oz. (30 ml) vials since its shelf life is very short.

Musk rose oil, besides being great for a massage,

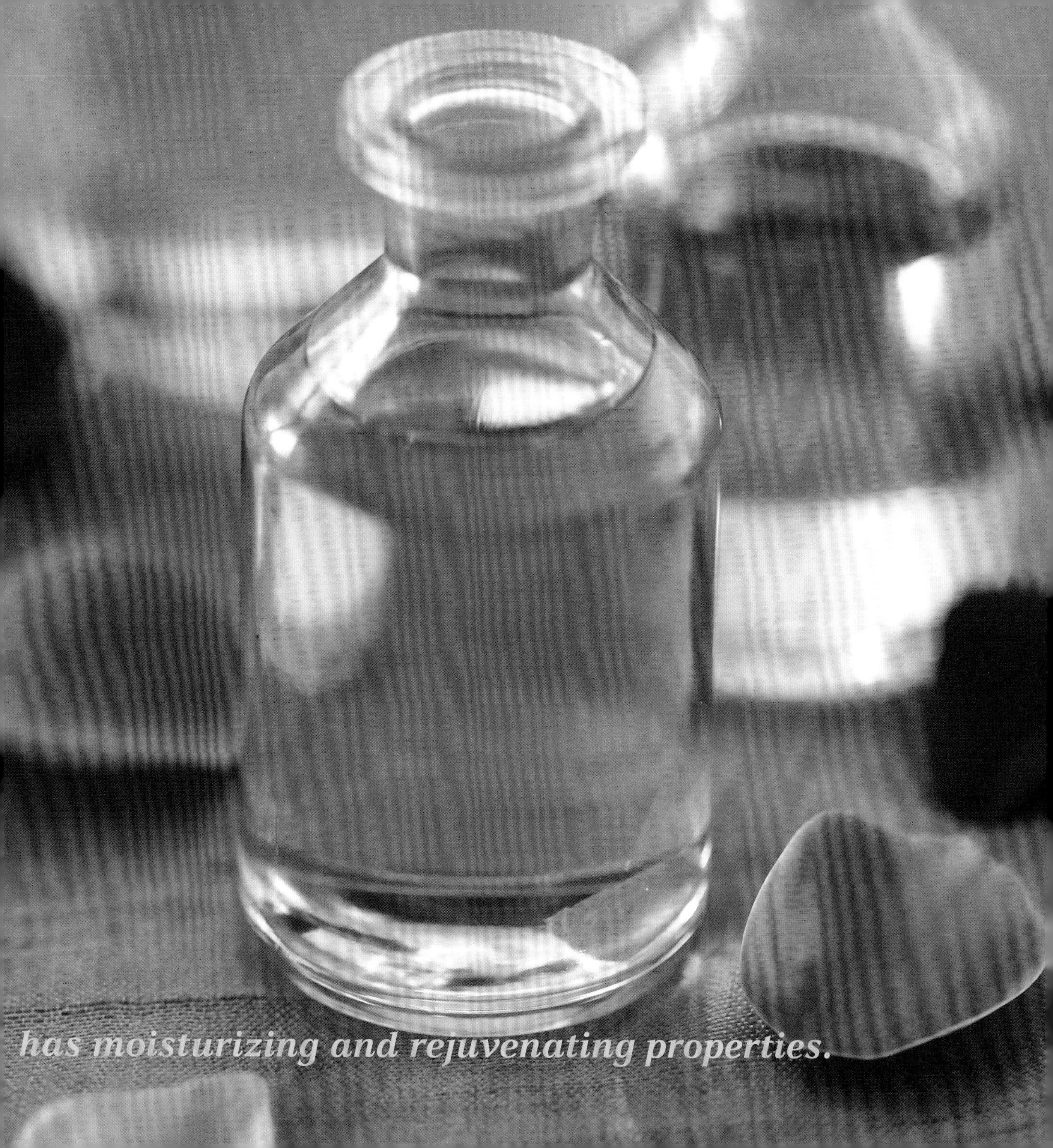

has moisturizing and rejuvenating properties.

Sesame Oil

Sesame oil is obtained by pressing the tiny white seeds of the plant. Its distinct aroma resembles the smell of nuts.

This oil is composed of 42% oleic acid, 44% linoleic acid, and also contains lecithin and sesamol, a natural anti-oxidant. Sesame oil is beneficial to numerous metabolic processes and is also a nervous system tonic.

In India, sesame oil is the oil par excellence for skin care and is never absent from massage oil blends.

This oil is especially suited for purifying facial massages since it contains substances that bind with heavy metal ions and causes them to be expelled from tissues. As a result, it has important regenerative effects and helps to delay and prevent aging of the skin. Sesame oil is very effective for sensitive and dry skin.

Sesame oil, due to its ability to increase blood flow, should not be used on inflamed skin.

Sesame oil is especially suited for sensual massage as it makes gliding your hands over your partner's skin much easier.

Oil of Primrose

The aroma of this oil, which is obtained from the small seeds of the primrose, also resembles the smell of nuts. Besides being beneficial for the skin, primrose oil positively affects both the nervous and immune systems.

It contains up to 60% linoleic acid and 14% gamma-linoleic acid. These are polyunsaturated acids and belong to the omega-6 family. They have an important effect on the regulation of hormones, particularly feminine sexual hormones, and are an important component of skin cells.

In addition, because of its polyunsaturated fatty acids, primrose oil is highly regenerative and stimulates skin cell division. As an authentic skin rejuvenator, it is highly recommended for both sensitive and aging skins and quickly shows visible results.

Primrose oil should be mixed in a one-to-five ratio with other bases. Buy it in small quantities, preferably in capsule form, since it has a short shelf life. Store it in a cool place.

Macadamia Oil

The macadamia is known as the "queen of nuts." Its oil is obtained by pressing the nut-fruit and results in a very valuable prime material for cosmetic use. It contains more than 50% oleic acid and up to 25% palmitoleic acid, which is surprisingly similar to the fatty acids of the skin. As such, the skin tolerates this oil very well and the oil penetrates the skin easily. Macadamia oil is greatly rejuvenating and contains vitamins A, B, and E. It is excellent for preventing aging of the skin. It is usually mixed with almond oil to make a massage blend.

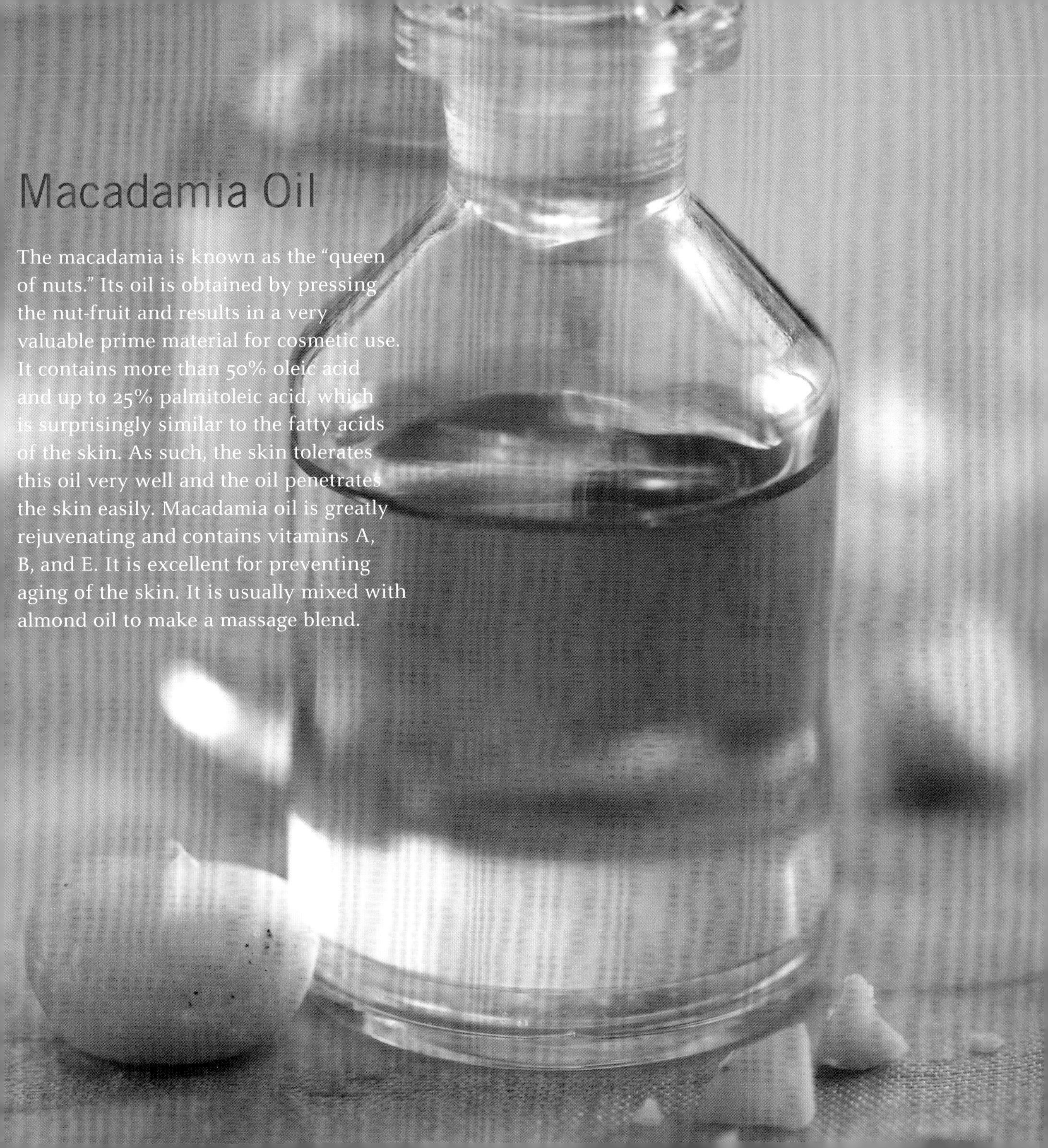

The Most Enticing Essences for

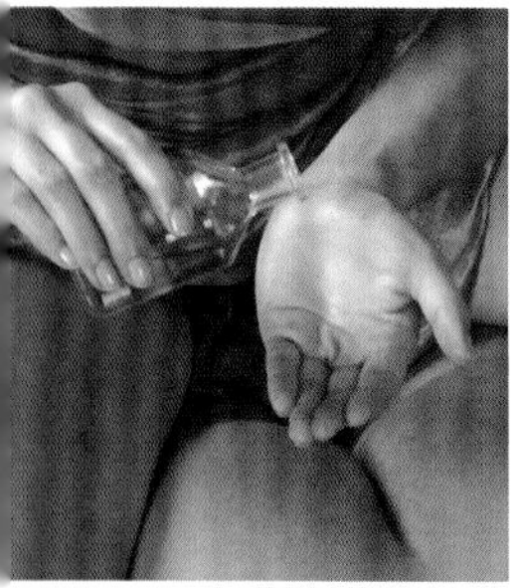

We will now suggest some oils we think are the most interesting to use for couple's erotic massage. We have chosen the ones that are most stimulating, exciting, and relaxing. We list them here with their specific characteristics.

Bergamot

(Citrus bergamia)

- **Evaporation:** Rapid.
- **Aroma:** A delicious fragrance of citrus. Its sweet aroma brings to mind fresh herbs and verdant flowers.
- **Properties:** Relaxing mood tonic.
- **Dose:** A good fit for sensual blends. Add 3 to 5 drops per 2 fluid ounces (50 ml).

Grapefruit

(Citrus paradise)

- **Evaporation:** Rapid.
- **Aroma:** Essence of fresh grapefruit, with a pinch of herbs, refreshing and bright, sparkling, radiating optimism.
- **Properties:** Excellent for cheering up and inspiring joy. It is also an excellent tonic for the skin and stimulates circulation.
- **Dose:** A good fit for sensual blends. Add 3 to 5 drops per 2 fluid ounces (50 ml) of base.
- **Close relatives:** Clementine, mandarin red orange, orange, and lemon belong to the same group.

Jasmine

(Jasminum grandiflorum)

- **Evaporation:** Medium to slow.
- **Aroma:**Exotic and heavy, sweet and floral, delicate, sensual.
- **Properties:** Exciting, provocative, stress-allaying, relaxing, physical tonic, notoriously erotic.
- **Dose:** Often diluted in alcohol for better coverage. You can add 2 to 3 drops for a sensual blend. If you want to use it by itself, add 1 drop to 2 fluid ounces (50 ml) of base.
- **Close relatives:** Magnolia champak, frangipani, and leaves and flowers of the magnolia belong to this group.

Essential oil of jasmine is ideal for an aromatic bath.

a Good Erotic Massage Oil

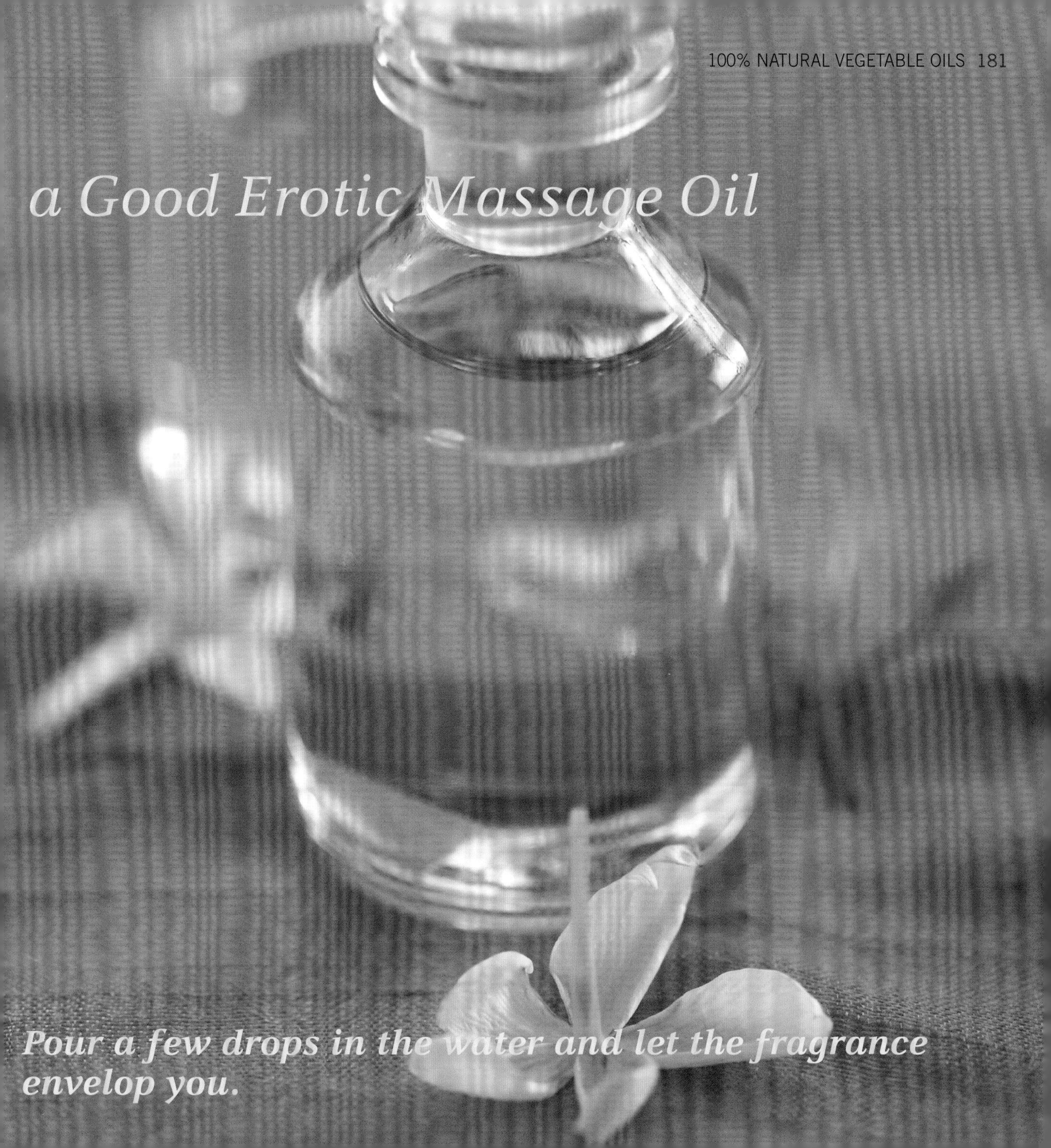

Pour a few drops in the water and let the fragrance envelop you.

Fine Lavender

(Lavandula officinalis)

- **Evaporation:** Medium.
- **Aroma:** Gentle, with a pure, refreshing note.
- **Properties:** Relaxing, calming, balancing. It revitalizes the skin, combats stress, and promotes harmony.
- **Dose:** Add 1 or 2 drops to 2 fluid ounces (50 ml) of base.

Sage

(Salvia sclarea)

- **Evaporation:** Medium.
- **Aroma:** Resinous fragrance, spicy, herbal. Somewhat clingy and soporific.
- **Properties:** Anti-depressive, balances and harmonizes, stimulates the senses, and regulates estrogen.
- **Dose:** Adds a touch of sophistication to sensual blends. Use 1 to 3 drops per 2 fluid ounces (50 ml) of base.

Neroli

(Citrus aurantium)

- **Evaporation:** Slow to medium.
- **Aroma:** Intense and sweet, a bit spicy.
- **Properties:** Highly anti-depressive and a nerve tonic. Acts as a physical and mental relaxant and relieves tension. A powerful aphrodisiac.
- **Dose:** Brings out the best in sensual blends. Use 1 to 2 drops per 2 fluid ounces (50 ml).

Rose

(Rosa damascene)

- **Evaporation:** Medium to slow.
- **Aroma:** Floral, rousing, fine and sweet, reminiscent of honey.
- **Properties:** Stimulating, a classic aphrodisiac, can mitigate emotional upset and lovesickness.
- **Dose:** Highly prized in sensual massage blends. You can mix it alone with the base, 2 drops per 2 fluid ounces (50 ml), or combine it with other essences (then use only 1 drop). If you dilute it in alcohol, use 2 to 4 drops.
- **Esencias cercanas:** Germanium rose and palmarosa oil. These two essential oils are highly valued and have very similar properties. They are also relatively inexpensive and can substitute for rose oil. Use 2 to 4 drops per 2 fluid ounces (50 ml) of base.

Sandalwood

(Santalum album)

- **Evaporation:** Slow.
- **Aroma:** Exotic, velvety, delicate with a hint of wood.
- **Properties:** A classic aphrodisiac, very sensual and restorative of mood. Stimulates the lymph system.
- **Dose:** 1 to 3 drops per 2 fluid ounces (50 ml) for sensual blends.

Vanilla

(Vanilla planifolia)

- **Evaporation:** Slow.
- **Aroma:** Soothing, sweet, and delicate.
- **Properties:** Brings about equilibrium and elevates mood, somewhat erotic.
- **Dose:** 2 to 4 drops per 2 fluid ounces (50 ml) for sensual blends. It combines well with essence of cacao and honey. These two can also substitute for it.

Ylang Ylang

(Cananga odorata)

- **Evaporation:** Medium to slow.
- **Aroma:** Exotic, intensely strong, and sensual. It is one of the most powerful of aphrodisiac oils. It is anti-depressive, regulates estrogen, and is a euphoriant.
- **Dose:** It is powerfully stimulating in sensual blends. Use 3 to 5 drops in 2 fluid ounces (50 ml).

Cedar

(Cedrus atlantica)

- **Evaporation:** Slow.
- **Aroma:** Resinous, harmonious, warm, soft, and soothing.
- **Properties:** Induces harmony, calmness, and serenity. For a man it helps boost self-confidence.
- **Dose:** This oil is especially recommended for massaging the belly/abdomen. Add 1 to 3 drops to 2 fluid ounces (50 ml) of any sensual blend.

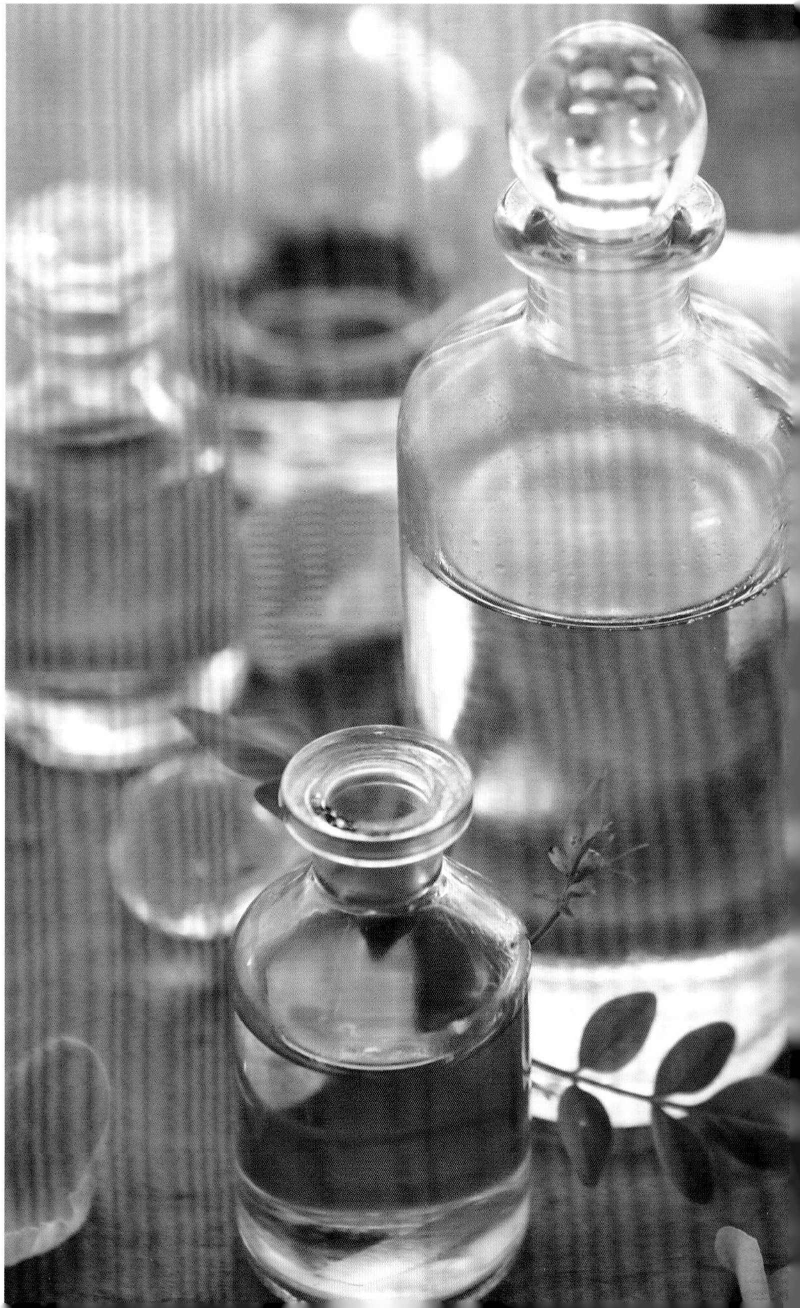

ALSO AVAILABLE

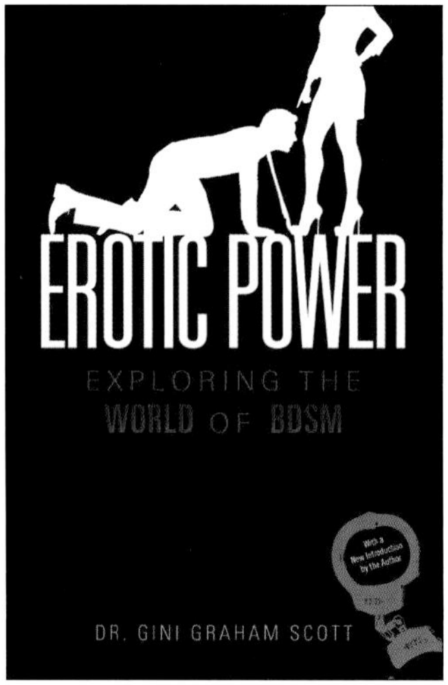

Erotic Power

Exploring the World of BDSM

by Dr. Gini Graham Scott

In *Erotic Power*, Scott delves into the psychological and sexual dynamics of the D&S power exchange through interviews with female dominants, their clients, various group participants, as well as her personal experiences. The many different kinds of D&S relationships, conflict between fantasy and reality, the public and private faces of the D&S community, and the commercial side of dominance are also discussed, with an emphasis on female dominance and male submission. This book will enlighten anyone who is beginning to explore the world of BDSM or curious about the psychology of varied sexual practices.

$14.95 Paperback • ISBN 978-1-62636-420-2

ALSO AVAILABLE

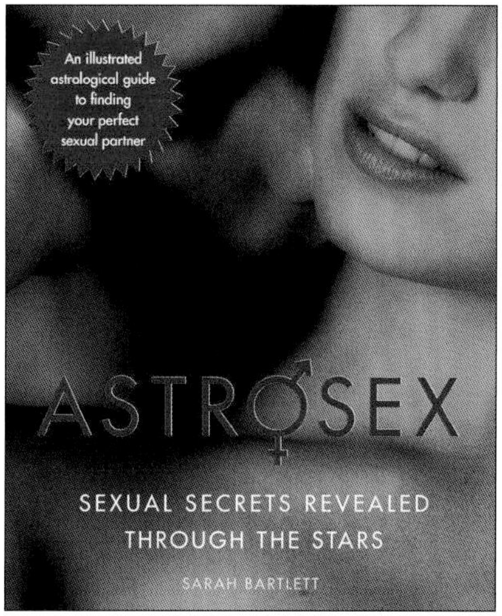

Astrosex

Sexual Secrets Revealed through the Stars

by Sarah Bartlett

We're all getting comfortable with the idea that men are from Mars and women are from Venus, but how many of us aware how much *all* of our sex lives are influenced by *all* of the planets *all* of the time? Perhaps the pick-up line "So, what's your sign?" is more important than most people in search of truly cosmic coupling may have realized.

Astrosex is the ultimate illustrated guide to understanding your own sexual desires and the sexual needs of your partner based on your horoscopes. Whether you want to unleash the lust of a Leo, tame a Taurus, seduce a Sagittarius, or break the ice with a Virgo, this sexy guide will help you navigate your love life using the stars.

The book includes a sexy introduction to the zodiac and how you can make it work for you. What then follows is an in-depth description of male and female sexual preferences for each star sign with tips on erogenous zones, preferred positions, and favorite fantasies. Illustrated with more than 350 atmospheric and sensual color photographs—including steamy sex positions—*Astrosex* provides a visually seductive and out-of-this-world experience.

$19.95 Hardcover • ISBN 978-1-62914-164-0

ALSO AVAILABLE

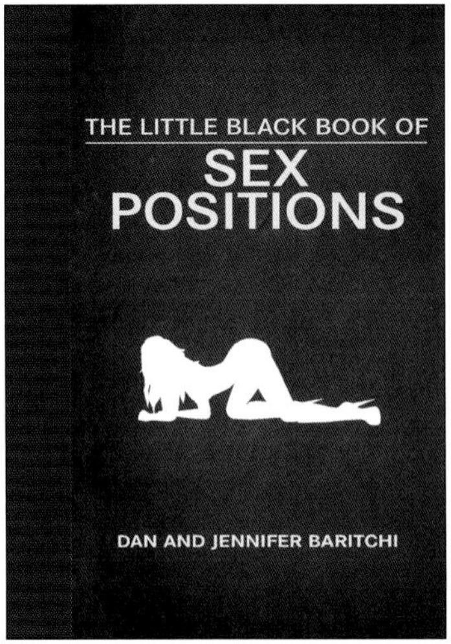

The Little Black Book of Sex Positions

by Dan and Jennifer Baritchi

If you think there are only three positions that get the job done, then it's time to get out of your sexual rut and start having a ball! *The Little Black Book of Sex Positions* exposes in glorious detail hundreds of sexy moves that can lead to mind-blowing ecstasy for you and your lover. The positions offered here are the next best thing to having an experienced partner right by your side . . . or behind, or face-to-face.

If your rolls in the hay have become a bit ho-hum, or if you just want to expand your spicy repertoire, this hot little how-to will having you flexing muscles you never knew you had with sexy positions you've always wanted to try like the YMCA, Forbidden Fruit, Pirate's Bounty, Rodeo, Deep Impact, and much more.

In a hardcover edition with full-color exciting yet tasteful illustrations, *The Little Black Book of Sex Positions* is handsome enough to keep on your nightstand, or to give to someone naughty and nice. You'll never think about "little black book" the same way again. Start stretching!

$16.95 Hardcover • ISBN 978-1-62087-611-4

ALSO AVAILABLE

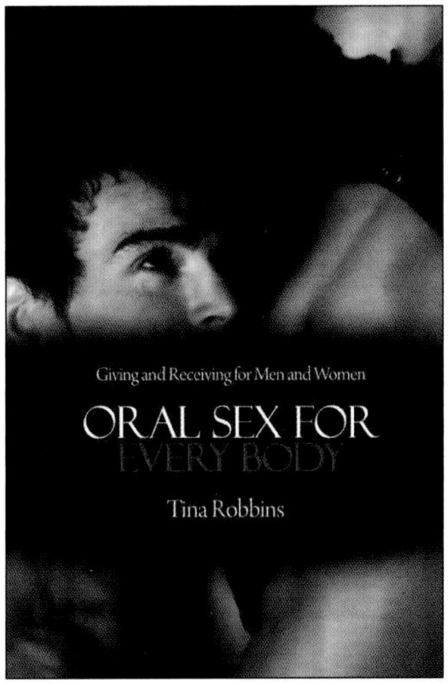

Oral Sex for Every Body

Giving and Receiving for Men and Women

by Tina Robbins

With clear and direct language, *Oral Sex for Every Body* is a practical, uninhibited guide to making your sexual relations more imaginative and pleasurable.

Oral sex has many variations (as many for her as for him), and you'll find all of them in this book. Let yourself be carried along and learn to enjoy invigorating oral sex, passionate cunnilingus, or an unforgettable sixty-nine. Let it free your imagination, forget about your fears, and prepare to surprise your lover as you never have before.

You will learn to discover and stimulate your partner's most excitable erogenous zones. Without haste, you will savor each vibration of their body and will find secret places that, along the way, will produce an intense, profound sexual experience.

ALSO AVAILABLE

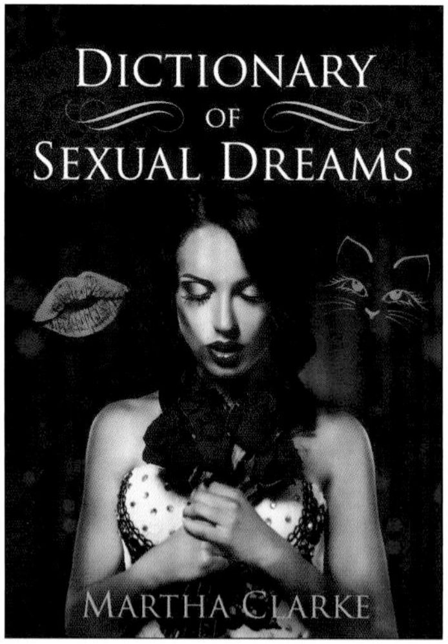

Dictionary of Sexual Dreams

by Martha Clarke

Approximately 8 percent of what we dream about has sexual connotations. Interestingly, authorities claim that sexual dreaming is often more intense than the physical act of sexual intercourse. *Dictionary of Sexual Dreams* helps us understand, as well as enjoy, these desires.

While we sleep, certain things take place that we would not necessarily pursue while awake: participating in an orgy, making love with someone of the same gender, or being intimate with our best friend's partner. From women who dream about making love with a stranger to men who dream about group sex, the fantasies that are revealed through dreams are symbolic, shedding light on our most profound impulses.

$14.95 Hardcover • ISBN 978-1-62914-477-1